Praise for Save Your Hands! ▪ 2nd Edition

"We've used **Save Your Hands!** in our program for many years. This expanded edition contains a wealth of accessible and well-illustrated career-extending, even career-saving, knowledge and advice regarding injury prevention strategies, ergonomics, conditioning, and other topics of critical importance for students and practitioners of massage therapy."

— **Lucy Liben, MS, LMT**, Dean for Massage Therapy, Swedish Institute of Health Sciences, NY

"I feel (**Save Your Hands!**) is an excellent work that should be required reading for every manual therapist, in or out of training. Furthermore, I think many other professionals including physicians, nurses, chiropractors, DOs and others ought to be familiar with its contents. I wholeheartedly endorse the book—it is a unique and valuable resource."

— **Emil Pascarelli, MD**, author, Dr. Pascarelli's Complete Guide to Repetitive Strain Injury, Emeritus Professor of Clinical Medicine, Columbia University

"**Save Your Hands!** provides excellent practical suggestions for improving safety of the provision of manual therapy services. The authors have been thoughtful and comprehensive in their approach and provide valuable information to the practitioner . . . "

— **Jeff Lau, PT, DPT, OCS, CMPT**, Program Director, PTA program, Provo College, Utah

"If this book does not help you prevent injuries as a manual therapist, nothing will. As one of the largest employers of manual therapists worldwide, the spa industry has unfortunately experienced many such injuries. If the advice in this volume were practiced industry-wide, it would save untold suffering, prolong thousands of careers and save spas a bundle in the bargain. Well done."

— **Steve Cappelini, LMT**, spa educator and author of Massage Therapy Career Guide, The Royal Treatment and Massage for Dummies

"**Save Your Hands!** has been a required textbook in our core curriculum for nearly a decade. It is a 'must read' for all massage students and practicing therapists to ensure injury-free longevity in their field."

— **Mary McDaniel, LMT**, Academic Director, Cumberland Institute of Holistic Therapies

"Quite simply, the book is excellently conceived and constructed, and is very well presented, and I highly recommend it."

— **Leon Chaitow, ND, DO**, author, Honorary Fellow, University of Westminster, London

"Anyone who plans a career in manual therapy should read **Save Your Hands!** first. Loaded with useful information, this book will prove a lifesaver for those looking for answers to hand and arm pain, and should be required reading in manual therapy training courses."

— **Deborah Quilter**, author, teacher & consultant, The Repetitive Strain Injury Recovery Book and Repetitive Strain Injury: A Computer User's Guide

"Employers in the spa industry have been in need of a guide to help them retain and care for highly skilled therapists as well as to reduce worker's compensation claims. My hope is that this text will be part of every massage school and training program and in the office of every employer of massage therapists."

— **Seraphina L. Ashe, LMT**, Spa Treatment Manager, The Spa at Sea Island, Georgia

"Students as well as seasoned practitioners will do well by arming themselves with insights from this thorough, well-organized, and well-illustrated text."

— **Leslie A. Young, PhD**, Editor-in-Chief, *Massage & Bodywork*, VP Communications, ABMP

"I found the revised version very easy to access and very informative. I value the organization and appreciate the reflective tone and positive approach to the topic of caring for the most valuable tools of the manual therapist. I especially appreciate the addition of physical conditioning, as it is a place where many practitioners do not attend to their self care and development. Bravo!"

— **Dawn M. Schmidt, LMP**, Director of Education, Cortiva Institute—Seattle

"I recommend to each of my PTA and massage therapy students to invest in this book and add it to their tool box. The book's illustration of correct and incorrect body mechanics along with the easy to read text that includes accessible captions, sidebars, and headings is an excellent resource for both the novice and the experienced manual therapist."

— **Ashlee Esplen, PTA, MS, CMT**, Associate Professor, ACCE PTA Program, Massage Therapy Program Coordinator, Butler County Community College

"*Save Your Hands!* is a necessary component to the curriculum for massage therapists and other healthcare occupations involving repetitive movements, that must include body mechanics training and safety education. DSM has required this book for our Introduction to Self-care and Professional Development course for many years. Well done!"

— **Nancy Dail, BA, LMT, NCTMB**, Director, Downeast School of Massage

"Taking care of ourselves while we care for others is a high priority! Your book offers an excellent overview of the issues related to MSDs, and how the treating clinician can work on self-awareness and self-modulation of positions and forces during patient/client care. I think it is a well-rounded look at ourselves and our environment, to keep us working in a healthy manner . . ."

— **Patty McCord, PT, OCS, FAAOMPT**, Evergreen Physical Therapy Specialists, PC

"This book is an invaluable resource for all manual therapists. From novice to expert, it is never too late to step back, evaluate your manual techniques, and incorporate changes that will prolong your career."

— **Sheila Yakobina, OTR/L, CHT** and **Stephanie Yakobina, OTR/L, CHT**

"I'm the Massage One instructor at the Palmer Institute and think your 2nd edition is fabulous. I always have recommended your first book to all my beginning students and will highly recommend this one as well."

— **Joyce Colahan, LMT**, instructor, Palmer Institute of Massage and Bodywork

Third Edition

Save Your Hands!

The Complete Guide to Injury Prevention and Ergonomics for Manual Therapists

Lauriann Greene & Richard W. Goggins, MS, CPE, LMP

with contributions by **Janet M. Peterson**, PT, DPT

ILLUMINATE PRESS
PHILADELPHIA, PENNSYLVANIA

Save Your Hands! The Complete Guide to Injury Prevention and Ergonomics for Manual Therapists, Third Edition

Published by Illuminate Press
2001 Hamilton St.
Philadelphia, PA 19130 USA
Email: hello@illuminatepress.com
Website: www.saveyourhands.com

Library of Congress Control Number: 2025909411

ISBN: 978-0-9679549-2-9

Originally printed and bound in the United States of America.

Cover and interior design by Shannon Bodie,
    BookWiseDesign.com with thanks to
    Olivia M. Hammerman, ochbookdesign.com
Copy editing by Shanna Germain
Indexing by Robert Saigh
Photography by Meryl Schenker
Illustrations on pages 34 and 319 by Valerie Rutley-Paine
Illustration on page 257 by Erica Beade
Illustration on page 255 by Harriet R. Greenfield
Illustration on page 36 from the Washington Department of
    Labor and Industries, Olympia, Wash.
Illustrations in Chapter 11 by Al Akib

Contents

Foreword by Ben E. Benjamin, PhD

Founder, Muscular Therapy Institute, Cambridge, Mass.
Author, *Listen to Your Pain*

Save Your Hands! is a book every massage therapist and hands-on health care practitioner should own and study. Its contents are broad, comprehensive, and research based. The valuable information within this book can help lessen the likelihood of injury among hands-on health care professionals throughout long-term careers.

Students who enter training to become manual therapists are intelligent, compassionate, and committed to making a difference in people's lives. What they do not know is that on average they will face a high risk of injury in their dream profession. One study found that 41 percent of massage practitioners were injured over a two-year period; another that 84 percent of chiropractors were injured during careers averaging only 11 years. Statistics such as these cited in *Save Your Hands!* are shocking and unfortunate.

Clearly, schools, students, and practicing professionals alike need the information in *Save Your Hands!*—how to listen to their bodies, how to recognize signs of poor movement habits, and how to establish working boundaries that acknowledge their personal limits.

I wish that *Save Your Hands!* had been available during my own training in therapeutic bodywork. Because I had personal experience with a career-threatening injury, I studied with leading manual therapists and physicians to learn as much as I could about the physical and emotional components of muscular tension and the body's pain responses. Simultaneously I studied several systems of movement education and brought these insights into my performance as a therapist. I wanted to learn how to provide the treatments my clients needed in a way that was, for my own body, efficient, effortless, pain free, and injury free. These are exactly the goals of *Save Your Hands!*

For example, I asked an Alexander Technique practitioner to observe my sessions so that I might become aware of poor alignment and alter ineffective, habitual movements into patterns of greater ease. Now, students in training, as well as professionals already in practice, can find this information in *Save Your Hands!*, including excellent illustrations and descriptions of the vulnerable areas in a working practitioner's body and detailed descriptions of how to stabilize and move the body to provide treatments with maximum effectiveness. I have long advocated smaller-width treatment tables as safer for practitioners; this practice is clearly explained here, along with other vital ergonomic concerns.

The authors also discuss another facet that I find quite important: recognition of the effects of our emotions on our work and strategies for setting boundaries that ultimately protect both our clients and ourselves. As a teacher who has long focused my students on their own self-care, I am impressed that this book also offers a comprehensive program of exercises that will help condition the practitioner's body in ways that lessen the risk of injury.

My own career in muscular therapy and sports medicine now spans more than 45 years, and I have rarely missed a day due to injury from my work. For me, a successful career is one that I enjoy, am inspired by, and can perform as long as I want to, knowing that I am doing everything necessary to protect myself from injury. Would you like your career to be like that? You will make an excellent start by reading and applying the principles found in *Save Your Hands!*

Foreword by Janet M. Peterson, PT, DPT

Member Emeritus of the National Board of Directors,
American Physical Therapy Association (APTA)
Contributor to *Save Your Hands!* 2nd Edition

I have spent over twenty years of my professional career evaluating clients as they work, assessing their risk for injury, and teaching them how to work with less risk. Sometimes this work involves evaluating their postures and work habits; sometimes it involves obtaining different equipment or using the equipment in new ways. Always, the client gets the most benefit when the advice and instruction is specific to their own work tasks. For current and future hands-on healthcare professionals, *Save Your Hands!* meets this need. It provides valuable ergonomics and injury prevention information that is specific to the particular risks and challenges these professionals face in their work. As the evidence presented in *Save Your Hands!* points out, health practitioners who perform manual treatment techniques are at considerable risk for injury as a result of the physically demanding work they do.

Comprehensive is the word that best comes to mind when describing this book. In this information-rich, yet easily accessible resource, you will learn why you are at risk, ways to reduce your risk and prevent injury from occurring in the first place, and how to most effectively approach treating injury if it does occur. While each of the professions represented here includes some of this information in their educational programs, *Save Your Hands!* presents a wide range of injury awareness, prevention and treatment topics and methods in one place, including important content you may not have received during your training. Physical therapists and physical therapist assistants, for example, may not have been introduced to all of the work-related risk factors and ergonomic principles included here. Some of the information on how nutrition and attitudes/beliefs about work affect injury risk may also be new to these practitioners. Lauriann Greene and Richard W. Goggins have done an excellent job in organizing the content of the book so that it flows logically when reading cover to cover, but can also be used quickly and easily as a reference. Well-placed sidebars, tables, and tips sections make it simple to find practical information and advice at a glance.

As a former member of the American Physical Therapy Association's (APTA) board of directors, I continue to look out for the interests of PTs and PTAs in all practice settings. The issue of work-related musculoskeletal injuries in our profession is not discussed enough; we tend to be so patient-focused that we sacrifice our own health at times. In the long view, we can be of better service to our patients/clients, and have longer careers, if we embrace the concepts in Save Your Hands! This is a book that will not collect dust on the shelf.

Preface by Lauriann Greene

When the first edition of *Save Your Hands!* was published in 1995, little was known about work-related injury among manual therapists. While a few books for massage therapists mentioned occupational injury, *Save Your Hands!* was the first book exclusively dedicated to understanding, preventing and treating work-related musculoskeletal disorders (MSDs) in these professions. After my own experience with injury during my massage therapy training, I wanted to help other hands-on practitioners protect their investment in their careers and their health. In the numerous injury prevention workshops I conducted in the U.S. and Canada, I met hundreds of massage therapy students and professionals, and heard them speak about their experiences with MSD symptoms and injury. While their stories provided anecdotal evidence of an elevated risk of injury in the profession, we had no real statistics on this subject. In addition, it seemed the risk of MSDs in this profession was a subject that few practitioners were willing to discuss openly. It became clear that there was a need to raise awareness of injury in the hands-on healthcare professions, and provide comprehensive, evidence-based information about injury prevention to practitioners.

In the time that has passed between the publication of the first edition and this third edition, many things have happened. The awareness of work-related MSDs in the general population has increased. Schools that train manual therapists have taken on more responsibility for alerting students of the risks of injury in these professions and teaching them prevention techniques, most notably how to improve their body mechanics in their treatments, one of many effective techniques used to reduce stress and overuse. Research has produced statistics that reveal the extent of the injury risk that manual therapists face in a number of fields, including physical therapy and chiropractic. Richard W. Goggins, MS, CPE, LMP and I published the first reliable statistics on injury among massage practitioners with invaluable assistance from American Massage and Bodywork Association (ABMP). That collaboration led to our decision to work together on the second edition of *Save Your Hands!*

Rick also had first-hand experience with injury. Already a Certified Professional Ergonomist for many years, Rick decided to train as a massage therapist to develop hands-on knowledge of the musculoskeletal system. But while working in the student clinic, he began to develop symptoms of an MSD. While I had lacked the knowledge of injury physiology, prevention and treatment that could have helped me overcome my injury, Rick's extensive ergonomics training provided him with an awareness of MSD symptoms and a knowledge of the appropriate steps to take to avoid serious injury. As a result, my injury became severe and chronic enough that, although I passed my state board exam, I was not able to continue working as a massage therapist; Rick, on the other hand, was able to immediately recognize the warning signs of injury, get effective treatment quickly, and attain his goal of becoming a professional massage therapist in addition to his work as an ergonomist.

Rick's and my personal experiences with injury illustrate the difference that awareness and knowledge can make when MSD symptoms begin. Written in consultation with a diverse group of healthcare professionals, *Save Your Hands!* is designed to arm manual therapists with the knowledge they need to take action to save not only their hands, but their backs, shoulders, neck, emotional well-being and, in some cases, their careers. As an ergonomist with more than 15 years experience at the time of the Second Edition, Rick brought to *Save Your Hands!* an important focus on ergonomics, which examines the physical and emotional aspects of the work that manual therapists do and many concrete steps they can take to prevent injury.

Having seen first-hand how painful, upsetting and disruptive a work-related MSD can be, Rick and I wanted to provide manual therapists with the comprehensive information they need to stay healthy in a profession dedicated to helping others. Now with the Third Edition, it is my sincere hope that the greatly revised and updated information in this book will provide you with the best information possible and be an invaluable resource for all manual therapists. I hope it will help you have a long, productive and healthy career.

Acknowledgements

Lauriann would like to thank: Richard W. Goggins, MS, CPE, LMT for his knowledge and skill in ergonomics and his expert collaboration, as well as his work with me on the 2006 Study of Massage Therapists with the ABMP (as well as his brother's help and expertise in statistics); Janet M. Peterson, PT, DPT, for her invaluable advice, informative preface and expert contributions; Ben E. Benjamin, PhD, for graciously accepting to write a foreword to the book; Dennis Homack, DC, CCSP for sharing the results of his survey of chiropractors; George Piligian, MD, MPH and Elizabeth Vucovik Gartlan, MS, RD for their help with the nutrition section; Kathy Rockefeller, PT, MPH, ScD for reviewing drafts, making helpful suggestions and forwarding research papers; Stephanie Yakobina, OTR/L, CHT and Sheila Yakobina, OTR/L, CHT for reviewing drafts and providing valuable input; Leslie A. Young, Ph.D. and *Massage & Bodywork* magazine for sponsoring our injury survey of massage therapists and publishing the results; Meryl Schenker for her superb photography; Zenith Supplies in Seattle for contributing equipment for our photo shoot; our wonderful models Aaron Brisbois, LMP, Katie Kelley, LMP, Kimmo Nissinen and Erica Newman Nash, LMP; Harriet R. Greenfield, Dawn Scott of Harvard Health Publications; Shannon Bodie and her team at BookWise Design for her outstanding cover and interior design, as well as Olivia M. Hammerman of OCH Design for her valuable contributions; Shanna Germain for her masterful copy editing and proofreading; and Robert Saigh for his skillful indexing.

Lauriann would also like to thank: my brother Robert A. Greene, MD, FACP, and sister-in-law Susan Presberg-Greene, MD, for their love, encouragement, medical review and valuable input; my niece and nephew, Stephanie Li and Jonathan M. Stewart, for their love and support; and my parents, Claire and David Greene, for their love, encouragement and unfailing support of everything I have ever accomplished.

Introduction

As a manual therapist, you have invested considerable time, effort, school and training expense, and work experience to become a professional in a demanding and rewarding healthcare field. Developing an injury as a result of your work can stall or even threaten the career you have worked so hard to create. *Save Your Hands!* provides the comprehensive information and proven methods you need to prevent injury, protect your investment in your career, and safeguard your health.

Save Your Hands! addresses the injury prevention concerns of massage therapists and bodyworkers, physical, occupational and hand therapists, chiropractors, osteopaths, nurses and athletic trainers—any practitioner who performs hands-on treatments. Manual practitioners can encounter symptoms or injury at any stage of their career, even during their training. If you are a student in any manual therapy discipline, *Save Your Hands!* can help you understand why and how injury happens, and show you how to develop good injury prevention habits and practices from the very start. For professionals, this book offers a comprehensive reference and practical guide you can refer to throughout your career, as your circumstances change and you encounter challenges that could increase your injury risk and cause symptoms to arise. Students and professionals alike will find a wealth of helpful tips and practical advice they can use every day to help them effectively manage the emotional and physical demands of their work. *Save Your Hands!* will help you protect your ability to have or continue to have a profitable, rewarding career in your chosen profession.

Preventing injury to your upper extremities, neck and back is the main goal of *Save Your Hands!* As manual therapists know from their own experiences with clients, it is certainly easier and more effective to prevent injuries from happening than to treat them once they have already occurred. One of the keys to prevention is to be fully aware of the injury risks you will face in the course of your career. You will find a thorough explanation of these risks in Part One of this book. Another key is to have effective strategies in place to deal with those risks. Part Two presents a multi-faceted plan of action, using methods that have been proven effective in preventing injury. Ergonomics is an essential part of this holistic approach to maintaining your health, and it is an important focus of this edition of *Save Your Hands!* By studying the workplace to find ways to take the most advantage of your strengths, ergonomics provides powerful tools you can use to reduce injury risk as a result of your work.

It is also possible, despite your best efforts, to find yourself developing symptoms; after all, who hasn't had aches and pains after a particularly hard day at work? How will you know when those symptoms signal that it is time to seek treatment, and which treatments work best for the injuries manual therapists most frequently encounter? In Part Three, you will learn about the typical symptoms and most common conditions manual therapists have been shown to experience, get an overview of effective treatment options, and understand the steps to take to keep symptoms from developing into chronic and possibly debilitating conditions.

Several appendices are included at the end of the book to further assist you in your prevention efforts. Massage schools and spas will find helpful recommendations in appendices written especially for them. In addition, the *Save Your Hands!* website is designed to be used in conjunction with the book. It is regularly updated with the latest news, information and links and includes a wide variety of injury prevention and treatment resources.

The message of *Save Your Hands!* is simple: there is a great deal you can do to protect yourself from work-related injury. Reading and proactively applying the information you find in these pages will help you develop an injury prevention strategy for your work. By making it part of your professional reference book collection, you will always have a source of evidence-based, proven information and advice you can refer to throughout your professional life. By doing so, you will be taking an important step toward protecting your health and well-being throughout your career as a manual therapist.

PART ONE

Why Manual Therapists Get Injured

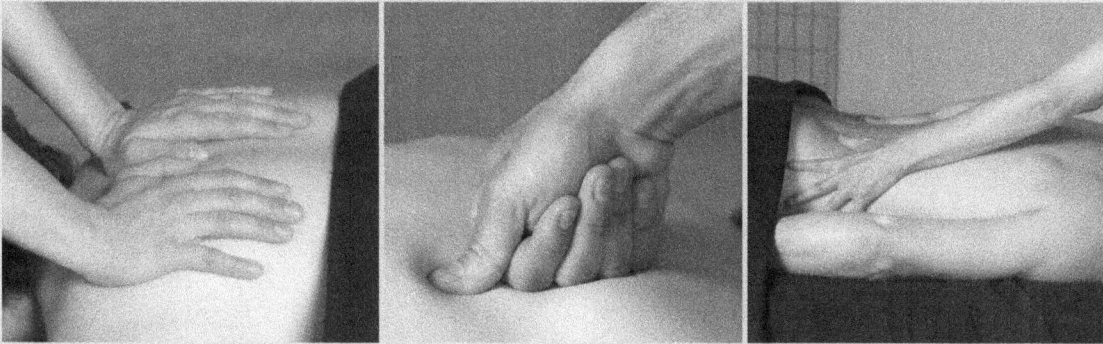

1

Raising Your Awareness
of Injury Risk

Anyone who has been a manual therapist for any length of time knows how physically demanding this type of work can be. Whether you're a massage therapist, physical therapist, chiropractor or any other type of manual practitioner, you use physical effort and skill to treat your clients' musculoskeletal systems. You use your hands and arms extensively to do these treatments; you stand much of the day; sometimes you bend over your client for long periods or have to lift a part of their body. Just like any professional who uses their body extensively in their work, manual therapists may experience certain unpleasant symptoms at the end of a long workday. Achy hands, tired forearms or a painful lower back are all indications of the toll that manual treatment work can take on the therapist's body.

Many manual therapists come to accept these feelings as part of the reality of doing their work. They concentrate primarily on relieving clients' symptoms, while enduring aches and pains of their own. Unless symptoms become severe or start to interfere with their ability to function at work, it can be easy to dismiss or disregard them. We all have busy lives, and taking the time to pay attention to and treat incipient symptoms can seem less important than the many other things we have to deal with each week. Also, not all manual therapists have developed the ability to maintain awareness of their own bodies' reactions to the work they are doing with a client or patient. The thought of becoming injured seems like a distant possibility, a rare occurrence and certainly something that couldn't happen to you.

Recent research indicates a very different reality. Statistics show that there is a substantial risk of work-related injury among manual therapists. To protect your own health, as well as your investment in your career, you need to be aware of the risk of injury in the work you do, and fully understand your own personal injury risk.

Looking at the Facts

Several recent surveys have produced reliable data on the incidence and causes of work-related musculoskeletal symptoms and injury among manual therapists (Table 1). The results of these surveys indicate that musculoskeletal symptoms and injury are common among these practitioners, who regularly perform treatments with their hands. These treatments can include soft tissue manipulation, therapeutic and/or relaxation massage, joint manipulation or mobilization, or resistive exercise, among others.

Although there were differences in the ways the surveys were designed and worded, each survey addressed the major issues of symptoms and injury in the profession for which it was intended. Despite these differences, there are obvious similarities in the results between the four surveys:

Musculoskeletal injury occurred frequently among the different manual professionals. One third or more of the practitioners in each profession reported injury within the past two years. The survey on injury among American massage therapists found that an alarming 77 percent of experienced practitioners reported

Musculoskeletal Disorders (MSDs)

Many different terms are used to describe non-traumatic, gradual-onset soft-tissue injuries. You have probably heard these injuries referred to as cumulative trauma disorders (CTDs), repetitive strain injuries (RSIs), or "overuse" syndromes. To avoid confusion, the more generic term "musculoskeletal disorders" (MSDs) is now commonly used to reference all of these injuries.

MSDs can happen suddenly, such as with a ligament sprain, or have a more gradual onset, such as with tendinosis that occurs due to overuse. MSDs and their related symptoms are very common in the general population. They are second only to colds and flu as a cause of missed work.

having some form of pain or discomfort due to their work during the previous two years. The survey also found that 64 percent of practitioners had symptoms serious enough to cause them to seek medical treatment, and 41 percent were diagnosed with a musculoskeletal disorder, such as overuse syndrome or tendonitis. A recent survey among Canadian mas-

Table 1. Injury and Its Causes Among Manual Therapists

Profession	Injury Diagnosis Rate	Parts of body most frequently injured	Most frequent injury types	Most frequent causes of injury
Massage Practitioners[1]	41 percent over a two-year period	Shoulder Thumb Lower back Neck Wrist	Overuse syndrome Tendinopathy Low back strain	Giving massage Applying pressure Standing for long periods of time Non-work related causes Positioning or holding client's limbs or head
Physical Therapists[2]	32 percent over a two-year period	Lower back Upper back Wrist/Hand Neck Shoulder	Muscle strain Ligament sprain Vertebral disc involvement	Transferring a patient Lifting Unanticipated patient movement Performing manual therapy Performing repetitive tasks
Physical Therapist Assistants[2]	35 percent over a two-year period	Lower back Upper back Shoulder Neck Wrist/Hand	Muscle strain Tendinopathy Tendinitis/ Tendinosis Ligament sprain	Transferring a patient Unanticipated patient movement Lifting Awkward or cramped position Maintaining a position for a prolonged period
Hand Therapists[3]	66 percent over course of career (~7 year avg.)	Thumbs Shoulder Neck Upper back Wrist	Joint injury Tendinopathy Tendinitis/ Tendinosis Myofascial pain	Poor work posture Massage/trigger point compression Cutting thermoplastics to make custom splints Mobilization Excess workload
Chiropractors[4]	84 percent over course of career (~11 year avg.)	Lower back Shoulder Upper back Wrist Neck	Strain Sprain Tendinopathy Tendinitis/ Tendinosis	Adjusting patient Gradual, non-specific onset Patient handling Working while fatigued Performing soft tissue treatment

sage therapists also found high rates of work-related pain and injury, with more than 60 percent of respondents reporting low back symptoms, and more than 80 percent reporting wrist and thumb symptoms. Low back and neck pain were reported more frequently by practitioners who had been practicing for fewer than five years.[5]

The types of injuries reported were similar. Muscle strains are the most common injuries reported across all of these professions, followed by tendinitis/tendinosis, ligament sprain and intervertebral disc injury.

Pain caused by tendon injury is often called "tendinitis." This term refers to inflammation in the tendon. More recent research has shown that, in fact, inflammation is not often found in the tissues of manual therapists with tendon pain and dysfunction. The term used now is "tendinosis," instead of "tendinitis." Therefore, for the chronic, slow-onset injuries like the ones manual therapists tend to experience we now use the term tendinosis. It is characterized by the degeneration of tendon fibers, not inflammation[7, 8]

The location of injuries was similar and directly related to the type of work being done. The lower back, upper back, neck, shoulder, wrist and hand were the most frequent injury sites for all professions, although the frequency of injury in these locations varied among the professions. Massage practitioners, PTs and PTAs who reported doing hand-intensive treatments were more likely to have thumb, wrist and arm injuries, although these practitioners also experienced back injuries. Low back injury appeared to be most common in PTs and PTAs working in a rehabilitation environment, possibly because they lift and transfer patients (or assist in doing so) who are unable to stand and walk without assistance. Back injuries were also common among nurses, nursing aides, and home health care workers who transfer patients manually, without the benefit of lift-assist devices. Back and shoulder injuries were common in chiropractors, and appeared to be primarily due to the physical demands of adjusting and handling patients. PTs who work in pediatrics reported more knee symptoms, perhaps because they spend more time kneeling and squatting to work with their clients.

The same types of manual treatments were cited as the main cause of injury. While the most frequent causes of injury appeared to be specific to each profession, practitioners in all of the professions reported performing massage, soft tissue treatment, manipulation or mobilization as the main causes of injury. It seems clear that performing manual treatments places the practitioner at risk for musculoskeletal injury.

The effects of injury on the therapist's work life were similar among the different professions. Many therapists reported changing the way they practiced in response to their symptoms. Chiropractors and physical therapists tended to change the way they treated clients. In a survey of Australian physiotherapists, one in six PTs reported either changing to a different type of practice or no longer performing hands-on treatment altogether in response to their symptoms.[8] The majority of PTs who made a change moved to a different (and one assumes less physically demanding) specialty within the field rather than leaving it altogether.

The Survey of Massage Practitioners at a Glance

- Web-based survey

- 1,000 e-mail invitations sent to Associated Bodywork & Massage Professionals (ABMP) members in the United States

- 601 respondents

- 89 percent rated their overall health 'good' or 'very good'

- 82 percent had received injury prevention training

- 77 percent experienced pain or other musculoskeletal symptoms related to massage work

- 64 percent sought medical treatment for symptoms

- 41 percent were diagnosed with a musculoskeletal injury

- Overuse syndrome and tendinopathy were the most common diagnoses

- Shoulders, thumbs and lower back were the most common injury locations

- "Applying pressure" was listed as the most common cause of work-related symptoms

- 19 percent had to reduce the amount of massage work they did due to symptoms

- 18 percent have considered leaving the profession due to symptoms or fear of injury

- 67 percent had ongoing symptoms

Massage practitioners also made significant changes to their practices in response to symptoms, with one in five cutting back on the amount of massage work they did. Similar to physical therapists, about one in five massage practitioners considered leaving the profession due to concerns about injury. According to the American Massage Therapy Association at the time, the average massage career was a little less than eight years. The relatively short time span of the average career in massage may be due in part to a burn-out factor from the physical demands of the work. In 2024, the Bureau of Labor Statistics acknowledged that massage therapy is physically demanding, making therapists susceptible to injuries.[9]

Speaking Openly About Injury

The survey results send another important message to manual therapists: you are not alone in your concerns about injury in your work. Everyone in your profession is dealing with the same risks, the same symptoms, and the same types of injuries. There is no shame in being vulnerable to injury. It is important for manual therapists to be able to speak openly about this important subject, promote awareness of injury in their profession, and do whatever they need to do to protect their health and their investment in their careers.

All of the survey statistics indicate that manual therapists have a high rate of injury. More recent studies[10, 11] have shown the same high prevalence of symptoms and injury in manual therapists. While their training, modalities and treatment methods may differ, there is a common risk among the various hands-on professions for upper extremity injuries, as well as injury to the low back and neck. Whether it's a massage therapist releasing myofascial tissues, a chiropractor mobilizing paraspinal tissues prior to making an adjustment, or a physical therapist performing cross fiber friction to break up scar tissue around a tendon, the demands on the practitioners' bodies, and the subsequent risks of injury, are similar. In the same way, a physical therapist helping to move patients who cannot stand on their own, a chiropractor supporting clients while lowering them to the treatment table, or a massage practitioner lifting a client's leg to bolster underneath are all at risk for back and shoulder injuries. Even though the professions are very different, the risk factors of doing manual soft-tissue work and lifting body parts are the same, so the same types of injuries occur.

Putting Injury Risk into Perspective

It is clear that manual therapists need to be aware of the risk of injury in their work. But many professions have inherent risks. Musicians, construction workers, truck drivers, people who type on a computer all day—workers in all of these professions, and many others, run the risk of MSDs as well as traumatic injury. Yet many people have successful, long-term, healthy careers in these professions.

The fact that injury can occur does not make it inevitable. There is a great deal you can do to prevent injuries from occurring in the first place, and to minimize their effects if they do occur. The surveys cited above enable us to begin to understand the injury risk manual practitioners face, and give us good reasons to find effective strategies and techniques to reduce that risk. The key to injury prevention is remaining aware of the risks and as you work taking the necessary steps to manage that risk. In the following two chapters, you will learn the specific risk factors inherent in a manual therapist's work, and find out which areas of the body are the most vulnerable to injury as a result of this work.

> **Maintaining awareness of the risk of injury and taking steps to manage that risk is the key to prevention.**

1. Lauriann Greene and Richard W. Goggins, "Musculoskeletal Symptoms and Injuries among Experienced Massage and Bodywork Professionals," *Massage & Bodywork*, 2006; Dec–Jan: 48–58.
2. Nicole L. Holder, et al, "Cause, Prevalence and Response to Occupational Musculoskeletal Injuries Reported by Physical Therapists and Physical Therapist Assistants," *Physical Therapy*, 1999; 79(7): 642–652.
3. Suzanne Caragianis, "The Prevalence of Occupational Injuries among Hand Therapists in Australia and New Zealand," *Journal of Hand Therapy*, 2002 Jul–Sep; 15(3): 234–241.
4. Dennis M. J. Homack, "Occupational Injuries to Chiropractors in New York State," (Masters' Thesis, Graduate School of Cornell University, 2004).
5. Wayne J. Albert, et al., "A Survey of Musculoskeletal Injuries Amongst Canadian Massage Therapists," *Journal of Bodywork and Movement Therapy*, 2007: 1–8.
6. K.M. Kahn, S.F. Bonar, et al, "Time to Abandon the Tendinitis Myth," *BMJ*. 2002 Mar 16;324(7338):626–627. doi: 10.1136/bmj.324.7338.626
7. Evelyn Bass, Int J Ther Massage Bodywork, 2012 Mar 31;5(1):14–17. doi: 10.3822/ijtmb.v5i1.153, "Tendinopathy: Why the Difference Between Tendinitis and Tendinosis Matters," https://pmc.ncbi.nlm.nih.gov/articles/PMC3312643/
8. Jean E. Cromie, et al, "Work-Related Musculoskeletal Disorders in Physical Therapists: Prevalence, Severity, Risks, and Responses," *Physical Therapy*, 2000; 80(4): 336–351.
9. U.S. Bureau of Labor Statistics website, https://www.bls.gov/ooh/healthcare/massage-therapists.htm
10. Lamprecht, A., Padayachy, K. The epidemiology of work-related musculoskeletal injuries among chiropractors in the Thekwini municipality. *Chiropr Man Therap* 27, 18 (2019). https://doi.org/10.1186/s12998-019-0238-y
11. Giles Gyer, Jimmy Michael, James InklebargerJ, "Occupational hand injuries: a current review of the prevalence and proposed prevention strategies for physical therapists and similar healthcare professionals" *Journal of Integrative Medicine* 2018 Mar;16(2):84-89. doi: 10.1016/j.joim.2018.02.003. Epub 2018 Feb 6. https://pubmed.ncbi.nlm.nih.gov/29526241/

2

Weak Links in the Body

In the survey results noted in Chapter 1, injury occurred most frequently in the same five parts of the body in each of the manual healthcare professions cited. This finding brings up an important question: why do some parts of the body get injured more than others?

The human body is at once both strong and fragile. Our bones are capable of withstanding enormous physical stress before breaking, and our muscles are capable of generating very high amounts of force before giving out. Yet, at the same time there are some "weak links" in the body that are particularly vulnerable and prone to injury, especially from repetitive, cumulative trauma. By understanding the vulnerabilities of these body parts and the mechanisms by which they can become injured, you will be better able to protect yourself.

For the most part, the weak links are the joints, the moving parts of the body. Movement can create instability or imbalance, which increases the risk of injury. Some of these weak links—for example, the lower back—are common sites of injury in the general population. Other weak links, such as the thumbs, are typically injured only when they are overused. The most commonly injured body parts among workers in general are the lower back, wrists and shoulders (in that order). Among massage therapists,

Table 2. Weak Links in the Body

Weak links	Vulnerable structures	Typical injuries
Thumbs	Carpometacarpal (CMC) joint, ligaments, tendons	Tendinopathy, osteoarthritis
Hands/wrists	Tendons, tendon sheaths and the median nerve as they pass through the carpal tunnel	Tendinopathy, carpal tunnel syndrome
Shoulders	Rotator cuff muscles and tendons (particularly supraspinatus), bursae	Rotator cuff tears and tendinopathy, bursitis
Neck/upper back	Paraspinal ligaments and muscles	Tension neck syndrome, myofascitis
Lower back	Paraspinal ligaments and muscles, intervertebral discs (particularly L5/S1)	Ligament strains, muscle sprains, disc degeneration, bulge or herniation

however, the survey found that one of the most commonly injured body parts is the thumb. In the survey of physical therapists, thumb symptoms were six times more likely among therapists who did more than 10 hours per week of manipulation and mobilization, compared to PTs who did not perform these techniques. Table 2 shows the parts of the body most frequently injured as reported in the surveys of manual therapists.

Some parts of the body, such as shoulders, backs and wrists, are highly vulnerable to injury in nearly any occupation. Throughout history, injuries to certain body parts have been associated with the type of work the sufferers do (e.g., washerwoman's thumb, miner's knee) or the sports they participate in (e.g., tennis elbow, baseball pitcher's shoulder). While these are inherently vulnerable structures, they typically become injured as a result of some form of overuse. In the case of the washerwoman, repeatedly wringing out rags caused the overuse, since this activity can damage the ligaments and tendons at the base of the thumb. The thumb is particularly at risk for injury among manual therapists because practitioners tend to use it repeatedly in their treatments.

For all of these parts of the body, it is usually a combination of their inherent structure and the long-term impact of the demands we commonly place upon them in our work that makes them prone to injury. A weak link can fail without external influence due to conditions such rheumatoid arthritis or osteoarthritis; these can also set the stage for MSDs to occur when doing manual therapy work. However, when discussing manual therapy work-related MSDs, we look most closely at the factors involved in doing that work. You'll read more about those factors in Chapter 3.

For the sake of simplicity, the following section discusses each part of the body individually. But we all know that the body works as a whole. Connective tissue and fascia are continuous throughout the body, and what you do with one part will influence others. For example, a restriction at your elbow will affect the movement of both your wrist and your shoulder. A practitioner who starts wearing a wrist support to help keep her wrists straight while she works can end up putting her upper arm into awkward positions. Keep in mind that, while it is important to pay attention to these weak links, it is just as important to consider how the entire chain moves and reacts.

All of the surveys indicated that MSDs experienced by manual practitioners happen most often in five parts of the body: the thumbs, hands/wrists, shoulders, neck/upper back and lower back. Of course, these are not the only weak links in the body. Elbows, knees and hips are also prone to injury, but manual therapists reported injuries less frequently at those sites. We'll discuss the five most often injured weak links in order from the most distal extremity, the thumb, to the most central part of the axial skeleton, the lower back. Keep in mind that each weak link is part of a kinematic chain that may include all of the other links.

Thumbs

You may think of your thumbs as your strongest and most useful digits for applying pressure. They are conveniently short, and unlike fingers, they have stabilizing muscles at their base to help support them. In fact, the unique structure of the thumb makes it particularly vulnerable to injury. Forces acting on the thumb are concentrated in the carpometacarpal (CMC) joint, the saddle joint at the radial end of the carpal bones that makes our thumbs opposable. As the muscles at the base of the thumb contract to stabilize the joints while pressure is applied with the tip of the thumb, the metacarpal bone is pulled down into the CMC joint and creates pressure there. For every pound of pressure that you apply with your thumb, there can be 10 to 12 pounds of pressure concentrated in the CMC joint.[1] If you use your thumb to apply 10 pounds of force to a stubborn trigger point, the result could be as much as 120 pounds of force at the base of your thumb. Your thumbs are already heavily used in your daily life: you use them every time you grip anything, send a text message on your cell phone, or hit the spacebar on your computer keyboard. All of this activity can lead to fatigue of the muscles around

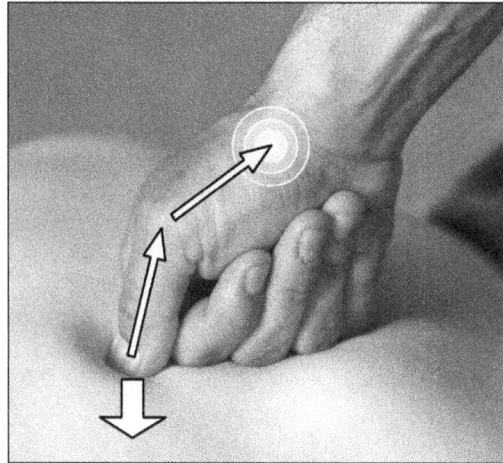

For every pound of downward force applied with the tip of the thumb, 10 to 12 pounds of force are concentrated in the CMC joint.

the thumb and damage to the ligaments, tendons and cartilage around the CMC joint, as well as subsequent damage to the joint. Be sure to keep the thumb relaxed when you use it, to avoid adding the risk factor of static loading.

Hands/Wrists

Unlike the thumbs, which are controlled to a great extent by nearby muscles in the thenar eminence of the palm and in the webbing between the thumb and index finger, the muscles that provide most of the movement of your fingers are in your forearms. The relatively strong flexor and extensor muscles start at your elbow, but stop mid-forearm and connect to your fingers through tendons. Most of these tendons pass through another weak link in your wrist: the carpal tunnel. The carpal tunnel is a small passageway between the carpal bones and the transverse carpal ligament. This passageway is shared by the nine forearm flexor tendons and the median nerve, which supplies sensation to your thumb and first three fingers.

Since the boundaries of the carpal tunnel are rigid structures, any hypertrophy occurring in the tendons or the sheaths that protect them will be contained within the carpal tunnel. This hypertrophy can put pressure on the median nerve. When you apply force to a client's tissues

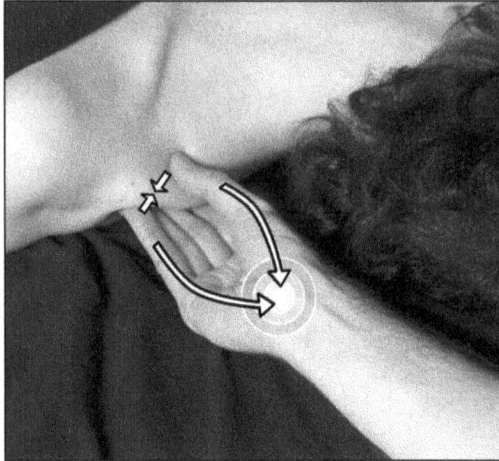

Gripping with the hand or applying pressure with the fingertips places stress on tendons and increases pressure in the carpal tunnel.

with your fingertips, you are also increasing the fluid pressure inside your carpal tunnel. When you work with your wrists bent (see photo, left), you are pulling your tendons through a narrower opening and creating friction, possibly irritating the tendons and sheaths, which results in more irritation and possibly degenerative changes to the tendons. These factors pressure can damage the median nerve as it passes through the carpal tunnel (see more about the carpal tunnel and carpal tunnel syndrome in Chapter 14).

The wrist is a complex mechanism with many moving parts in one small area, so it is also vulnerable to injury outside of the carpal tunnel. Tendons on the extensor side of the wrist can become irritated by tight muscles rubbing across them. The extensor carpi ulnaris muscle which attaches to the fifth metacarpal and produces extension of the wrist toward the pinky finger, is the most often affected.[2] The median nerve can even be damaged as it exits the carpal tunnel at the base of the palm.

Shoulders

The shoulder has the greatest range of motion of all the joints: its shallow ball and socket joint allows flexion/extension, adduction/ abduction, internal/external rotation, and circumduction. The downside of this flexibility is the potential for awkward working postures, joint instability and injury. We rely on the muscles around the shoulder, especially the rotator cuff, to stabilize the shoulder during movement. The rotator cuffs are made up of fairly strong, thick sheets of muscle. As we age, these muscles become thinner, and the connective tissue in them becomes less flexible. The rotator cuff has a relatively poor blood supply, so injuries such as tendinosis and partial tears are slow to heal.

Poor posture can pull the joint out of its normal, healthy position and place additional stress on tissues in the area. All of our daily activities are performed with our hands in front of us—eating breakfast, driving a car, working at the computer, and treating clients. Over time, these habitual postures can result in shoulders that are rounded forward, tight chest muscles, and stretched and weakened back muscles.

Consider also that two of the strongest muscles that attach to the upper arm, the pectoralis major and the latissimus dorsi, are both internal rotators. You can end up overdeveloping and shortening these muscles through both work and exercise. If this happens, the muscles can overpower the external rotators and pull the shoulders into constant internal rotation. This combination of poor posture and imbalanced musculature can pull the shoulders forward

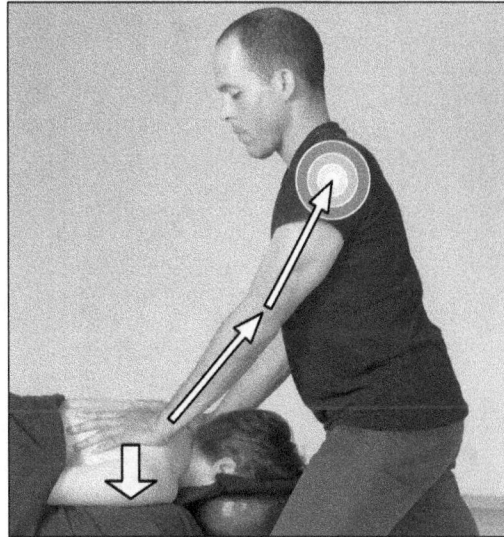

Applying downward pressure with the arms concentrates forces in the shoulder, placing stress on weaker muscles such as the rotator cuff.

in their sockets, placing stress on the rotator cuff and irritating tendons and ligaments. When you use your arms to apply pressure, particularly while reaching away from the body, the additional stress can cause injury.

Neck/Upper Back

The area of the cervical spine contains a number of complex and vulnerable structures that are exposed to greater stressors than one might imagine. Balanced on top of your cervical spine is your head which, when combined with the musculature that attaches to it, weighs an average of 10 to 12 pounds. That's as much as a bowling ball! When your head is not centered over your spine, such as when you look up or down or tilt your head to the side, the muscles alongside your cervical spine have to work harder to hold up that weight. If you look down the entire time you are assessing and treating your clients, this sustained contraction of the neck muscles can reduce blood flow and lead to chronic tightness and soreness of the muscles. Many of us already suffer from "tech neck" to some degree: neck strain and tension due to staring at a computer screen or looking down at

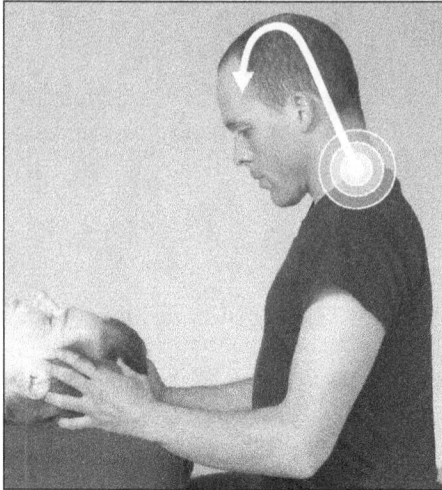

When the head is not centered over the spine, its considerable weight stresses the neck muscles, intervertebral discs, and cervical ligaments.

your mobile phone for hours at a time. Tipping your head away from a neutral position also changes the curvature of the cervical spine, placing stress on ligaments and intervertebral discs. Over time, this posture can lead to irritated ligaments and bulging discs. The consequences of neck disorders can extend into the head, shoulders, and upper back, since the musculature of the neck is connected to these other regions. Compression of nerve roots in the cervical spine can cause symptoms in the shoulders and down into the arms, as well as migraines, along the nerve pathways.

Lower Back

Low back disorders are very common. Eight out of ten adults will experience at least one episode of back pain in their lifetimes,[3] and half of them will go on to have at least one more episode.[4] Low back pain is the second most common pain condition after headaches among the general population. Low back disorders are a common reason that people seek care from manual therapists, but they are also a common complaint among practitioners themselves.

Causes of low back pain are as diverse as they are common, and include everything from arthritis to kidney problems, but the most prevalent causes of low back pain are musculoskeletal in nature. As with the CMC joint of the thumb, forces tend to concentrate in your lower back (lumbar spine), specifically in the L5/S1 region which is the base of support for all movement of the back. These forces can be very high: as much as 60 percent of a man's body weight is in his upper body, and women typically have close to 50 percent of their weight above the hips.[5] Every time you lean forward without supporting yourself with your arms, the the core stabilizer muscles of your body have to hold up at least half your body weight. For example, your work may require you to bend forward when working with a client on the treatment table, a position that requires a considerable amount of activity in the erector spinae and other spinal stabilization muscles. When you stand upright with your vertebrae stacked neatly on top of each other, pressure is distributed evenly through the intervertebral discs. When you bend forward, you disengage the bony and ligamentous structures of the posterior spine, transferring the load to the discs themselves. Because the pressure is now on the anterior portion of the disc, holding this position or repeatedly moving into it can damage the connective tissue of the discs over time. Weakened discs are more prone to bulges and herniations.

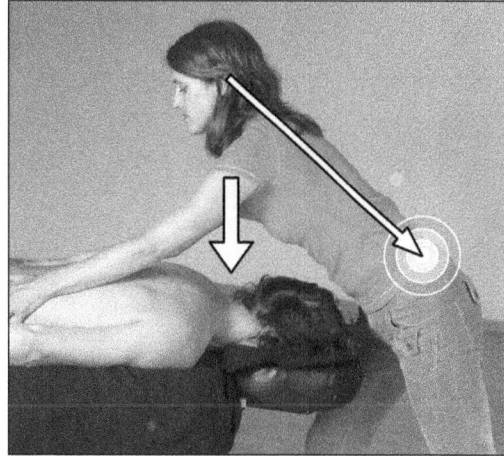

Most of the body's weight is in the torso. The force required to hold up or lift the upper body concentrates in the lower back.

Protecting Your Weak Links

You can see that many musculoskeletal injuries occur as a result of the nature of the structure of the weak link combined with the physical demands to which it is exposed. While you cannot change the vulnerability of the weak link, you may be able to avoid or reduce the demands you place on it. To continue the chain analogy: if you know there is a weak link in a chain, you can avoid putting that part of the chain under a high load (such as hoisting a heavy object with it) or repeatedly stressing it (such as using it to tow a boat). One of the strategies manual therapists can use to avoid MSDs is to protect these weak links as much as possible from overuse and misuse. By understanding the specific factors that increase your risk of injury, you will be able to identify specific steps you can take to reduce that risk.

1. Thomas Trumble and Carol Recor, University of Washington Orthopaedic Grand Rounds: Hand and Wrist Arthritis, University of Washington Medical Center, Seattle, Wash., July 22, 2003. *University of Washington Television Web site*, http://www.uwtv.org/programs/displayevent.aspx?rID=2451&fID=443.
2. Drs. Mark E. and Jason S. Pruzansky, HandSport Surgery Institute, https://handsurgeonsnyc.com/extensor-carpi-ulnaris-tendinitis-ecu-tendinitis/
3. Handouts on Health: Back Pain (National Institute of Arthritis and Musculoskeletal and Skin Diseases, National Institutes of Health, U.S. Department of Health and Human Services, Bethesda, MD, September 2005).
4 National Research Council and the Institute of Medicine, *Musculoskeletal Disorders and the Workplace: Low Back and the Upper Extremities* (Washington, D.C.: National Academies Press, 2001; 43.)
5. Don B. Chaffin, Gunnar B. J. Andersson and Bernard J. Martin, *Occupational Biomechanics, 3rd Edition*, (New York: John Wiley and Sons, 1999).

3

Risk Factors for Musculoskeletal Disorders

You have probably heard fellow practitioners, as well as some authors, proclaim that a certain method or technique will prevent injury for manual therapists. Learning "good body mechanics," for example, has been touted for years as a sure-fire method for preventing MSDs. Exercising to strengthen muscles is also often mentioned as the best way to avoid injury. It certainly would be wonderful to find the "magic bullet," a fast, easy method to avoid work-related MSDs. But decades of research have shown that reliance on just one tactic, such as using good body mechanics, focusing on posture, or building strength, is rarely effective in preventing these types of injury.

Taking a single approach to injury prevention assumes that there is only one factor that causes these injuries. Except in cases of traumatic or sudden injury, there is no single factor that causes musculoskeletal disorders. Unlike a traumatic injury (you stub your toe, it swells, it heals, and you're better), with MSDs it is rarely possible to point to a single event and a single cause and say, "This is the moment I became injured and this is why it happened." The gradual-onset MSDs that manual therapists experience have more insidious, complex causes, which can make preventing these injuries, as well as diagnosing and treating them, quite challenging.

A Multifaceted Approach for a Complex Problem

There are many factors that contribute to work-related MSDs, and only by taking all of these factors into account can one truly understand this complex issue. Even people who are in fantastic condition and have excellent body mechanics, like professional athletes, still get injured when the wrong combination of factors come together. Rotator cuff injuries are fairly common among baseball players, especially pitchers, in part because of the susceptibility of the rotator cuff to injury, but also because pitchers overuse their shoulder joints over the course of throwing thousands of pitches in a season. While

> **Injury prevention starts with awareness of your body, its vulnerabilities, and how it responds to the many different kinds of stress placed upon it.**

manual therapists do not necessarily push their bodies to the extremes that baseball pitchers do, the nature of the work creates the potential to overuse body parts that are susceptible to injury. A multifaceted approach to injury prevention begins with awareness of your own body, its vulnerabilities, and how it responds to the many different kinds of stress placed upon it.

To be able to take action to protect yourself from injury, it is important to first understand the many factors that contribute to causing injury. In occupational health, we refer to these as "risk factors." The term risk factors is used in the same way it is used by public health professionals when discussing health issues such as risk of heart disease. You may have heard that smoking, excess weight and high blood pressure are risk factors for heart disease. That doesn't mean that someone who smokes, is overweight, and has high blood pressure is going to have a heart attack. It does mean that having those risk factors places that person at an increased risk when compared to someone who doesn't have them.

The same concept holds true for risk factors for MSDs. For example, in a job that involves work-related risk factors like repetitive motions, forceful gripping and bent wrists, such as a construction worker fitting pipes, a small percentage of workers will develop hand or wrist injuries, even though all of them are exposed to the same risk factors.

Figure 1 illustrates the many risk factors that have been shown to contribute to musculoskeletal injury. Most of these risk factors are direct causes of musculoskeletal disorders, particularly the ones that are highlighted in bold in the diagram. Other risk factors, such as depression, can play a role in causing injury or may be symptoms of injury. Depression can reduce your awareness of how you are using your body; it is also easy to imagine becoming depressed if an injury keeps you from working or enjoying your hobbies.

Musculoskeletal injuries most often occur when a combination of the different risk factors shown in Figure 1 are at play. Since multiple factors are usually involved in developing MSDs, it is highly unlikely that a single method would be effective in preventing them. For the same reason, it has been difficult to find a single treatment method that is effective in resolving symptoms once they occur. Treatment methods tend to focus exclusively on the physical symptoms and disorders, while there may be psychological factors that are playing a partial role in creating or exacerbating the symptoms. To be effective, treatment needs to include reducing the physical and psychological risk factors to which the patient is exposed at work and at home (see more about treatment in Chapter 15).

Because multiple risk factors are often involved, it can be difficult to isolate the ones that are primarily responsible for injury. A group of

Figure 1. Risk Factors for Musculoskeletal Injury. The risk factors most strongly associated with injury are shown in bold.

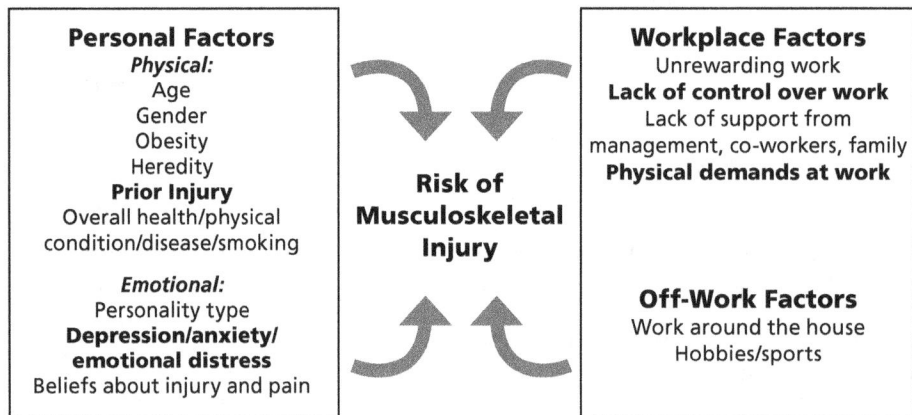

Personal Factors
Physical:
Age
Gender
Obesity
Heredity
Prior Injury
Overall health/physical condition/disease/smoking

Emotional:
Personality type
Depression/anxiety/ emotional distress
Beliefs about injury and pain

Risk of Musculoskeletal Injury

Workplace Factors
Unrewarding work
Lack of control over work
Lack of support from management, co-workers, family
Physical demands at work

Off-Work Factors
Work around the house
Hobbies/sports

people may be exposed to the same physical risk factors through their work, such as the construction workers mentioned above, but some of these workers may have additional risk factors, such as prior injuries or a lack of control over how they do their work. This would help explain why some individuals get injured and others don't, even though they do the same type of work.

Off-work activities can also contribute to injury. Gardening, which entails a good deal of bending, kneeling and use of hand tools, can contribute to lower back, knee and upper extremity conditions. Sport-specific injuries like tennis elbow (lateral epicondylosis) can occur from a combination of poor technique, force, and overuse of muscles and tendons.

Although risk factors outside of work play a role in injury, they present a much lower risk for injury than workplace factors do. Part of the reason may be that we have greater control of our off-work activities. Think about a hobby or sport in which you participate. If that activity starts to cause pain or other symptoms, you stop and rest, or change your approach to relieve your symptoms. If you get injured, you avoid that activity for a while until you are completely recovered. Most of the time, you don't have anyone's expectations to meet except your own. You probably don't have that luxury at work. Coupled with a physically demanding job, lack of control in your work can cause injury.

Work-related risk factors like these are the primary reason that manual therapists have such a high rate of MSDs. For this reason, much of this book will deal with risk factors specific to the work of manual therapists. Remember that workplace factors are modifiable, so you can influence and change them. In Part Two, you will learn how to modify the risk factors you encounter in your work so you can prevent injury.

Some risk factors, like prior injury, are not modifiable, but are still important to consider when evaluating your overall risk of injury. These factors increase your susceptibility to other risk factors and affect your body's ability to cope with the physical demands of your work. If you know that you have one or more of these non-modifiable risk factors, you may need to find ways to adapt the modifiable risk factors in your situation in order to protect yourself.

In the following section, you will learn about the different risk factors and how they can increase your susceptibility to injury. The discussion begins with personal risk factors, characteristics that are inherent to your own physical and emotional makeup. Work-related risk factors are then examined in more depth, along with similar exposures to risk factors outside of work.

The key to managing risk factors is to reduce your exposure as much as possible by modifying the risk factors that you can, and maintaining awareness of and developing coping strategies for those you can't.

Personal Risk Factors

Each individual has a unique set of personal characteristics. Some of these characteristics can be risk factors, making you more susceptible to MSDs. These physical and psychological factors do not cause injury in themselves, but, when combined with external factors associated with work, sports and hobbies, they can increase the potential for injury.

Your Physical Characteristics

Inherent physical characteristics that help determine your risk of injury include your age, gender, heredity, prior injuries, weight, smoking and your overall health. While the first four characteristics are not modifiable, the last three are under your control. The benefits of maintaining a healthy weight, avoiding smoking, and paying attention to your overall health go well beyond preventing MSDs.

Age

As we age, we naturally experience a gradual decline in muscle mass, lose connective tissue elasticity, and undergo a thinning of the cartilage between joints. Healing slows with advancing age, while at the same time the body is dealing with a lifetime of accumulated soft tissue damage, and for some people, osteoarthritis. As a result, we tend to become more prone to musculoskeletal disorders as we get older. While some decline in physical abilities is inevitable, you can keep or restore a lot of your strength and flexibility though exercise. Another bit of good news—it's never too late to start. Our bodies benefit from exercise at any age. You can also reduce the likelihood of damage from cartilage loss by following the principles of joint protection in Chapter 9. You can find helpful injury prevention tips for older practitioners in Chapter 8.

Gender

All other factors being equal, studies show that women are more likely to suffer from MSDs than men.[1] There are many theories that attempt to explain why women are more prone to MSDs, including differences in hormones, body structure and strength levels. Another factor to consider is that, for the most part, the world has been designed by men, for men. The heights of desks and countertops, the diameter of tool handles and the force required to operate them are often designed for the size and capabilities of men. In this male-oriented environment, women often have to adopt awkward postures and use a higher relative amount of strength to accomplish the same tasks as men. It is also important to take into account that women may have higher reported injury rates because they are generally more likely to seek medical care for their symptoms than men.

Heredity

Some disorders, such as osteoarthritis, occur more often when there is a family history of the condition. Degenerative disc disease and carpal tunnel syndrome may also have genetic components. Inherited musculoskeletal abnormalities can also increase susceptibility to injury; for example, the presence of a cervical rib or an elongated transverse process on the C7 vertebra can both increase the likelihood of developing thoracic outlet syndrome. This does not mean that some people are destined to have MSDs. These hereditary traits do not cause MSDs by themselves; there is typically a triggering event that causes an MSD, either cumulative trauma to tissues or damage that results from a sudden injury.

Prior Injury

One of the risk factors most consistently associated with MSDs is a previous injury, either to soft tissue or bone. A broken wrist, for example, may heal with more scar tissue or reduced space in the carpal tunnel, increasing the risk of wrist tendinosis and carpal tunnel syndrome. A motor vehicle accident may cause whiplash to the neck, creating complex soft tissue and nerve damage that is slow to resolve. A muscle tear in the lower back may heal with scar tissue that lacks the functionality of the original tissue, weakening the muscles in that area.

Scar tissue may also cause adhesions to develop that restrict the flow of blood and lymph and keep individual muscles from operating independently of each other. These adhesions can cause irritation and pain; they can also cause muscles to fatigue easily and weaken over time. Other muscles, less well suited to the task at hand, may be recruited in place of the fatigued ones.

All of these factors increase the risk of further injury to the muscles, tendons and joints in the area of the prior injury. Acute trauma (much less commonly seen in manual therapists) and the inflammation it provokes may cause lesions to articular cartilage, including thickening of the bone at either end of the joint, bone spurs and thinning of the cartilage, the classic characteristics of osteoarthritis.

Obesity

Being a little overweight is certainly healthier than obsessing about your weight or abusing your body through crash dieting. However, being considerably overweight, to the point of obesity, definitely has health consequences, including an increased likelihood of MSDs. Obesity can cause diabetes, which affects both the nerves and blood vessels, particularly in the extremities. Excess body weight also places additional stress on the lower back, hips and knees, which can damage connective tissue and increase the risk of conditions such as osteoarthritis. People who are obese are also more likely to have atherosclerosis (clogged arteries), which can reduce circulation and slow healing.

Smoking

In addition to all of the other ways that it can negatively affect your health, smoking constricts the arteries, increasing your risk of peripheral vascular disease. Reduced blood flow can result in ischemia, muscle pain and slower healing following trauma. Smoking greatly increases the likelihood of low back pain by reducing circulation and depleting the body of vitamin C. This vitamin is an important component in the formation of collagen, which in turn is critical in the repair of damage to intervertebral discs and blood vessels.

Overall Health

Poor overall health increases your chances of developing a chronic injury. People who are in poor health may have a disease, such as diabetes or thyroid disorders, that increases their risk for musculoskeletal injury. They may have poor eating, sleeping or lifestyle habits (including alcohol, caffeine or tobacco use), which have degraded their overall health. They may lack the physical conditioning necessary to withstand the physical demands of their work. As a result, they can be easily fatigued, their bodies do not repair damage as quickly or as thoroughly, and injury becomes more likely. In Chapter 10, you will find information on maintaining your overall health. For guidelines on physical conditioning for manual therapists, see Chapter 11.

Your Emotional Makeup

Psychological factors play a role in increasing the risk of MSDs. Some of these factors are modifiable with counseling, medical treatment, biofeedback and other techniques. Of course, it is normal to have emotions. But emotions that interfere with normal daily functioning are often part of a clinical condition that can increase the risk of injury. Psychological risk factors include depression, anxiety, distress and fear-avoidance behavior. Your overall personality type and your attitudes about your work also come into play in determining your injury risk.

Anxiety, Stress and Depression

One of the main symptoms of anxiety is increased overall muscle tension, which places additional stress on connective tissues and joints, and may result in reduced circulation and ischemia. Increased muscle tension is also a common side effect of emotional distress, often referred to as stress. Stress may also alter one's perception of pain through changes to the autonomic nervous system, resulting in an increased sympathetic response, which inhibits relaxation.

The link between pain and depression is well documented, but not fully understood. Many chronic pain sufferers report feelings of depression, and antidepressant medications have been shown to be effective in reducing pain for some people. While it seems obvious that chronic pain would cause feelings of depression, it also appears that feelings of depression make us more sensitive to pain, especially in the head, back, neck and limbs. Depression may also affect posture and body mechanics. Picture two people as they walk away from a competition. One is slumped forward, chest caved in, shoulders rounded forward, head forward and looking down. The other is standing tall, chest raised, shoulders back and head held high. It is clear which person won and which one lost. Emotion can change our posture, and our posture can reinforce our emotions. Depressed individuals who become injured may take a passive approach to their medical care, thereby slowing the healing process. Persons experiencing anxiety, stress and/or depression may also be less attentive to avoiding risk factors as they work.

Fear-Avoidance Behavior

Some people avoid movement when they have sub-acute or chronic injuries, fearing that the movement may cause pain and further injury. Fear of activity that causes pain, and avoidance of that activity, are very natural, protective reactions. But this fear and avoidance may extend to any activity, even if the activity is beneficial, and lead to a decreased level of function. Movement increases circulation and maintains flexibility and muscle tone. The tendency to self-prescribe rest for minor injuries may actually work against the healing process, resulting in muscle guarding, loss of range of motion, and eventually, atrophy of underused muscles. For non-specific low back pain, for example, studies have shown that an early return to normal activities and exercising in a pain-free range of motion every day are much more effective in aiding recovery than bed rest.

For any injury, the amount of rest prescribed and the moment chosen to return to activity should be part of a treatment plan developed by a qualified healthcare professional. Patients who learn to confront their apprehensions about pain and movement are better able to take an active role in their recovery, and tend to have a gradual, but steady, decrease in symptoms.

Personality Type

Our personalities greatly influence how we approach our work, and how we deal with symptoms of injury. A perfectionist or an overachiever may work too hard or try to accomplish too much in each treatment session. They may tend to focus on pleasing their clients, and pay less attention to the fatigue and soreness they are experiencing. An individual with this type of personality (commonly referred to as "Type A") will tend to use more effort and generate more muscle tension when applying the same amount of force than a person who is more relaxed. Another personality type is the stoic, who chooses to suffer symptoms in silence rather than seeking medical attention. Awareness of your own personality type and the potential consequences it can have on your work and your health can help you recognize and hopefully correct behaviors or attitudes about your work that can lead to injury.

Work-Related Risk Factors

You saw in Figure 1 that two of the principal causes of musculoskeletal disorders are related to the workplace. Stressful aspects of your work have an emotional impact that can lead to physical symptoms, while the direct impact that physically demanding work has on the body is more readily apparent. Work that is both emotionally stressful and physically strenuous creates an even greater risk for injury than either would alone.

Since these factors play such an important role in the development of musculoskeletal disorders, it is important to identify your personal exposure to them. To help you assess your own injury risk, you will find a worksheet in Appendix A for you to write down the risk factors to which you are exposed at work and elsewhere. There is also space on the worksheet to write down the strategies that you learn, from this book and other sources, for reducing your exposure to these risk factors.

Emotional Stress at Work

Emotional distress, anxiety or stress caused by your work can increase your risk of developing an MSD. Stressful risk factors at work can include:

- Lack of control over how work is scheduled or the type of work you do
- High work demands
- Unrewarding work
- Lack of support from management or co-workers.

Some of these risk factors, such as high work demands, may result in greater physical exertion as well as excessive psychological burdens. There is some evidence that working for demanding and unsupportive management may actually cause workers to change their movement patterns, using awkward movements and more force than is required by the job.

If you have ever driven a car in bad traffic, you have probably experienced an interaction of emotional stress and changes to your movement patterns. You may grip the steering wheel more tightly, hunch your shoulders, and clench your teeth. The movements you make to turn the steering wheel or turn your head to check the lane next to you may not be as smooth as usual. After a long drive in these conditions, you may feel increased tension in your neck, shoulders and lower back. Your work can be just as stressful, and result in the same types of muscle tension and awkward movement patterns.

Pressure at work can also be self-imposed. Imagine this scenario: it is your first week working at a clinic. You believe you need to make a good impression on your boss in order to keep this job. After the fourth client of the morning, your hands start to hurt. You try not to think about it—maybe it'll go away. So you ignore the pain that first day, and the next, and the next. You do a great job, and the boss loves you, but now you are in pain every day and it is getting worse. What do you do now?

Working under this kind of pressure to perform, whether external or self-imposed, will put you in a precarious situation. You are too tense to pay attention to things that may be interfering with your performance, including the signals your body is sending you that it is overtaxed. If you are a student, you may feel that to get a good grade you have to show your instructor that you are comfortable with a technique that makes your wrists hurt. If you are working professionally, your body mechanics may suffer because you are too preoccupied with giving your clients great treatment so they will sing your praises to your supervisor. Perhaps you are your toughest critic, and it is your own excessively high standards that must be met at all costs. Whatever the source of the pressure, it has the same result: it overpowers your awareness and your ability to change your behavior to protect yourself from injury.

Clinic or group practice settings can produce stressful situations. You may find that you have conflicting responsibilities, or that you have to deal with peer pressure to take on more work than you feel is healthy. Whether you work for someone else or for yourself, it is important to have a workload that allows you to work at your optimum level. You will experience stress if you have too much work, since you will not get enough rest and recovery time. Even if you are physically capable of handling that much work, the mental strain of overwork can eventually cause burnout. At the very least, you won't be giving each client the effort and attention they deserve. On the other hand, not enough work can be at least as stressful, since it brings with it worries about insufficient income, and self-doubt about your choice of career or your abilities as a practitioner. All of these factors can increase your risk of injury on the job. You will learn more about how to manage the pressure of different types of work settings in Chapter 4.

The Physical Demands of Your Work

We know that risk factors due to physical work demands are a direct cause of MSDs. In the survey results, you saw that the injuries manual therapists are at risk of developing are strongly related to the nature of the physical work they do. What is it about performing hands-on treatments that causes the "weak links" of the body to fail?

Physical work-related risk factors are present in many professions. Warehouse workers can injure their backs by repetitively lifting heavy boxes in the same way that manual therapists can injure their backs by lifting parts of a heavy clients' body. While the type of work, the setting, and what is being lifted are all different, the strain on the back is the same.

Ergonomics researchers have studied MSDs in different workplaces and identified the most common physical workplace risk factors[2] (Table 3). You can see that these risk factors exist in many of the common activities involved in manual treatment. Notice also that many of the risk factors come into play in activities you do outside of work as well as during your workday. The cumulative effect of exposure to risk factors during work and outside of work increases your overall injury risk.

Repetitive Motions

Soft tissue massage, manipulation and mobilization often include repetitive movements of your upper extremities. Although there may be some variety to the movements themselves, they often involve using (and possibly overusing) the same muscles and joints repetitively. Overuse can cause small tears in muscle, tendon and ligament fibers; this microtrauma, without adequate healing time, can cause degeneration of these tissues and further injury. One of the parts of the body that is most prone to injury from repetitive motion is the thumb, a common injury site among manual therapists. Practitioners tend to apply pressure with the thumb over and over during treatments; they also tend to friction or knead tissue with the thumbs, using small, repetitive movements. Repetitive movement can be a cause of injury in other parts of the body as well. Repetitively bending at the waist contributes to low back injury, repetitive gripping can cause wrist tendinosis and forearm muscle strain, and repeatedly kneeling on the ground, as in the case of pediatric PTs, can cause knee injuries. Note that repetitive movement by itself may not cause injury. It is noted here as a risk factor because it is most often combined with force and awkward postures.

Hand Force

Force (or pressure) applied with the hands can result in microtrauma to muscle and tendon fibers in much the same way that repetition can. Hand force in soft tissue work is generated either through pressure applied with the fingertips or palm, or through grasping or gripping, either with the whole hand or with the tips of the fingers and thumb. Applying force with the hands is one of the principal risk factors for upper extremity MSDs.

The stronger the muscle, the less risky it is to use it to exert gripping force. For example, a strong muscle-tendon unit like the forearm flexor group is capable of generating much higher forces without incurring dam-

Table 3. Risk Factors for Musculoskeletal Disorders in Manual Treatment Work

Risk factors	Examples from manual therapy treatment	How they cause injury
Repetitive motions	Most effleurage, petrissage, percussion and friction techniques. Typing and mouse use at the computer (when combined with poor ergonomics and/or overgripping of the mouse).	Frequent movements, often in combination with force and awkward postures, result in microtrauma to connective tissues. Trauma accumulates over time due to lack of recovery, and results in degeneration and scar tissue formation.
Hand force	Gripping a part of the client's body with the whole hand or pinching tissues between the tips of the fingers and the thumb, especially when holding the grip for long periods of time.	Hand force is generated either through applying pressure or gripping. Gripping places strain on both the flexor and extensor muscles and tendons, and increases pressure in the carpal tunnel.
Awkward postures	Bending the wrists when applying pressure. Reaching out to treat a client at the center of the table. Bending forward when leaning over a low treatment table. Twisting at the lower back. Bending at the neck to observe a client during treatment. Kneeling or squatting to work with a client at floor level.	Bending the wrists increases the likelihood of damage to tendons and tendon sheaths in the wrist, as well as increasing pressure in the carpal tunnel. Reaching out places the muscles and tendons in the shoulder, especially the rotator cuff, in a position that is likely to damage tendons. Tendons can also rub on bursae, and muscles can impinge nerves and blood vessels. Bending the back or neck causes forces to concentrate in the spine as the muscles work to hold up the weight of the upper body and head. It also compresses the intervertebral discs asymmetrically. Kneeling and squatting cause pressure behind the kneecap, which can damage the cartilage. Kneeling can also cause inflammation in the bursae.
Static loading	Holding one position for a long period of time, especially in an awkward posture, such as bending over a treatment table. Maintaining force, such as gripping and holding, or applying downward pressure to treat trigger points.	Tension in contracted muscles can exceed blood pressure in the capillaries that supply oxygen and nutrients. Localized decrease in blood flow (ischemia) and build-up of metabolic byproducts results in fatigue, pain and increased muscle tension.
Contact stress	Pressure from hard or sharp surfaces on soft tissues, such as pressing the fingertips against bony structures, or using a hand tool that places pressure on the palm of the hand.	Compression of soft tissues can damage nerves and blood vessels; for example, pressing the fingertips against bony structures or using a hand tool that puts pressure on your palm.

Table 3. *(Continued)* **Risk Factors for Musculoskeletal Disorders in Manual Treatment Work**

Risk factors	Examples from manual therapy treatment	How they cause injury
Lifting	Lifting a treatment table or other equipment. Lifting a client's torso, limb or head.	Heavy lifting, and lifting in awkward postures (bending, twisting), place stress on muscles, tendons and ligaments in the shoulders and lower back, and on the intervertebral discs in the spine.
Carrying	Carrying a treatment table or other equipment with a mobile practice.	Carrying can place the same stress on the body as lifting, but with an increased likelihood of fatigue due to static loading.
Pushing and pulling	Pushing down while performing compression. Pulling to traction a client's limb or head.	Pushing and pulling can concentrate high forces in the shoulders and lower back. Pulling is more likely to cause back injury than pushing.
Fatigue	Doing a number of treatments in one day, especially ones that require deep work.	Fatigue results in failure of the stronger muscles, placing additional strain on smaller muscles, tendons, ligaments and joints.
Vibration	Vibration to the hands, arms, or entire body.	Vibration to the hands and arms can increase muscle tension in the forearms and damage nerves and blood vessels. Vibration to the entire body can increase tension in the back muscles and cause degeneration of the intervertebral discs.

age than a much smaller group like the thenar and hypothenar muscles in the hand. Your grip is four to five times stronger when using the whole hand (with the thumb in opposition) than when you hold something with just the tips of the fingers and thumb.[3] Think about the difference in effort you feel in your hand and forearm when you lift a client's arm with a comfortable grip around their wrist versus when you pinch their upper trapezius between your thumb and fingertips (see Figure 4 in Chapter 6).

When you apply pressure through your fingertips, the forces concentrate in the carpal tunnel, which acts as the fulcrum to the relatively long lever arm created by the metacarpals and phalanges. As pressure in the carpal tunnel increases, the likelihood of damage to the tendons or tendon sheaths that pass through it also increases. This increased pressure can also impinge the median nerve, potentially damaging the nerve itself, as well as the blood vessels that supply it. Applying excessive pressure with the fingertips also places a great deal of stress on the smaller distal interphalangeal (DIP) joints in the digits.

Gripping involves one of the most potentially overused muscle and tendon groups in the body: the forearm flexors and extensors. While the flexor muscles provide the gripping force, the extensor muscles are co-activated to stabilize the fingers and wrists. Repeated or sustained gripping, particularly when a good deal of force is utilized, can cause microtrauma to the tendons and tendon sheaths, particularly at the carpal tunnel. Pinching is an even bigger risk factor than gripping with the whole hand, not only because pinching involves smaller muscles, but also because it places stress on the ligaments, muscles and tendons of the thumb.

The hand and wrist are not the only parts of your body at risk when you apply hand force. Applying pressure with any part of your upper extremity transfers forces further up your arm to the stabilizing muscles of the shoulder, potentially straining the muscles of the rotator cuff.

Awkward Postures

It is common for manual therapists to work in positions that entail bending or twisting at the waist, elevating the arms and shoulders, and bending the wrists. These awkward postures can become habitual, or are stressful to the body because they require significant muscle activity to maintain. They also place additional pressure on joints and ligaments, constrict blood vessels, and compress nerves.

However, the opposite of "awkward posture" is not necessarily "good posture." The term "neutral posture" is used to describe positions that require the least amount of muscle effort to maintain, and place the least amount of stress on joints. While understanding neutral posture is important, the problem with the concept of postures—good, neutral or otherwise—is that they tend to be static. Since we cannot escape the pull of gravity, any posture you hold is going to include some amount of static loading (see next section). Your goal should be to move through a variety of near-neutral postures as you work. You will learn more about these concepts in Chapter 5.

A Bit of Biomechanics

Ergonomists frequently use the principles of biomechanics to study the effects of work on the human body. In simple terms, biomechanics is the application of fundamental concepts of physics to human movement. One of the central concepts of musculoskeletal biomechanics is leverage. A lever consists of a fulcrum and a lever arm, with resistance at one end of the lever arm, and force applied at the other end to overcome the resistance.

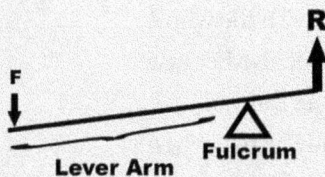

Think about using a pry bar. It has a curve near one end (the fulcrum), with a short hook that you place under an object, such as a nail, that you are prying up (the resistance) and a longer end that you push down (the force). The long end gives you leverage, or mechanical advantage, multiplying the force that is applied at the short end.

Now think about turning the pry bar around and prying up the nail while holding the short end instead. You would have to apply a great deal of force just to generate a little bit of force at the long end of the bar, because you are now at a biomechanical disadvantage.

In the human body, the musculoskeletal system can be viewed as series of levers. The joints are the fulcrums, the long bones are the lever arms, and the muscles apply the force to overcome the resistance at the other end. To feel this yourself, pick up an object and hold it in your hand, palm up, forearm parallel to the floor. The weight of the object creates resistance, which travels up the lever arm formed by your ulna and radius to the elbow, which is the fulcrum. Here, your brachialis and biceps muscles contract to generate force in order to overcome the resistance created by the weight of the object in your hand. Notice that these muscles attach to the bones in your forearm, quite close to the elbow, while the object in your hand is much further away. Your upper arm muscles are at a biomechanical disadvantage: they have to generate quite a bit of force to overcome the weight of the object and raise it.

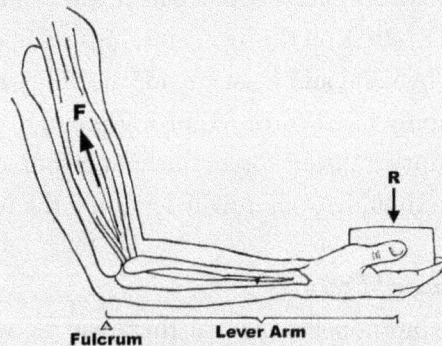

In fact, most of the musculoskeletal system is at a biomechanical disadvantage. While this may seem like a bad design, it actually allows the parts of your body to move longer distances with short muscle contractions, giving you speed of movement. A relatively short contraction of your elbow flexors will move the hand holding the weight quickly through a fairly long arc, but the force generated by that muscular contraction must be much higher than the resistance in your hand.

Because of this inherent biomechanical disadvantage, it is best not to rely on your upper body strength alone to do your work—you need to use the strength of the large muscles in your lower body and torso to overcome this disadvantage.

Static Loading

Static loading is sometimes referred to as sustained exertion. Essentially, static loading is an isometric muscle contraction that is maintained for more than a few seconds at a time. Grasping and holding a client's limb, leaning over and holding up the weight of your own upper body against gravity, or maintaining pressure with your fingers or thumbs are all examples of static loading.

As you contract a muscle, the fluid pressure inside that muscle increases. With a strong enough contraction, the pressure inside the muscle can exceed blood pressure in the capillaries that supply those muscles with oxygen and nutrients. At maximum effort, the fluid pressure inside a muscle can be up to four times higher than the pressure of the blood in the capillaries. This pressure prevents blood from flowing to the muscles, resulting in ischemia. Even a moderate level of muscle contraction

The Effects of Static Loading

Try this exercise: Hold a light weight, 1 to 3 pounds, in each hand (use 1-liter bottles of water or juice if you don't have weights). Raise one arm straight out in front of you to shoulder level and hold it there. Raise the other arm to shoulder level, then lower it back to your side and repeat, using a slow, steady motion. See which arm gets tired first. Was it the arm you expected?

may be enough to reduce blood flow to that muscle, depriving it of oxygen.[4] If the contraction is held for more than a few seconds, the lack of oxygen in the muscles creates metabolic byproducts, which are acidic in nature, to build up. Insufficient blood flow to the area impedes the swift evacuation of these byproducts from the muscles, causing pain. Pain tends to increase muscle tension, which further reduces blood flow and perpetuates the cycle of ischemia, which can lead to injury. If you have ever felt a sudden twinge in your lower back when you straighten up after bending forward for any length of time, you have experienced the effects of static loading on your muscles. Muscles in spasm due to ischemia are more likely to fatigue quickly, placing them, and the structures around them, at risk for injury.

Figure 2. The Ischemic Cycle

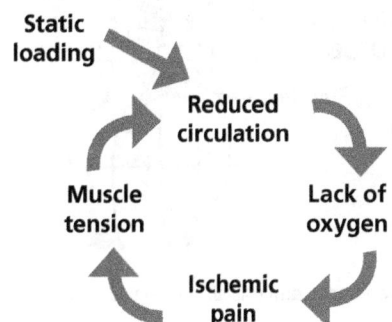

Static loading → Reduced circulation → Lack of oxygen → Ischemic pain → Muscle tension → (back to Static loading)

Lifting

Lifting is one of the most common causes of low back injury. The forces generated during lifting tend to concentrate in the lower back. When you lift, your lower back—particularly the L5/S1 region—acts as a fulcrum, and the force of the lift is generated by muscles that run very close to your spine, including the erector spinae. If you lift while leaning forward or reaching out, the force created by the object you are lifting (and by the weight of your own upper body) is multiplied by the long lever arm formed by your spine. In order to lift a 10-pound weight held away from your body, your paraspinal muscles have to generate at least 100 pounds of force.[5] It is no wonder that physical therapists and nurses who lift clients manually have a high incidence of back injuries. In fact, there is no safe way for one person to manually lift another. Even when two practitioners lift a 110-pound person together, they still generate forces in their lower backs that exceed the strength of the intervertebral discs and thereby increase their risk of injury. While lifting a lighter weight, like a client's limb or a treatment table, results in much lower force, repeated lifting of moderate weights like these, particularly while bending or twisting, can also result in injury.

Lifting with your arms outstretched, especially above shoulder height, can place considerable stress on your shoulders and your lower back. The same concepts of leverage apply, but in this case your arms are acting as long levers and your shoulder muscles have to provide the high forces to counteract the weight in your hands.

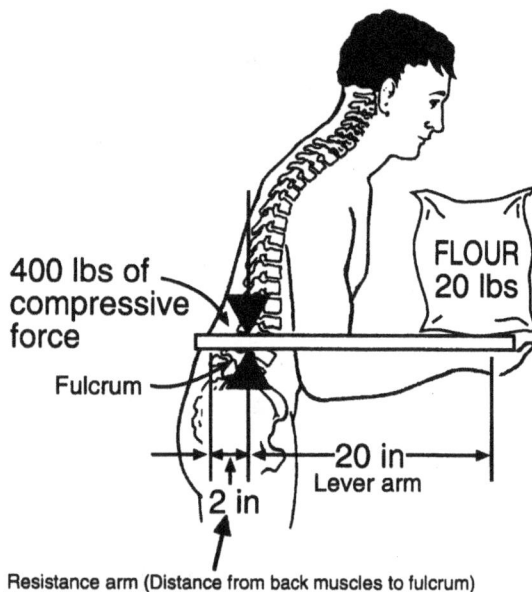

400 lbs of compressive force

Fulcrum

FLOUR 20 lbs

20 in Lever arm

2 in

Resistance arm (Distance from back muscles to fulcrum)

Carrying

Your work may require you to carry equipment, linens or machines during your workday. If you have a mobile practice, you may find yourself carrying a heavy, bulky treatment table or other equipment into clients' homes or offices. The same effort is required to lift the object while carrying, but it is sustained over a longer period of time.

This prolonged effort is another type of static loading that can fatigue your muscles, making the other structures of your back, such as the discs and ligaments, more vulnerable to injury. Carrying can also fatigue your arm muscles, particularly the forearm muscles involved in gripping. By the time you start your treatment, your muscles are already fatigued and some amount of microtearing may have already taken place.

Pushing or Pulling

Pushing or pulling can also cause back and shoulder injuries. To move the same amount of weight, pushing or pulling require less effort than lifting or carrying. These movements are therefore less likely to cause injury.

Force vs. Effort

The terms "force" and "effort" are often used interchangeably, but they are actually two different concepts. You create force when you apply pressure, for example, to a trigger point. Force is the end result. Effort is what you experience in your body as you generate that force.

There are many ways to reduce the effort you experience in doing your work. By recruiting large, strong muscles, such as those in your upper arms and chest, you will use less effort to apply the same amount of force than if you used the smaller, weaker muscles in your hands and forearms. In a neutral posture, you can apply force with less effort than you can in an awkward posture. When you have a good deal of experience using a particular technique, you can often generate more force with less effort than when you were first learning that technique.

Emotional tension can make you feel that you need to use more effort than a task truly requires. If you are apprehensive about working with a particular client, nervous about impressing your boss, or stressed about something going on outside of work, these feelings can generate a high level of overall muscular tension. When you work, that tension will increase your level of effort without actually generating any more force. If you can remain relaxed, you will experience less overall effort while accomplishing the same amount of work.

Pushing is the easier of the two, since it allows you to use the large muscles in your legs, hips and chest, along with your body weight, to move objects forward. Pulling requires you to use the relatively smaller muscles in your back, particularly your erector spinae muscles, so it tends to concentrate forces in the lower back in much the same way that lifting and carrying do.

Contact Stress

Contact stress is a technical term for a very straightforward risk factor. When the soft tissues of the body come into contact with hard, sharp or narrow surfaces, damage can occur to vulnerable structures such as nerves, blood vessels and tendon sheaths. A common example when working with clients is using the fingertips to hold pressure on a trigger point in a thin sheet of muscle over bone (such as the infraspinatus over the scapula). Contact stress can also occur when using hand tools that end in the palm of the hand, where the tool handle can compress the median nerve at the point where it exits the carpal tunnel. Contact stress is also common among computer users who rest their wrists on the edge of the desk as they type.

Fatigue

While technically not a risk factor by itself, fatigue can make you more susceptible to injury when combined with other risk factors. Physiologically, a muscle is "fatigued" when it reaches the point where it can no longer contract. The biochemistry of muscle fatigue is complex, and is not due to accumulation of lactic acid as once thought, but may instead be due to leaking of excess calcium into the muscle fibers. Fatigue can actually help protect muscles from damage that could occur from over-contraction. But once a muscle fails and stops contracting, it can no longer support and protect the other structures in that area (like joints, ligaments and intervertebral discs). As a result, even a low level of fatigue can increase the likelihood of injury.

As some muscle groups fatigue, others can be recruited, but those muscles are typically smaller and less well conditioned to the movement. These smaller muscles will, in turn, fatigue more quickly. Using these smaller muscles may pull tendons across bones or bursae, causing friction and irritation.

Muscle fatigue may also diminish coordination, increasing the risk for injury. Fatigue, whether muscular or mental, can also reduce your attention to proper positioning and technique. When you are tired, you do not react as quickly to stimuli like pain that may signal you to stop or change what you are doing.

Vibration

Vibration can be a very serious risk factor. Although manual therapists are not often exposed to vibration in their daily work life, they can encounter it in their off-work activities. Prolonged exposure to high-frequency vibration, such as when using power tools, can damage blood vessels and nerves in the hands and forearms. Vibration also causes involuntary contraction of the muscles, known as tonic vibration reflex, which can increase muscle tension and ischemia. Whole body vibration, like the low frequency vibration your lower back endures when driving, can cause muscle fatigue and degenerative changes to intervertebral discs. These effects of vibration can sometimes take hours to subside, and need to be taken into consideration if you use power tools for yard work or home projects. You should also be careful about lifting just after driving, when the combination of whole body vibration and static loading from sitting in one position can make your lower back susceptible to injury.

Risk Factors Outside of Work

All manual therapists have a life outside of their main job, with personal activities and responsibilities. These may be hobbies or sports that you love; they may also be responsibilities or second jobs that you may dislike or find stressful. These activities outside of work tend to add to the negative effect of the activities you do at work, rather than creating injury themselves. As far as your body is concerned, it doesn't matter if the risk factors come from work, home or elsewhere. Even though you may have a break between your time at work and the time you spend working around the house or playing sports, you may still have enough cumulative exposure during a single day and over time to cause injury. For this reason, it is important to remain aware of the additional stress that off-work activities can place on your body and mind.

Mobile Phone Use

Nearly everyone owns a mobile or cell phone. While these devices are now an integral part of our lives, they carry with them some exposure to injury risk factors. There is an MSD now referred to as "Texter's Thumb," also known as de Quervain's thumb, which occurs when the thumb is used excessively to send text messages. There's also "cell phone neck," a variation on tension neck disorder, caused by bowing your head for extended periods of time to look down at your phone.

It is possible to adjust the way you use your cell phone so you can avoid these MSDs. Take frequent breaks from texting, perhaps limiting your texting to 15 minutes at a time. Of course, if you start to feel pain or discomfort in your thumb, you should stop immediately. To avoid "cell phone neck," never look at your phone while it's on your lap or below your waist. It's best to bring your phone up nearly to the level of your eyes to read and send texts. In this way, you are only slightly bending your head to read and send texts, or to look at anything else on your phone. Use a phone stand or a "pop socket" to lean your phone on as high a surface as possible, or to hold it with your hand at a level that requires bending your head no more than 20 degrees downward. For both texting and holding your phone, limit the time you are bowing your head, while away from work and certainly while you're at work!

Hand-Intensive Activities and Hobbies

There are many jobs and hobbies that involve intensive use of the hands and arms. Playing an instrument, building furniture and gardening are all hand-intensive activities. Activities of daily life, like opening jars or lifting heavy bags of groceries, also place additional stress on your body. All of these activities can have the same risk factors as your manual treatment work, and when they are combined with those work-related risk factors, they can increase your overall risk enough to cause injury. If you already use your fingertips to apply pressure to your client's tissues, playing an instrument that requires pressing and holding strings or keys will increase your overall exposure to the risk factors of repetitive movement and static loading. If you love to garden and spend every weekend pruning your bushes and trees, the stress of gripping the pruning sheers in addition to the risk factors already present in your work can get you injured. Exercising or participating in sports can be very beneficial to your overall health, but some of these activities can have risk factors very similar to the ones you are exposed to at work.

In Chapter 9, you will find tips on avoiding additional stressors or risk factors in your daily life. Chapter 11 contains a conditioning program designed specifically for manual therapists to help you stay in shape without creating additional stress to already overworked parts of your body. Since most people spend some amount of time working on a computer in their daily life, Appendix B provides ergonomics guidelines that can help you minimize risk factors involved in computer use. With a profession that places considerable demands on your musculoskeletal system, you may wish to reconsider engaging in other activities that carry the same risk factors, or reduce the amount of time you spend doing those activities. At the very least, be particularly aware of your increased risk and be ready to react quickly to any signs or symptoms that may develop.

Risk Factor Exposures that Lead to Injury

All of this discussion about compressive forces, microtrauma and cumulative damage might have you worried about your career choice at this point. But before you put your practice up for sale, remember that simply being exposed to a particular risk factor does not necessarily mean you will become injured. Working for 15 minutes per day in an awkward posture is not particularly harmful, and neither is lifting something weighing 10 pounds if you are in a good posture. A moderate level of stress and strain on the body can actually be good for you. If you never lifted anything, you would be as weak as a newborn kitten, and if you never got into an awkward posture, you would spend your entire life in a static posture, which is worse. Too little activity can be just as harmful as too much activity, and a little bit of lifting, bending and reaching in everyday life, when done properly, actually helps maintain strength and flexibility.

The human body has a remarkable ability to adapt to the physical activities to which it is subjected. Depending on the nature of the activities, that adaptation can either be positive or negative. Some of the benefits of having a physically demanding profession include stronger muscles, tendons and bones, as well as increased endurance and improved movement patterns. Negative effects of this kind of work can include overstretched and weakened muscles, chronically tight and painful muscles, shortened ligaments and tendons, and tendons that rub across bony surfaces or bursae, all of which can lead to injury. Whether your body will adapt positively or negatively to the physical demands of your work depends on which of the risk factors you frequently encounter, and to what extent you are exposed to them.

In reality, risk factors, whether at work or away from work, do not result in injury unless you are exposed to them:

- For longer durations
- At greater intensities
- With higher frequencies of exertion
- Or particularly when multiple risk factors are combined at once.

Duration

The amount of time you are exposed to risk factors can significantly increase your likelihood of injury. A busy manual therapist can easily be exposed to risk factors like repetitive motion and awkward postures for several hours every day. The exposure does not need to occur all at one time, either. The cumulative effect of multiple exposures of several minutes at a time, without adequate time for recovery, can also result in injury. It doesn't matter to your body whether you get all of your exposure from your manual treatment work, a second job, work around the house, hobbies, or a combination of these.

Intensity

The higher the intensity with which you apply hand force, or perform activities like lifting or carrying, the more likely your risk of injury will be. All other things being equal, work done with low intensity hand force is less likely to result in injury than work done with high intensity hand force. "Low" and "high" are relative terms, and depend on how much of your body's capacity is being used when you apply pressure or grip something. When lifting, the heavier the object and the further it is from your lower back, the greater the potential for injury.

Frequency

Frequent exertions increase your risk of injury by increasing your overall duration of exposure. But they can also produce fatigue while reducing the opportunity for your body to recover from the previous exertion. If you do not get adequate rest or allow enough healing time between exertions, the result can be cumulative trauma. When your exertions are frequent and closely spaced—for example, during repetitive movements like percussion or kneading—the muscles that are recruited do not have a chance to fully relax between efforts. This rapid muscle firing causes a constant state of contraction and a high level of static loading and resulting ischemia.

Combining Risk Factors

Any of the risk factors discussed in this chapter can cause injury to your musculoskeletal system. So it is not surprising that combining two or more factors at once will increase your risk of injury that much more. Hand and wrist injuries are often the result of exposure to several risk factors: tendonitis and carpal tunnel syndrome, for example, are much more likely to occur when hand force is combined with repetitive motion and awkward postures. By combining risk factors,

Figure 3. Injury Threshold and Patterns of Exposure

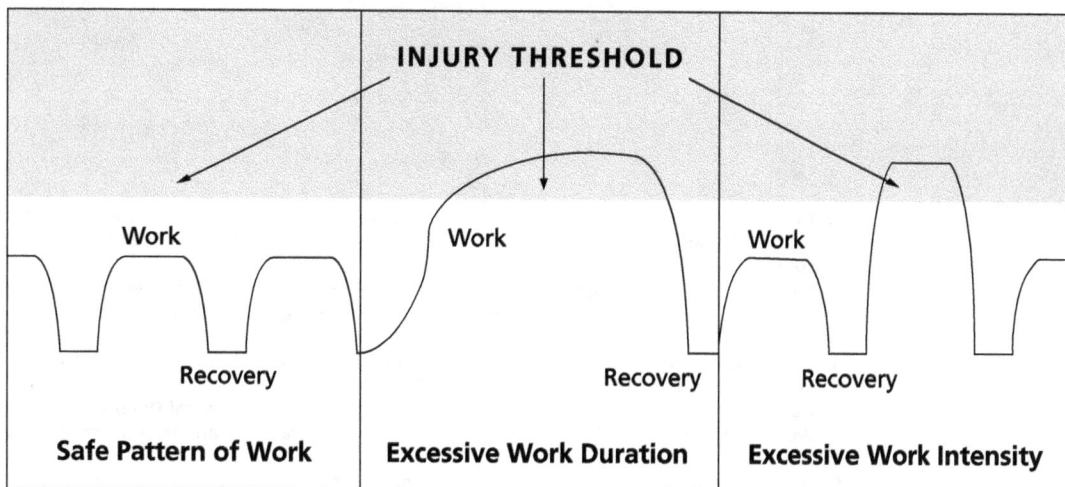

your risk of injury may be more than 10 times higher than it would be otherwise. In Figure 3, you can see how excessive work duration or intensity can push you past a safe balance of work and recovery and over the threshold of injury.

Assessing Your Injury Risk to Prevent Injury

Becoming aware of the risk factors to which you may be exposed is the first step in preventing injury. Use the information in this chapter, as well as the worksheet in Appendix A, to help you objectively assess your own risk and become conscious of the specific risk factors that are most at play in your particular situation. Armed with this knowledge, you can start developing an injury prevention strategy that you can put into practice in your work and daily life. In Part Two, you will learn practical, proven injury prevention methods you can use every day to stay healthy in your career.

1. Laura L. Tosi, Barbara D. Boyan and Adele L. Boskey, "Does Sex Matter in Musculoskeletal Health?: The Influence of Sex and Gender on Musculoskeletal Health," *Journal of Bone & Joint Surgery*, 2005; 87:1631-1647.
2. National Research Council and the Institute of Medicine, *Musculoskeletal Disorders and the Workplace: Low Back and the Upper Extremities* (Washington, D.C.: National Academies Press, 2001; 85-183).
3. Virgil Mathiowetz, et al, "Grip and Pinch Strength: Normative Data for Adults," *Archives of Physical Medicine and Rehabilitation*, 1985; 66(2): 69-74.
4. National Research Council and the Institute of Medicine, *Musculoskeletal Disorders and the Workplace: Low Back and the Upper Extremities* (Washington, D.C.: National Academies Press, 2001; 204).
5. Don B. Chaffin, Gunnar B. J. Andersson and Bernard J. Martin, *Occupational Biomechanics, 3rd Edition*, (New York: John Wiley and Sons, 1999).

PART TWO

Preventing Injury

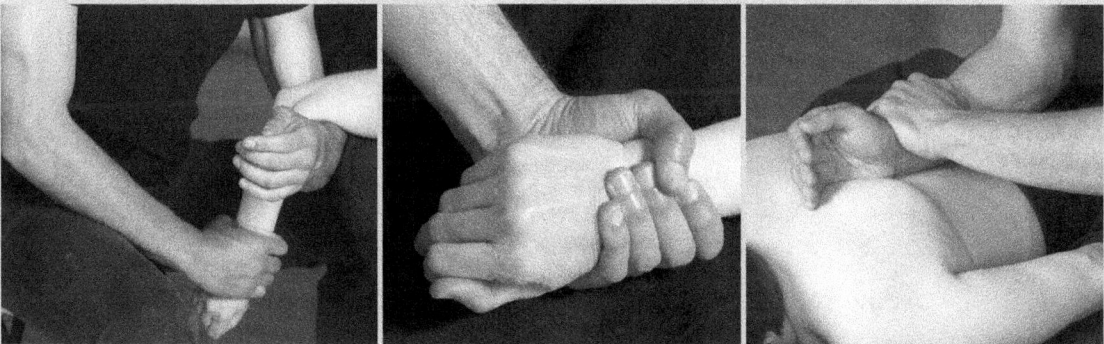

Preventing Injury

While injury is common among manual practitioners, it is certainly not a foregone conclusion that it will occur. There is a great deal you can do reduce your risk of becoming injured. Proven methods exist to lower the incidence of work-related injury. Many of them involve making simple but important changes to your activities, both at work and elsewhere; others will take more thought and practice to apply. But taking the necessary steps to prevent injury is much easier and less disruptive to your career and your life than dealing with an injury once it has occurred.

Since multiple factors are involved in causing work-related injuries, some on the job and some outside of the workplace, a successful prevention strategy must address all of the potential causes. Any single approach to injury prevention, like changing your work methods, developing good body mechanics, or doing conditioning exercises, may not be enough by itself to keep you from getting injured. In combination, these tactics can be very effective in helping you maintain a long and healthy career.

A Six-Step, Holistic Approach to Injury Prevention

1. Maintaining awareness of the risk of injury in your work
2. Understanding how risk factors cause injury
3. Developing awareness of your body as you work
4. Reducing risk factors through ergonomics
5. Developing good body mechanics and work practices
6. Taking care of your general physical and emotional health, including physical conditioning designed specifically for manual therapists.

4

Using Ergonomics in Your Work

Because the work of a manual therapist is so physically demand-ing, workplace risk factors play a primary role in causing MSDs among manual practitioners. While some risk factors, like your age or previous injuries, are realities that you cannot change, risk factors in your practice are modifiable to a great extent. Ergonomics is a proven and remarkably effective way of addressing workplace risk factors and reducing injury risk.

The main goal of ergonomics is to find ways to make the work environment better fit the worker. Think about sitting in a comfort-able chair at home. Now, think about how you felt the last time you were in an economy class seat on an airplane. That's the difference between an environment that fits you well and one that doesn't. Unlike an uncomfortable airplane seat, a poorly fitting job or workplace can cause more than just discomfort. MSDs can occur when the physical demands of a job exceed the capabilities of the worker in it, or when a poorly fitting workplace puts the worker in an awkward position for hours at a time. For example, tasks that require working overhead for long periods of time, such as painting ceilings, tend to result in rotator cuff injuries. Finding ways to adapt your work or workplace to better fit your body can reduce your exposure to work-related risk factors and help you stay healthy in your career.

Body Mechanics is Not Ergonomics

You may have learned to develop and use good body mechanics while you were in school, in continuing education classes or through on-the-job experience. While using good body mechanics is certainly an important part of injury prevention, it is not enough in itself to prevent MSDs. It is also not the same things as ergonomics. Ergonomics is about adapting the work to fit you; body mechanics is about you adapting to fit the work.

Working with good body mechanics can help you work more efficiently and with less stress. You will find a detailed discussion of body mechanics in Chapter 5. However, experience has shown that working with good body mechanics does not, by itself, prevent injuries from occurring. You can still overuse your hands and wrists even if you keep them in the best possible position as you work. There will always be situations in which it is not possible to use good body mechanics. In a poorly-designed workspace—for example, a treatment room that does not have adequate space around the treatment table—you will end up working in awkward postures involving twisting or reaching. Lifting and carrying a portable treatment table is always an awkward exercise under any conditions, given the large size and unwieldy shape of the table. There are a number of other aspects of a manual therapist's work that are inherently risky, simply due to the repetitive, physically demanding nature of the work itself.

Ergonomics goes beyond body mechanics to:

- design a worker's equipment, tools, and physical workplace to support their use of good body mechanics
- plan work schedules and breaks to allow adequate recovery from the physical demands of work
- observe work methods to find alternative techniques with fewer physical risk factors
- examine the impact that work has on emotional states, with the understanding that emotions can also affect health.

In this chapter, you will learn some fundamental principles of ergonomics, and see how various aspects of your work can be adapted or changed to help you prevent injury on the job.

Equipment, Tools and Workspace

The primary piece of equipment used by most practitioners is the treatment table. While a manual therapist may concentrate on features such as price, color and client comfort when choosing a table, the features that ergonomists would consider most important are weight, table dimensions (especially width), and adjustability.

Weight is a particularly important consideration for students and for practitioners with a mobile practice. They may have to lift their tables several times a day, often out of an awkward location, such as the back of a car. Tables are difficult to carry because they are large and need to be carried either with one hand or on one shoulder. To compensate for the increased load on one side of the body, the muscles of the lower back on the opposite side have to contract more. This asymmetrical loading around the lumbar vertebrae can result in disc damage.

A key ergonomics principle is to lighten the load when lifting and carrying. That means buying the lightest table you can find, and placing face cradles, bolsters and other equipment in another bag that can be lifted and carried separately. It is a good idea to use a cart to transport even the lightest table. Several manufacturers offer small carts specifically built for transporting portable tables. Look for large diameter wheels, which will roll easily over obstacles and can make going up and down stairs easier. If you don't think a cart will work for you, at least use a carrying case with a shoulder strap long enough to cross over to the opposite shoulder. By slinging the case across your body, you can take some of the weight of the table onto your shoulder and hip. Alternate the shoulder on which you carry the table to avoid overusing one side of your body.

Table Dimensions and Adjustments

The most important non-adjustable table dimension to consider is width. With the population getting larger all the time, it may be tempting to buy the widest table available to provide more room for your clients. Some modalities may involve placing your knee up on the table or sitting next to the client, and for those techniques, a wider table

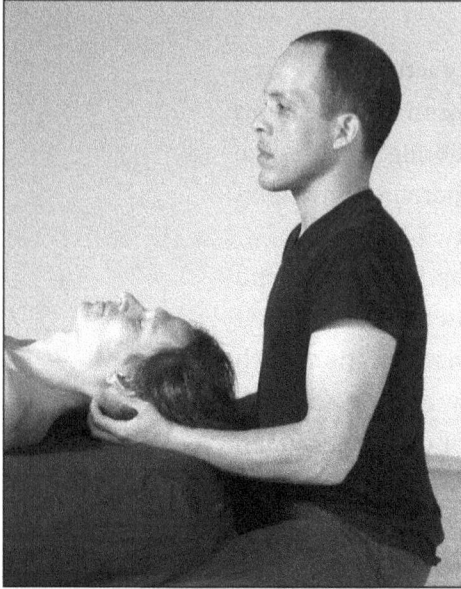

For seated work, set the table height a few inches above the height of your elbows to perform precision work.

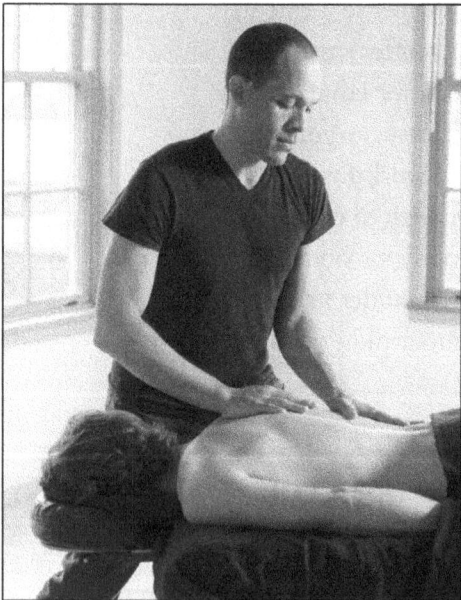

Stand up and set the table a couple of inches below elbow height to perform work that requires more pressure or larger movements.

makes sense. However, for most treatment work, a wide table can lead to bending over, twisting and reaching out, particularly for shorter practitioners. These awkward postures increase stress on the shoulders and lower back. A narrower table will be lighter and less bulky to lift, and will provide better access to the mid-line of the client. Side extensions are available for some narrow tables for use with larger clients. There are also tables available that are wide at the shoulders and feet, but narrow through the center. These tables better match most clients' body proportions, and provide the practitioner with better access to the lower back and hips, which are typically a major focus of hands-on treatment.

Along with width, the height of the table is very important to your working posture. There is no one table height that is appropriate for all types of work. Here are some general ergonomics guidelines for positioning your work based on the amount of force and type of movements involved:

- Small, precise, and low-force movements of the hands should be done at or a little above elbow height while seated in a neutral posture (a more detailed description of neutral posture can be found on page 79).
- Work involving larger movements and moderate amounts of force should be done several inches or more below elbow height while standing, also in a neutral posture.
- As a general rule, for light to medium work, your knuckles should just brush the top of your table when you swing your arm out in front of you.

- As the force requirements of the work increase, the height of the work surface should drop, so that body weight and larger muscle groups can be used to apply the force.
- When working with bigger clients, you will need to lower the table as necessary.

Given that most practitioners do a combination of different techniques with each client, nearly all manual therapists would benefit from using a power-adjustable table, although obviously this is not an option for a mobile practice. In some hands-on health professions, using power-adjustable tables is the norm. In other professions, particularly massage and physical therapy, many practitioners work with tables that cannot be readily adjusted during a treatment session. While power-adjustable tables do cost more than other tables, the benefit of being able to adjust the table as you move from technique to technique is well worth that investment in your long-term health, particularly if you work full-time as a manual therapist. Using a power-adjustable table is not only better for you as a practitioner; it is also better for your clients, since the quality of the treatment you provide is bound to improve when you can easily adjust the table. If you work in a group practice or clinic, it's worth speaking with your supervisor or the owner about the advantages in the short- and long-term of using power-

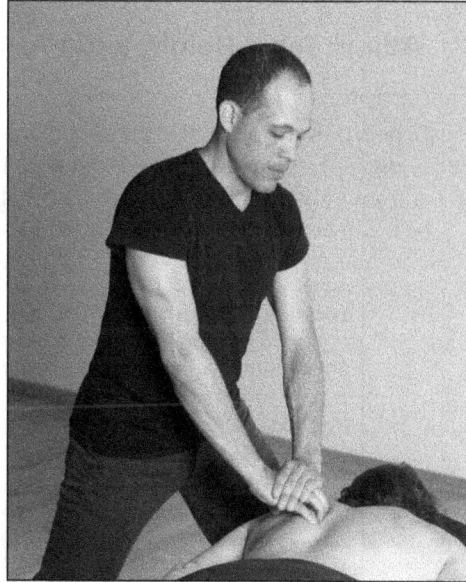

Drop the table several inches for deep work requiring more downward force.

Five Good Reasons to Use a Power-Adjustable Treatment Table

1. They are easier to adjust in height than standard treatment tables, so you are more likely to adjust them for every client.

2. They often have a greater adjustment range than manually-adjustable tables.

3. You can change the height for different techniques, such as moving from light to deep work during a session.

4. When you reposition your client into a side-lying or seated position, you can lower the table to account for the change in the height of the client's body relative to you.

5. You can raise or lower the table to allow mobility-impaired or shorter clients to more easily get on and off.

Adjust Table Height and Working Position Based on Your Symptoms

To help prevent injury, fine tune your table height and your position at it based on any symptoms of discomfort you may be experiencing. Making small adjustments to the height of your table and your position while your symptoms are still at the level of discomfort (rather than pain) can help you avoid more serious symptoms later on. Here are some examples:

Location of Discomfort	Possible Cause of Discomfort
Shoulders, especially in upper trapezius	Table may be too high
Both sides of lower back	Table may be too low
One side of back	Too much twisting
Back of neck	Too much looking down while working

adjustable tables to see if they may consider making this investment. You can refer them to this section of the book to support your request.

For practitioners who are happy with their current manually adjustable tables and do not want to invest in a power-adjustable table, retrofit kits are available that attach to an existing table and provide height adjustment through a hand crank or power unit.

Sitting and Standing as You Work

Sometimes, the choice of whether to sit or stand as you work is obvious. Standing as you work is the clear choice if you move frequently to cover large areas of the client's body, or have to lift a client's limb. Sitting is the logical option when working on the head, neck or other delicate areas. Sometimes, it can be unclear whether you should sit or stand for certain techniques or in specific situations. To help you decide when to sit or stand, Table 4 lists some of the pros and cons of each position.

Alternating Sitting and Standing

Since standing and sitting each have their benefits and downsides, it is helpful to alternate between the two while you work. Standing allows

Table 4. Standing vs. Sitting

Working While Standing		Working While Seated	
Pros	Cons	Pros	Cons
• Better for larger movements, longer strokes • Ability to lean in with upper body weight • More mobility • Easier to involve larger muscles of lower body	• Can be tiring • Stressful to lower extremities • Can cause low back fatigue and soreness • Can result in venous pooling in lower legs, varicose veins	• Better stability for small, precise movements • Rest and recovery for the lower extremities • Easier to change height (with a height-adjustable stool) relative to the client	• More stressful to the lumbar spine than standing • More likely to isolate the upper extremity for generating force • Can result in reaching from the shoulder to cover larger areas

you to use the larger muscles in your legs, hips and core to generate force, and to use a wider variety of motions. But standing continuously can be fatiguing, not only to the leg muscles, but also to the lower back.

Sitting allows you to rest your legs, and lowers your position relative to the table, so you aren't bending or stooping. Sitting also provides more stability and precision as you work on delicate structures of the neck, face or hands. At the same time, sitting creates more strain on the lower back than standing upright, and it tends to limit you to using the muscles in your upper body.

Most treatment sessions should offer opportunities to switch between the two positions. How much time you choose to spend in each position will depend on your own level of physical conditioning and how much fatigue you are feeling at that moment, as well as the specific techniques you are using.

Try to sit during at least one-fourth of the time in any treatment session, to avoid fatigue from prolonged standing. For a 60-minute session, try to spend at least 15 minutes of that time seated.

Floor Surfaces and Footwear

Standing while you work can be very fatiguing, particularly when you are on hard surfaces like tile, stone, concrete or thin carpet over concrete. Prolonged standing in place on surfaces like these without much movement can result in conditions such as varicose veins in the legs. Blood tends to pool in the veins in the legs without the pumping action of the muscles to help it return to the heart. Standing on hard surfaces can also aggravate foot injuries, such as plantar fascitis, and cause low back fatigue. Better surfaces for standing while you work include traditional wood flooring (laminate floors over concrete do not have enough "give"), carpeting with a cushion backing or underlay, and foam-backed vinyl flooring.

Choosing an Adjustment Range When Purchasing a Treatment Table

To choose an adjustment range when you are buying an adjustable table, you will need to consider both your height and the type of work you will be doing. Most adjustable tables have at least a 10" (25 cm) height adjustment range. If you start with a height range appropriate to your stature, you should be able to adjust the table to accommodate different size clients as well as different modalities. Power-adjustable tables often have a much greater adjustment range than manually adjustable ones. General guidelines for table adjustment ranges based on practitioner height may not work for everyone, since body proportions vary from person to person: for example, some people are long-legged, while others are long-waisted. Arm length can vary quite a bit as well, and practitioners with relatively long arms for their height would need a slightly lower adjustment range.

Try this method for picking a table height range for most types of treatment work: Stand in neutral posture, arms hanging comfortably by your sides, while wearing the shoes you would typically wear when working. Measure up from the floor to your first (MCP) knuckle. For most massage work, for example, you should have about 1/3 of the height adjustment above this point, and about 2/3 below it. In other words, if your floor-to-knuckle height is 28" (71 cm), you would want a table that adjusts up to about 32" (81 cm) and down to about 22" (56 cm). As mentioned earlier, if you do a good deal of deeper work, you may want a table with a lower adjustment range; if you mostly do lighter work, you will want a slightly higher range. If you use a wide variety of modalities, look for the table with the widest adjustment range. PTs, chiropractors and osteopaths may need even lower table heights for techniques such as lumbar manipulations. Techniques such as shiatsu, craniosacral, and reflexology have their own unique requirements for tables. If the above guidelines do not seem to fit with the type of work you do, or place you in awkward working positions, contact your school, professional association or colleagues for additional guidelines.

If you do a considerable amount of your work at the head or foot of the table while seated, you should also pay attention to how the ends of the table are constructed. A solid brace attached to the table legs may add stability, but it may also prevent you from sitting with your legs under the table. This can lead to a considerable amount of forward flexion and reaching when working on a client's head, neck or feet. Look for a more open construction on the ends to allow you to work in a neutral posture while seated.

If you work on hard floors, anti-fatigue mats are available. Good mats are about half an inch thick; they are just soft enough to provide some give under your feet, but not so soft that you sink in and have trouble moving around. The outside edges of mats should be beveled to prevent tripping. Place them on all sides of the treatment table so you have consistent footing. While this can be an expensive option, the mats offer the additional benefit of providing cushioning if a client ever falls from your table.

A less expensive alternative is to use visco-elastic insoles in your shoes, or "outsoles" that are made from the same materials as anti-fatigue mats. In addition to being more affordable, these options have the added advantage of staying with you wherever you go during your workday.

Wearing the right footwear is also very important. The shoes you wear should offer cushioning and support, without binding your feet in any way. Good options include cross-trainers or light hiking shoes, both of which can offer good lateral stability and room around the toes. If your work requires more formal footwear, look for uniform shoes made for people who spend a lot of time on their feet, such as nurses or postal carriers, or dress shoes that are made by manufacturers of walking shoes. Shoes that are designed in the shape of your foot, with more room for your big toe, will be more comfortable than shoes that narrow at the toes. The heels should be no more than one inch (2.5 cm) thicker than the rest of the sole, so you can stay centered over your ankles to maintain your balance, rather than shifted forward.

If you have significant issues with your feet—fallen arches, over-pronation or supination—you may want to see a podiatrist, rehabilitation therapist, or other qualified practitioner to have custom orthotics made. Your feet are your base of support, and problems with them can result in altered gait, as well as hip and lower back discomfort.

Maintaining Adequate Space in Your Work Area

Without sufficient space in your treatment room, it is likely that you will get into awkward, constrained or stressful positions as you work. To work most efficiently, you need enough room around the table to allow you to stand in whatever place is most comfortable for any given technique. If you are comfortable, you will be more likely to assume relaxed, efficient, naturally-aligned postures while you are working.

Arrange your treatment area to create as much space as possible around the table. As a general rule, maintain at least 3 feet (1 meter) of open space around all sides of the table. With this amount of space, you will be able to take a wide stance when necessary, or roll a stool or exercise ball around the table to sit on when working on your client's hands, neck or other areas that require precision rather than force. Given that the typical treatment table measures approximately 7 feet by 2.5 feet (2 meters by 0.75 meters), an appropriate workspace would need to measure at least 14 feet by 9 feet (4.25 meters by 2.75 meters). If you currently work in a cramped room, monitor yourself carefully to avoid unhealthy positioning and distorted body mechanics. Remember, if you don't adapt your workspace to your body, your body will adapt to your workspace. To be sure that your body adapts in a positive way, do whatever you can to make your workspace as comfortable as possible.

Hand-Held Tools

Another type of equipment you can consider adding to your practice is hand tools. A number of tools are available for performing hands-on modalities, particularly for applying sustained or deep pressure. You may believe that all soft tissue work should be done with your hands alone, so you can palpate and feel what is happening in your clients' bodies. Your hands, and particularly your fingertips, are indeed very sensitive, because

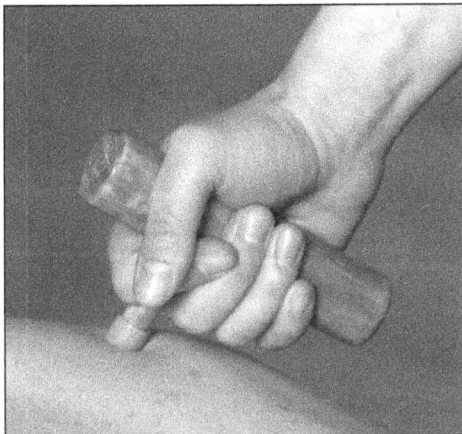

Tools with a large diameter handle can be held with a loose grip.

the nerves run very close to the surface. For this same reason, they are easily affected by pressure. Applying sustained pressure with your fingertips can result in localized compression of the nerves and the small blood vessels that nourish them. In the short term, this can lead to inflammation, reduced circulation, and a loss of sensitivity that can take some time to resolve. Over time, repeated damage to nerves and blood vessels in the fingertips without adequate time for healing can result in a long-lasting reduction in sensitivity. Pressure applied with the fingertips has also been shown to increase pressure in the carpal tunnel, increasing the likelihood of damage to the median nerve, which supplies sensation to most of the fingers.

Rather than lose the ability to use one of your most important tools—your hands—consider using them only to locate trigger points, adhesions, or other conditions needing treatment, and then using a small hand tool to apply pressure. If you use a good tool carefully and sensitively, your clients often will not even realize that you are using a tool instead of your hand. You can always rest a couple of fingers of your other hand on either side of the tool, so you can regulate the pressure you are applying and feel for changes in the tissues.

When evaluating hand tools, look for ones that:

- Allow you to keep your wrist straight as you apply pressure.
- Do not place pressure at the base of the palm where the median nerve exits the carpal tunnel.
- Allow you to grip comfortably using all of your fingers and your thumb; avoid tools that you would have to hold primarily with your fingertips, since the idea of using a tool is to take pressure off the fingertips. Gripping with just a few fingers is more risky than gripping using the entire hand.

Tools are useful for more than just compression and trigger-point work. Cupping tools can be used to lift tissues in place of repetitive techniques such as petrissage and skin rolling. Percussive tools and power massagers like the "massage gun" can be used in place of your hands for percussion techniques or tapotement, or to provide general relaxation to groups of muscles. Graston® tools can help you provide deep tissue or cross-fiber friction with less stress to your hands and arms. These are just a few of the many tools available to you to make your work life easier.

Using tools does not avoid all problems. While tools may help take some of the stress off your hands and wrists, using them improperly can place your upper arm in awkward positions, increasing your risk for shoulder injury. Repetitive gripping is also a risk factor for MSDs, and gripping a tool can become a problem for some manual therapists. For others, gripping causes fewer adverse effects than using their thumbs or fingertips. Most of the hand tools out there are fairly inexpensive, so it is easy to experiment with different tools to find out whether they work for you.

Using tools is not a good practice for every practitioner, every client, or every technique. In fact, tools should be used in a fairly limited way in your practice. They can help you reduce the effort required for a number of situations, allowing your hands to rest and be more available for those techniques where tools are not appropriate.

Even if you choose not to use tools with your clients, you should consider using them to massage your own tissues. They can give you

Using Hand-Held Tools Safely

Following some basic safety guidelines can help make your use of tools a positive experience for you and your clients.

- Since tools can allow you to use larger muscles, you can apply more force with less effort, sometimes a good deal more force. Keeping this fact in mind, be careful to not exert more force than you intend to when using tools.

- Practice with tools on yourself to get a sense of how much pressure you are applying. Compare a tool in one hand with using your fingers on your other hand to apply equal force on your quadriceps. Compare the effort with the tool hand to the finger hand.

- Check in frequently with your client to make sure they do not experience any discomfort as you use tools. Be sure to get their feedback on the level of pressure you are using.

- Go easy with tools until both you and your clients are used to them.

- Keep a few fingers around the tip of the tool to help gauge your pressure.

- Some tools are designed primarily for applying direct downward pressure, and

should not be used for lateral motions such as cross-fiber friction or muscle stripping.

- Check tools before each use for cracks or nicks that could cause them to break or could tear the client's skin.

- Do not use tools on the elderly or anyone else with fragile skin that could tear easily.

- Do not use percussive tools directly over the kidneys or other delicate organs.

- Use tools primarily in areas that are less sensitive, such as the larger muscles of the back and hips. Use them carefully on sensitive areas, such as the IT band, the pectorals, the rotator cuff muscles, etc. Do not use them at all over delicate structures such as floating ribs, the xyphoid process, or around any sites of potential endangerment.

- Put tools down when you are not actively using them. Holding on to them while performing other techniques can place your hands in awkward positions or cause static loading from continuous gripping.

- Sanitize tools after use with each client.

more leverage for self-massage, and allow you to apply pressure to trigger points without having to assume awkward postures.

Other Equipment

You may have other tools or equipment in your practice that could use a little ergonomics attention as well. If you use heavy pieces of equipment, like ultrasound machines or hydroculators, pay attention to how you store and lift them. Try not to place too many tools in one container, to keep the weight down, and make sure the container has good handles to make lifting easier. Store heavy or frequently used equipment in a location between knee and waist level so it can be lifted without bending or reaching. Better yet, use a cart so the equipment can be wheeled about rather than lifted and carried.

Nearly all practitioners use a very common piece of equipment that can contribute to MSDs: a computer. You will need to examine your computer workstation to make sure that the chair, keyboard and monitor are set up in a manner that promotes neutral posture. Appendix B provides a diagram and guidelines for computer workstation set-up. There are also some very good, free resources on computer workstation ergonomics available on-line (see *www.SaveYourHands.com* under Resources for links to these Web sites).

Managing Your Work Schedule

How you schedule your treatment sessions during your workday is a critical ergonomic consideration in protecting your musculoskele-tal health. Leaving adequate time between sessions to recover from the physical demands of your work is essential to preventing injury. Giving your body adequate recovery time between sessions and after your work-day allows your circulatory system to flush out metabolic by-products of muscle use, reduce inflammation, and replenish energy and electrolyte stores. Recovery time also allows the body to repair microtrauma and strengthen connective tissues that have been exposed to stress.

To allow enough recovery time between sessions and not overload your body, be sure to limit the total number of manual treatment sessions you do each week. For massage practitioners, whose work primarily consists of extensive hands-on treatment, a full-time workload is considered to be about 20 hours of hands-on massage per week. Other manual therapists, who alternate intensive manual treatments with other modalities, examinations and client education, may be able to do more hours of treatment per week. Bear in mind that, in general, the more treatments you do, the greater your risk of injury. Listen to your body, and keep the number of work sessions you do to a level that allows you to feel good at the end of the week, not exhausted and overloaded.

The goal is to have a consistent, manageable workload from day to day and week to week. If you find yourself with a slow week, take advantage of the free time to stay physically active to maintain your level of work conditioning.

Manual therapists in practice may find that their workload varies from week to week, or month to month. You may see 20 clients one week, then have a slow week with only 8 clients, and then suddenly find yourself with thirty clients the week after. It can be difficult to say "no" to a clinic manager who schedules too many clients for you, or to tell clients you have worked hard to acquire that you cannot see them. At the same time, you need to balance these considerations with the increased potential for injury from taking on too much work all at once.

In addition to limiting the number of sessions in a week, make sure that your daily work schedule also remains reasonable. Pace yourself throughout your day, and avoid taking on "walk-in" or unexpected clients at the end of the day when you may have already worked to your capacity. Avoid back-to-back scheduling of clients who require deep or extensive treatment, and if possible, avoid scheduling too much deep work in the same day. Remember that it can take more than 24 hours for your body to recover from microtrauma after vigorous work.

Checking in With Yourself During Your Workday

When you begin your workday, you probably check your schedule and make sure that your treatment room and equipment are set up properly. To be truly prepared for the day ahead, you need to also assess your physical and emotional state before your first session. Athletes are taught to assess their own physical condition to see if they need some extra warm-ups or special exercises before they start a training session or competition. Taking a few minutes to take stock of your physical and mental readiness for your work will allow you to adapt yourself and prepare for whatever challenges you will face that day.

Take a few minutes to check in with yourself. Take a few deep breaths—this will help you be present in the moment and help reduce any tension you may be feeling. Ask yourself: how do I feel today? Do my hands, arms or back hurt or ache, do they feel tight or weak, or do they feel good today? What is my energy level? Am I tired or rested, full of energy or sluggish, warm or cold, peaceful or anxious, happy or down? Note any factor that could increase your risk of injury that day, and make a quick plan of how you will deal with those factors during the day so they do not increase your injury risk.

If you are tired or sluggish, perhaps you can find a time between clients to take a short nap or a walk to recharge. Think about keeping a spray bottle filled with water and lemon slices in your workspace, and spraying a fine mist over your face to refresh yourself as you work. If you are seriously tired and not feeling up to seeing many clients that day, perhaps you can consider rescheduling one or two for a different day. If you are anxious or unhappy, try to do something that will relax you and put you at ease. Spending 5–10 minutes, comfortably seated and concentrating on breathing deeply, can be quite refreshing. Doing some vigorous exercise for fifteen minutes to half an hour could be very calming, and will also get your circulation going if you feel cold.

Before you start to work, warm up your muscles and increase your circulation. Think of the first few minutes of each treatment session as an extension of your warm-up routine. Keep your techniques easy and light, to get blood flowing into the tissues of your hands and arms at the same time as you do the same for your client's tissues. Begin to do deeper, more stressful techniques only when your hands are warm and you feel energized.

Make time to relax, stretch and breathe consciously throughout the day. No matter how good your technique or body mechanics are, periods of physical and mental work should be balanced with periods of rest, relaxation and exercise if you are to remain healthy. See Chapter 11 for specific recommendations for warming up as you start your workday, and exercises and stretches you can do during breaks from work. You'll also find information about Mindfullness Based Stress Reduction

(MBSR) in Appendix C. MBSR is an important and proven practice that can be very calming for both you and your clients or patients.

Try to maintain this level of awareness throughout the day. Be consistent, and this way of working will quickly become second nature. Expect that you may have to compensate for changes and surprises as the day unfolds. You will probably feel different at 3 p.m. than you did at 9 a.m. Adjust the way you work for each client, just as you adjust your table height to accommodate each client's body and the different techniques you use. Flexibility is a healthy quality that will allow you to adapt to new and changing circumstances in your work and help prevent injury.

Leaving Time Between Sessions

The amount of time that you should leave between clients will vary by the type of work you do and your body's ability to recover. A good break should allow you enough time to get up and walk around, perform a few stretching or relaxation exercises, drink some water, and mentally let go of the previous client so you can prepare yourself for the next one. A good guideline would be to leave a minimum of 15 minutes between clients. If you have time only to chart your previous client and wipe down the table, you are not giving yourself an adequate break. Activities that involve repetitive motions, like surfing the Internet, responding to e-mail, or doing strength-building hand exercises are best avoided during breaks. If you know that a particular client is going to require deep or physically taxing work, you may want to consider taking a longer break than usual following that session. Scheduling a session of especially physically-demanding work just before your lunch break can be a good strategy.

As a general guideline, if your muscles still feel noticeably fatigued after a session, it is too soon to start another session. Experiencing some mild, cumulative fatigue is normal if you are doing several hands-on sessions in one day. But if your muscles are giving out, your hands are trembling or aching, or you are feeling uncoordinated, you need to take a longer break or stop working entirely for the day.

Building Rest and Recovery into Your Treatment Sessions

In addition to leaving an adequate amount of break time between sessions, it is also important to find ways to build short recovery pauses into each of your sessions, particularly those that are intensive, like deep tissue or sports massage. It may be easier for practitioners in certain manual treatment professions to take a pause during a session than others. A physical therapist, for example, may be able to break up hands-on time with modalities like exercise instruction. Chiropractors can use traction devices to provide "hands-off" treatments. Massage therapists, on the other hand, often keep their hands in constant contact with their client's bodies, using manual techniques that involve repetitive movements and pressure while the client remains completely passive and motionless. The practitioner gets to rest only during the brief time when the client turns over. Doing a massage that involves an hour or more of unbroken activity offers little opportunity for recovery and can be very demanding on the practitioner's body.

Some techniques can provide a natural break from the repetition and hand force that are often required in hands-on treatment. A positional release technique that involves gentle movements, like Strain-Counterstrain, can provide effective treatment that is easier on both the client's and the practitioner's bodies. Instead of vigorously compressing trigger points or stretching muscles against their tendency to resist, the practitioner moves parts of the client's body into their "position of ease," typically shortening muscles while monitoring their trigger points with light pressure. Positions are often held for up to 90 seconds to give the muscle time to release and adapt neurologically to being free of the trigger point. In addition to providing a little recovery time for the practitioner, this kind of technique may prove to be more effective for clients who are not responding to trigger point compression, or find trigger point work too unpleasant or painful.

Building recovery time and short breaks into a treatment session is not as critical a consideration for massage therapists who do light relaxation massage exclusively, as long as they don't stay in static postures for more than a few minutes at a time. Using a variety of strokes applied with different motions and parts of the body and moving around the client as you work are nonetheless important. But for more physically demanding types of work, such as deep tissue massage, manual therapy and other more clinical types of treatment, it is important to find frequent opportunities for recovery during the treatment session. Intense work without periods of rest is hard on the practitioner's body, and in most cases, clients respond better to intense treatment when it is performed for a short period with the opportunity to rest afterward.

Don't think of giving yourself a break as being selfish in any way. All healthcare professionals strive daily to balance their own needs with the needs of their clients. Setting limits in this way is a very healthy and necessary process. The less fatigued you are, the better you will be able to treat this client, and the rest of the clients you will see today and the rest of the week. Use the following strategies to help you find the time you need within your treatment sessions to pause and recover from the physically intensive work you do.

Get Clients Actively Involved

Encouraging your clients to actively participate in their treatment can give you another opportunity to pause during a treatment session. Massage therapists in particular learn to keep a client as passive as possible during relaxation massage, but this passivity is not always appropriate for treatment work. Allowing the client to remain totally passive throughout the treatment session may actually hinder their healing process. Recent studies have found that people with neck and back injuries who seek passive treatment are more likely to experience depression related to their injuries, and may be more likely to develop a chronic condition. Get your clients involved in their own treatment by incorporating both active and passive range of motion exercises or resisted movement techniques like muscle energy technique in your treatments, and by using assessment methods like active range of motion or gait analysis in addition to passive treatment. As you take an occasional breathing break for yourself in the presence of your client or patient, you can encourage them to breathe with you. It's likely you will both feel more present in the moment, and experience reduced muscular tension and a feeling of relaxation.

Incorporating stretching and active movements into your sessions may also help clients re-learn healthy movement patterns following treatments that address trigger points, adhesions, and other causes of pain and dysfunction. A combination of passive stretching followed by active stretching can improve trigger point treatment results by demonstrating to the client that the treatment has helped them move the affected part of the body without pain or restriction.

Give Clients Time to Experience Treatment Results

Build more recovery time into your sessions by giving your clients time to experience the results of a treatment before moving on to the next technique. If you have just worked on a client's shoulder, give them time to move the shoulder and compare it to the other one, before treating the other shoulder. You can even have clients stand and walk around after treating their hips, legs or lower back, so they can see the difference the treatment has made to their gait. In this way, your client will integrate the work you have done while you get a mini-break. Even the small amount of time you gain by taking mini-breaks really does make a difference, as it decreases muscle tension and allows your tissues to flush out metabolic byproducts created by intensive muscle use.

Vary Your Use of Modalities

Many manual therapists regularly combine a number of modalities into a single treatment session. In doing so, they limit the total amount of time they use their hands for any one client. Therapists who currently do nothing but manual techniques with their clients can help save their hands by introducing other modalities into their work. Hydrotherapy, aromatherapy and passive stretching are just a few of the modalities that can be used to treat specific complaints and enhance relaxation. These methods require less physical exertion and are often just as effective for the client.

For example, you may spend ten minutes manually massaging a client's lower back in an attempt to make hypertonic muscles more pliable. You can spare your body the physical work of softening these muscles by applying moist heat for the same amount of time, to warm the tissue and help increase circulation to the area. Increased circulation not only eases muscular tension; it may also make trigger point work go faster. Since the ischemic compression used to treat trigger points is thought to be effective due in part to the rush of blood into the area as compression is released, it makes sense to have plenty of fresh blood in the area to help with this process.

Aromatherapy can be used in conjunction with hydrotherapy to enhance relaxation. You may be able to relieve a client's headache by administering a warm, lavender-scented footbath, placing a cold pack on the forehead, and laying a warm, moist compress on the neck. Gently massaging scented oils or topical analgesics, such as Chinese liniments or lavender essential oil, into the skin in areas of tension or pain can be both soothing and therapeutic.

Other techniques can also take some stress off your body, as long as they are within your scope of practice. Percussive massage tools like deep massage "guns" can help break through muscle guarding and reach deep muscles. Paraffin baths can be used to thoroughly warm the extremities prior to mobilization. These treatments are not only easier on your body; they can also be quite enjoyable for the client. Offering spa services, such as body wraps or facials, to your clients is another way to add modalities that are not as hand-intensive while also enhancing your practice.

Gradually Increasing Your Workload

Starting a new job, graduating from school, or taking on a vacationing colleague's clients are just a few of the situations that can increase your workload. If the increase is gradual, your body will be able to steadily build the strength and endurance necessary to withstand the increased demands you are placing on it. If you suddenly increase the amount of work you do and don't give your body the time it needs to adapt to the additional workload, you can become injured.

A runner would not run a marathon without first gradually increasing the distance in training sessions. Be sure to increase your own endurance for your work by gradually increasing the number of treatment sessions you do in any given day or week. If you sell a large number of gift certificates at Christmas, be aware that you may end up with a very heavy workload in January when all the recipients schedule sessions with you. Also be particularly cautious with taking on continuing education opportunities that involve a good deal of hands-on practice. Taking a weekend workshop to learn new techniques in addition to your regular workload may be good for your career, but it can overstress your tissues and cause an MSD. It is common to use too much effort or poor body mechanics when learning new techniques, which also increases your injury risk. Limit yourself to no more than one hands-on workshop per month, decrease your regular workload around the time of the workshop, and be on the lookout for any symptoms that may develop.

Choosing Your Work Situation

So far, we have been talking about ergonomics as it applies to setting up your workspace and your work schedule: the physical aspects of your work. But ergonomics also considers the way people react emotionally to their work environment. What we refer to as "working conditions" includes both your physical and your emotional experience of your work environment. All aspects of your working conditions combine to determine not only how happy you will be at work, but also your MSD risk.

As a manual therapist, you have the freedom to choose the type of work situation that best suits you. You can be self-employed, or work full- or part-time at a group practice or clinic. You can work from your home, at your clients' homes, or in a professional office or facility.

Your choice of work situation will depend on your personality type and your need and desire for different levels of social interaction, support, independence and lack of distractions. Some practitioners may feel lonely and isolated working for themselves, while others may find the pressure of meeting the expectations of others makes working for someone else difficult or intolerable. Since issues such as lack of support at work, anxiety and stress can all impact your risk of injury, it is important to carefully consider the advantages and disadvantages of each type of work situation. If your current work situation does not suit you, leaving it can lower your risk of injury. Changing work situations creates its own anxiety, but only for a short time, while staying in a bad work situation will continue to cause stress and anxiety that can lead to injury.

Working for Others

There are many reasons that manual therapists decide to work for someone else. If you need more financial and job security, you may find working for someone else to be less stressful than working for yourself. However, when you work for someone else, you risk giving up some control over your working conditions, schedule, and possibly even what types of clients you see and what types of treatments you are asked to do. Without control over your schedule, you can easily find yourself overloaded and unable to take adequate breaks.

Keep in mind that these issues are negotiable when you are interviewing for or starting a new job. If you are looking for a position at a clinic, take the time to interview the management about their attitudes toward their employees, and ask what they do to create an ergonomically sound, safe working environment. Ideally, you will be able to find a situation that offers good working conditions and personal control over your work.

Some employers may have unreasonable expectations of their employees. It will be up to you to set very clear limits. Make your employer aware of your personal work capacity when you first start your job. If you are new to your profession, the number of treatment sessions you are able to do in a day or week may be fairly low. Tell your prospective employer that you would like to start out with a small number of sessions and slowly, gradually increase that number as you are able to do more. Impress upon your boss that you need his or her help to work toward developing a schedule that will be profitable for the company and healthy for you. Your company needs you to stay healthy and productive, so it is in their best interest to help you avoid becoming injured.

If necessary, educate your employer about the prevalence of work-related injury among manual therapists and the need to create working conditions that help keep employees healthy. Capture their attention by telling them that they can reduce expensive employee turnover by implementing simple, inexpensive injury prevention methods. Make them aware that workers' compensation insurance claims for injuries sustained on the job can cost employers a great deal of money. Get your fellow employees together and suggest a meeting with the employer to discuss optimizing working conditions.

If your employer does not have the time or inclination to meet with you, write a group proposal for the changes you would like to suggest. Set limits for the number of treatment sessions practitioners perform per day and per week. If there is more work than the present number of therapists on staff can handle safely, suggest hiring more therapists. Make suggestions for improving the physical conditions of your work place: rooms big enough so the therapist can move comfortably around the table, or installation of power-adjustable tables. Suggest hiring an ergonomist to do a formal evaluation and present professional ergonomics recommendations. Be positive, enthusiastic and firm, and your employer may very well adopt your suggestions.

Here are some tips to make working for someone else easier on you:
- Negotiate with management the number of hands-on hours per day and time between clients.
- Avoid the temptation to pick up extra hours by filling in for co-workers or taking walk-ins when you have already worked a full schedule.
- Take the opportunity to learn the business side of running a clinic, group practice or spa. Ask management if they would be willing to let you work part-time in an administrative or managerial capacity.
- Be prepared to move on if your interactions with management continue to be stressful, or if your working conditions otherwise resemble any of the descriptions of risk factors you have read in this book (lack of control over working conditions, over-scheduling, lack of support, etc.).
- Keep in mind that if you value independence, you may want to work for yourself or in a partnership, rather than as an employee.

Working for Yourself

Manual therapists who work for themselves may also be at risk for injury due to stress and over-scheduling. You may end up taking on too much work to make a sufficient income to pay loans or overhead. For the same reasons, you may hesitate to turn away clients. You may overestimate your own ability to handle a heavy workload. It may seem attractive to schedule many sessions each week, to make the most money possible in the shortest amount of time. While this strategy may produce more income at first, your long-term financial prospects will suffer if your career is cut short by an injury.

Setting Limits with Clients and Employers

It is important to learn to say "no" to clients, to avoid taking on too much work and increasing your injury risk. Whether it is due to a strong work ethic, an overachiever's personality, a strong need for approval, or an overdeveloped sense of professional responsibility, some manual therapists can fall into the trap of never saying "no" to their clients' requests. When those requests are for additional deep work when you are already tired, a lengthy session at the end of an already busy day, or other demands that could exceed your capacity, your inability to set limits could result in injury.

Setting boundaries with clients sometimes means limiting the types of treatments you provide. For example, you would not provide treatment that is outside your scope of practice or that you do not have the necessary training to provide. You would decline, because providing that service would not be in either your or your client's best interest. For the same reason, you should decline to provide treatment that places you at risk for injury. By setting limits and protecting yourself, your clients will have the benefit of a healthy therapist who can continue to provide them with good ongoing treatment, rather than a therapist who is burnt out or unable to practice due to injury.

Use the ergonomic scheduling principles in this chapter to set a manageable schedule for yourself. Maintaining a consistent, moderate workload will allow you to preserve your strength and endurance while limiting your risk of overloading yourself. Occasionally, you may have to put clients off until the following week, or tell them you cannot take them and refer them to a colleague. Keep a list of colleagues to whom you can refer clients if your schedule is too full that day or week, or if you are not feeling physically capable of handling any more clients. If these clients have a pressing need for treatment, they will appreciate the referral. Tell them you hope they will call you again in the future, and you will likely keep their business.

You may also want to leave free time in your schedule each week for clients who are in urgent need of your services, rather than seeing them in addition to an already full workload. Maintaining clear boundaries and learning to say "no" when it is best for you to do so can keep you from needing treatment for your own injury.

Here are some tips if you work for yourself:

- Don't overload yourself and take on more work than you can really handle. Think in terms of career longevity rather than trying to get as much business as possible early in your career.
- Don't exhaust yourself with every client. Pace yourself throughout your day and your week so you don't end up physically drained.
- Leave adequate time between treatment sessions for rest, stretching exercises, and to mentally let go of one client and prepare for the next.
- If you know you have a tendency to take on too much work, decide in advance how many treatments you will do per week, and then commit to that number.
- If you are frequently stressed about your ability to run a business by yourself, you may need the security of a partnership or a position working for in a clinic or other setting where you are working for someone else.
- Avoid social isolation, and the depression and anxiety that it can create, by staying active in your professional association, attending meetings of your local chamber of commerce, or frequently exchanging treatments with peers. Having a good support system is important and can help you avoid isolation, burn out and lack of perspective, as well as injury.
- Find a mentor, someone more experienced in your manual therapy profession who can offer support to you in your career. You can turn to your mentor if you have questions or if issues or symptoms arise. Your mentor can also periodically watch you work and point out ways you can work with more ease.

Using Ergonomics to Help Your Clients

Ergonomics can be a valuable tool to add to your practice, enhancing the way you treat and advise your clients. Most of your clients work, either at a formal job or around the house or both. For these clients, the better part of their waking hours is spent getting ready to go to work, at work, or commuting to and from work. Since work is such a big part of your clients' lives, it makes sense to learn more about what your clients do on

Risk Factors for Intake Forms

At work, do you regularly do any of the following:

- Bend forward, to the side, or twist at the lower back?

- Tip your head forward, backward or to the side?

- Reach overhead repeatedly, or hold you hands overhead?

- Bend your wrists more than just a little in any direction?

- Kneel or squat for more than a brief amount of time?

- Stand or sit for prolonged periods with little movement?

- Grip with the whole hand (such as holding power tools) with more than a light effort?

- Pinch objects between the tips of the fingers and thumb?

- Repeat the same or similar motions every few seconds?

- Lift even moderately heavy (20-pound or 9-kilogram) objects from below the knees, above the shoulders, or while reaching out?

- Lift objects frequently (more than once per minute)?

- Lift anything weighing 50 pounds (23 kg.) or more?

- Carry objects more than 3 feet (1 meter) at a time?

- Push or pull objects with more than a light effort?

- Work with vibrating power tools?

- Operate machinery that transmits vibration or impact to your body?

- Use your hand as a hammer, such as pounding parts into place?

- Come into contact with hard or sharp edges with your hands, wrists or arms?

- Work at a computer for more than 4 hours per day?

the job. Understanding your clients' work will help you determine the factors that may be causing the musculoskeletal issues they ask you to treat.

You may already ask some questions on your intake forms about your clients' work, and during interviews you probably get some details from them about specific work tasks that may have caused the symptoms that initiated their visit. You can take your intake forms one step further by asking about their exposure to specific risk factors. In the box, above, you will find some specific questions about work exposures that you can add to your intake forms. You can also use the risk factors in Table 3 on page 31 as a good general guideline. Remember, though, that a little exposure to risk factors is typically not harmful. You will need to ask how often and for how long they are exposed before making any assumptions about how these risk factors may be contributing to injury.

Ask your clients to describe or demonstrate any tasks they do frequently at work, so you can get a sense of which muscles might be overused or overstretched during these activities. This discussion can help you focus your treatments and help your clients understand which repeated exposures might be responsible for their muscle hypertonicity, pain or injury.

Since there can be considerable differences in the way people work within a certain type of job, ask your clients to be as specific as possible in their responses. Even office work can vary quite a bit. One person might spend most of their day entering data, repetitively typing at the keyboard, while another looks up information on the Internet, and spends most of their time reaching out to use the mouse. You would expect that the client who does data-entry would have symptoms in their hands and wrists, and perhaps also in their neck and upper trapezius muscles if they are looking down while entering data. Meanwhile, the person who frequently reaches to the mouse may have all of their symptoms on that side of the body, especially in the shoulder and wrist.

While office workers always have their share of musculoskeletal discomfort, most other professionals have higher exposures to risk factors and report more work-related injuries. Nurses and nursing assistants who are involved in direct patient care have a high rate of musculoskeletal injuries. Moving patients and bending over frequently to provide patient care takes its toll on their backs and shoulders. Construction workers also suffer from the physical demands of their jobs, particularly heavy lifting, working in awkward postures, and using vibrating power tools. These activities result in injuries to the neck, back, upper extremity, knee and hip.

Knowing what your clients do on the job can help you focus your treatments to specific parts of the musculoskeletal system, or to find underlying conditions that might be contributing to the conditions that led them to seek treatment. Clients who work in physically demanding jobs involving a great deal of movement will typically require soft-tissue work in the more injury-prone areas of the back, shoulders and wrists. On the other hand, more sedentary workers may require focused treatment on the parts of the body that tend to be overused, such as the neck and upper extremity for computer users. Massage therapists can combine this focused treatment with a relaxation massage for the rest of the body, to help restore circulation and loosen muscles that are sore from lack of use.

In addition to providing focused treatment based on your clients' occupations, you can also help them prevent future discomfort by educating them about the principles of ergonomics. While it takes years of education and experience to become a good ergonomist, manual therapists have enough background in anatomy and physiology to be able to explain how musculoskeletal disorders occur at work, and to discuss some possible solutions with their clients. Given a little awareness of risk factors and some ergonomics information, most people are able to figure out solutions for themselves. Another way you can help your clients is to point them to some ergonomics resources, whether on the Internet or through a local organization.

Remember that many of the risk factors listed above can lead to more serious conditions than just discomfort or minor injury. Gripping vibrating power tools for long periods can result in a condition known as hand-arm vibration syndrome, or vibration white finger, where nerves and blood vessels in the hands are severely damaged. Jobs such as assembly line work, which involve a combination of repetitive motions, hand force and bent wrists, often have a high incidence of tendon injuries and carpal tunnel syndrome. Workers who repeatedly use the palm of their hand as a hammer can suffer from a condition known as hypothenar hammer syndrome, where the nerves and blood vessels on the ulnar side of the palm become damaged from the repeated pounding.

Bear in mind that you may be the first health professional that workers come to when they begin experiencing symptoms. Symptoms you see in your clients may be the result of more serious conditions that require referral to a physician or occupational health specialist.

5

Developing Good Body Mechanics

Now that you have used the principles of ergonomics to adapt your workplace to your body, you need to reinforce those principles by using your body properly in that workplace. We use the term "good body mechanics" to describe the principles of using your body effectively and efficiently as you work.

Good body mechanics and good ergonomics go hand in hand. You won't be able to use good body mechanics in a workspace that is poorly designed and doesn't fit your body. If your table is not at the right height for your body and your techniques, for example, your posture will suffer no matter how much you try to focus on working in the proper positions. On the other hand, if you don't use good body mechanics when working at your table, you won't be getting the full injury prevention benefit of having an adjustable table and setting it to the proper height. The best results occur when you use ergonomics principles and body mechanics principles simultaneously in your work.

In addition to helping you avoid awkward postures, good body mechanics often help you reduce your overall level of effort. By using your body more efficiently, you will use muscles that are best suited for the work and avoid fatigue and stress to your tissues. Occasionally, there are situations in which using good body mechanics requires more effort; for example, bending your knees to lift something requires more effort than bending from the waist, but it is much better for your back. Overall, using good body mechanics will make your work easier, and allow you to take another step toward reducing your risk of injury.

Defining Good Body Mechanics

We can define good body mechanics as the use of positions, postures and movement patterns that allow you to distribute stress evenly throughout your body as you work. By using good body mechanics, you avoid accumulating stress in any one area of your body and potentially injuring the structures in that area. Practicing good body mechanics allows you to use the strength and momentum of the entire body to create motion, rather than using smaller, more fragile parts of your body that are more easily injured. Because your body moves as a unified whole, your movements can be more flowing, even, relaxed and controlled.

For a manual therapist, the practice of good body mechanics concentrates on the three main physical aspects of your work:

- Your breathing
- Your posture, or the way you align the different parts of your body as you work
- Your movements, including your techniques and how you position your body in relation to your client's body

When you practice good body mechanics, these three components work together, supporting and building on each other. Your body will be aligned in a posture that places the least amount of stress on your musculoskeletal system. Most of your movements will be within a comfortable range around that posture. Your breathing will help you maintain this posture as you work and reduce muscular and emotional tension that can disrupt your awareness of your posture and movements. This approach will help you move in ways that are the least likely to damage the most vulnerable parts of your musculoskeletal system: the weak links you learned about in Chapter 2.

As you read through this chapter, it may initially seem difficult to imagine that anyone could consistently follow the recommendations for maintaining proper posture and using good body mechanics in their daily work life. It may seem impossible that anyone could really stand as straight as suggested and always work in ideal positions, while consistently remembering to breathe deeply from the diaphragm. Remember that the goal is to use good body mechanics, not

> **The goal is to use good body mechanics, not "perfect" body mechanics.**

"perfect" body mechanics. Your body mechanics should not be just another source of anxiety or stress about your performance on the job. In the real work world, no one uses perfect form at every moment. The idea is to continue to use your body in a natural and efficient way, while doing your best to maintain an approach that maximizes your strength and avoids overloading your weak links.

Breathing

Deep, regular breathing is an essential, and often overlooked, component of good body mechanics. It is important to be aware of your breathing, and to train yourself to breathe regularly and deeply as you work. In general, people have a tendency to hold their breath or breathe shallowly when they're anxious or nervous, concentrating, or exerting themselves physically. Catching yourself breathing shallowly or holding your breath are often the first indications that you are also not using good body mechanics and tension is building in your body.

Your posture can have a positive or negative effect on your breathing. Poor upper body posture can make deep breathing difficult: rounding the shoulders and caving in the chest prevent the lungs and rib cage from fully expanding. Some work positions will cause you to tighten your lower torso or collapse your chest, preventing you from taking a deep breath. See postural stretches in Chapter 11 to improve your posture.

Poor breathing is often the result of unconscious physical tension caused by emotional stress; for example, anxiety about your job performance or the stress of working with a difficult client. Tension and stress often cause shallow breathing. Concentrating intensely on a new or complex technique can also cause shallow breathing: you may even hold your breath at times without realizing you are doing so.

Shallow breathing and breath holding have a number of negative effects. As you saw in Chapter 3, accumulated tension contributes to static loading in the tissues. Emotional tension interferes with overall body awareness. Shallow breaths tend to be rapid, around 12 to 19 per minute, as opposed to a more relaxed breathing pattern of 6 to 10 breaths per minute. Deeper, slower breaths have been shown to help invoke the relaxation response of the parasympathetic nervous system, slowing your heart rate, reducing your blood pressure, and reducing muscle tension.[1] Slower breathing may actually release more oxygen into the blood stream. To get a better idea of a slow pace of breathing, count slowly to 5 when breathing in, pause for a second, then count to 5 as you breathe out, and pause again for a second before your next breath.

Shallow breathing directs the breath more into the upper chest than deep into the lungs. As a result, the scalene muscles are often overused in order to help create space underneath the clavicle bones for the lungs to expand. The scalenes are much smaller muscles than the large and powerful diaphragm, and are quicker to fatigue and go into spasm. They then pull up on the first rib, bringing it up into the already crowded thoracic outlet, through which the brachial nerves and arteries pass on their way to the arms. Stress-related breathing patterns, while not likely to be the primary cause of

Learning to Breathe from the Diaphragm

To test whether you involve your scalenes more than necessary in breathing, lie flat on your back on your treatment table or bed. Place your fingers at the base of your neck, in the hollow between your clavicle and the anterior aspect of your upper trapezius. Take a few deep breaths as you normally would. You may be able to feel the tissues superior to your first rib (the scalenes) rising and falling as you breathe in and out. If you do, focus on initiating your next few breaths with your diaphragm, pulling it down deep towards your belly. It may help to place your other hand over your navel to feel the rise and fall there, comparing it to the space above your first rib. With practice, you should be able to re-learn diaphragmatic breathing, and reduce scalene involvement in your breathing.

conditions like thoracic outlet syndrome, can be a contributing or aggravating factor.

As you work, make a conscious effort to remain aware of your breathing. In fact, doing some deep breathing is a great way to start your work day, or to refresh yourself during a treatment. As you are working, if you catch yourself breathing shallowly or holding your breath, ask yourself if you are emotionally stressed or physically tense or tired. If you are emotionally stressed, try to figure out why and then use coping techniques to let go of the stress. If physical tension is the problem, examine your body mechanics and see if your posture or technique may be the cause. If so, adjust them as necessary to allow you to breathe fully and deeply.

Try to find as many opportunities as you can during your workday to take a moment to breathe deeply. The more often you do, the more it will become a habit or even an automatic reflex that becomes a natural part of your work. There are any number of opportunities during the day when you can take a deep breath: as you reach for a tool; while you're getting more oil or cream; or while you're adjusting your table or other piece of equipment. Taking these short "breathing breaks" may only involve taking a few deep breaths and blowing them out, but you will be surprised how effective taking these few seconds to think of yourself can be to release any physical or emotional tension and feel refreshed.

If you let it happen, deep breathing in this way can also put you in touch with how you are feeling in general: tired, anxious, happy, annoyed, etc. Once you have this awareness, you can try to adapt your work accordingly. This self-care technique is easy to do if you remind yourself that the client or patient is not the only person involved in the treatment—you are working as a team, and your wellness also counts. It's good for your self-esteem and your well-being. It's one of the first steps in developing the "injury prevention mindset" you will need for a long, healthy career.

In either case, consciously taking a deep breath from the diaphragm and blowing it out slowly will almost instantly counteract both emotional and physical tension. Conscious breathing has the benefit of relaxing both you and your client. Your breathing cues your client to breathe regularly and deeply, encouraging relaxation and reducing muscle guarding. If your client is less guarded, your work will be easier. See Chapter 11 for exercises that can help you learn (or review) how to breathe slowly and deeply.

Posture

Your posture is the starting point for your work. Principles of good body mechanics focus on maintaining good overall posture and using the entire body effectively as a whole unit. It is common for manual therapists to be taught to use the lower body to generate force, but your upper body must be in a posture that allows you to transfer that force to your upper extremities. If you are creating force and trying to transfer it to your client with your joints in a poor position, those joints will be at risk for injury. Although we tend to discuss posture in terms of its individual components, such as where your elbows

Finding a Centered Balance Point

In addition to maintaining a neutral posture, you need to work from a balance point where your weight is centered over your core and hips. Once your weight is balanced in this manner, you can move easily without placing unnecessary stress on postural muscles such as erector spinae or rectus and transverse abdominus. This point of balance is your "center." To help get a sense of this balance point, stand with your eyes closed and relax your body. If your balance is unsteady, you may want to do this exercise in a door frame so you have something to grab on to if necessary. First, tip a little bit side to side, just until you feel off balance. Slowly make the movement smaller and smaller until you feel centered. Next, make the same movements front and back, again making smaller motions until you are centered. Now, make little circles with your body, first counter-clockwise, then clockwise, slowly spiraling in to the center. Once you feel centered, you can ask someone else to check your posture from the front and from the side.

Long-term postural deviations can cause a change in proprioception, throwing off our sense of where center is. As we get older, the sense of balance can diminish, so it's good to challenge your balance regularly by doing this kind of exercise.

Ergonomics Principle—Use Larger Muscles

A muscle's strength is related to its size or, more technically, its physiological cross-sectional area (PCSA). Simply put, if you added up the area of all of the fibers that make up a muscle at their thickest point, you would have the PCSA for that muscle.

Take a look at the pad of muscles in your thenar eminence at the base of your thumb. These muscles flex, abduct and adduct your thumb, as well as bring it into opposition across your palm. Because you work with your hands, the muscles in this area are probably fairly well developed. Now compare the size of your small thenar eminence with the much larger wrist flexor muscles in your forearm. You can generate 4 to 5 times as much force by using these much larger forearm muscles to grip with the whole hand than by using the smaller muscles of the thenar eminence when you use a pinch grip.

Now compare your forearm flexors to the muscles in your upper arm, which are even larger. Compared to your very large deltoid and pectoralis major muscles, though, all of your arm muscles are relatively small and weak. And all of the muscles in your upper body are downright puny compared to the muscles in your core, hips and legs.

If you have a bathroom scale, place it on your treatment table with the table set approximately at hip height. Place a folded towel on the scale for padding, and push down on it with your palms, keeping your elbows bent so you are using only your arm muscles. How many pounds of force are you able to generate, and how much effort did you use?

Now lower the table so that your fingertips just touch it when you stand next to the table with your arms at your sides. Place the scale on it, but this time apply pressure

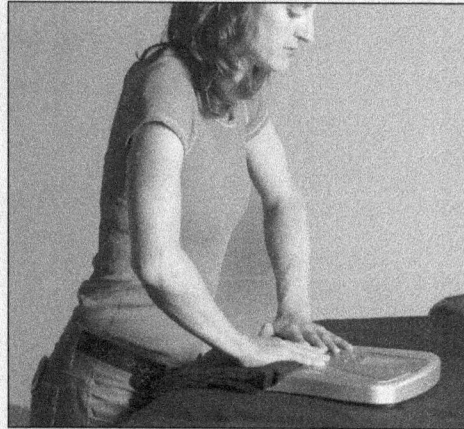

How many pounds of force are you able to generate when the table is too high?

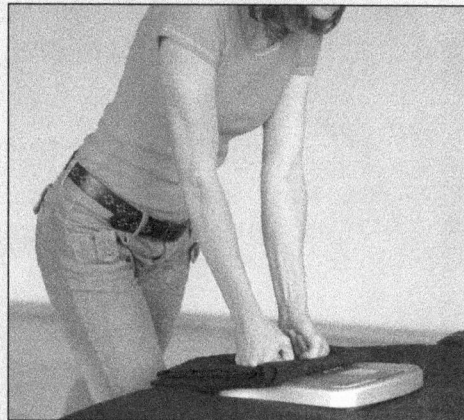

Lower the table and lean in using body weight. Are you able to generate the same amount of force with less effort?

with loose fists, with your wrists straight and your elbows straight but not locked. Lean in using body weight, stabilizing your arms with your deltoids and pectorals, as well as with the many back muscles that attach to your scapulae. Were you able to generate the same amount of force with less effort?

should be or how to line your feet up with your movements, keep in mind that everything in the body is connected. One of the first steps in developing good body mechanics is learning to move your body as a whole unit as you work. Disciplines such as T'ai Chi, Alexander Technique or The Feldenkrais Method® emphasize holistic movement patterns, and can help you develop the feeling of moving your body as a unified whole.

Starting From a Neutral Posture

You are in a "neutral posture" when your joints are aligned so that your muscles can move in their mid-range of motion, the position in which they can generate the most force. In this posture, your joints and muscles work most efficiently and your nerves, ligaments and blood vessels are not compromised. As you work, try to keep most

---

Tips for Finding Your Neutral Posture

Try these activities to help you find your neutral posture:

1. Stand in front of a full-length mirror and make sure that:

   - Your head is straight, not tilted or jutted forward

   - Your shoulders are level and not rounded forward

   - Your pelvis is level

   - The space between your arm and your body is equal on both sides

   - Your kneecaps and toes are pointing straight ahead

2. Ask a friend to take a full-length photo of you from a side view. If you are standing in a neutral posture, you should be able to line up:

   - the middle of your ear with the tip of your shoulder

   - the middle of your hip with your knee and ankle

   The most common postural problems are a forward-head position and shoulders that are rounded forward. If these are problem areas for you, you may want to try the Chin Tuck and Backwards Shoulder Circles exercises in Chapter 11.

---

of your movements within a comfortable range around a neutral posture. This approach is the foundation for learning to use good body mechanics as you work.

By aligning your joints, your skeleton will bear most of your body weight and take the stress off your muscles and tendons. In manual treatment, the arms are often used in a weight bearing capacity;

> Neutral posture should be your starting position as you begin each session, and you should return to it as your rest/recovery position during your sessions.

for example, when you lean in with your upper body weight to apply pressure. By keeping your wrists and elbows straight, you will transfer the load up through the skeletal system to the larger muscles of your chest and shoulders. These muscles are stronger and better suited to applying force than smaller muscles. All things being equal, you can apply the same amount of force with less effort when you use larger muscles. Large muscles have a greater capacity for generating force, so when you use them to perform tasks requiring moderate force (like those that manual therapists do in their work), you are using a smaller percentage of the available strength of those muscles. They will be less likely to fatigue and become injured than smaller muscles, which would be working at or near their full capacity to generate the same force.

Before you begin to work, it is important to identify and get into your starting neutral posture. This posture will be your starting position as you begin each session, and it will be your rest/recovery position during your sessions. It will form the basis of your body mechanics and you should return to it as often as possible during your treatment sessions. Once again, you are not looking for "perfect" alignment or "perfect" posture: for many people, their bodies have adapted over the years and it is difficult for them to get into a textbook neutral posture. The goal is to get a feel for what neutral posture looks and feels like for your body, and to stay as close to that posture as possible as you work. Take a look in a mirror so you know what neutral posture looks like for you, and try to familiarize yourself with what your neutral posture feels like.

Standing Neutral Posture
To familiarize yourself with standing neutral posture and experience

what it feels like, stand in front of a mirror with your feet roughly at shoulder width, with your knees straight but not locked back. Make sure your major joints are aligned:

- Ears over shoulders
- Shoulders over hips
- Hips over knees
- Knees over ankles

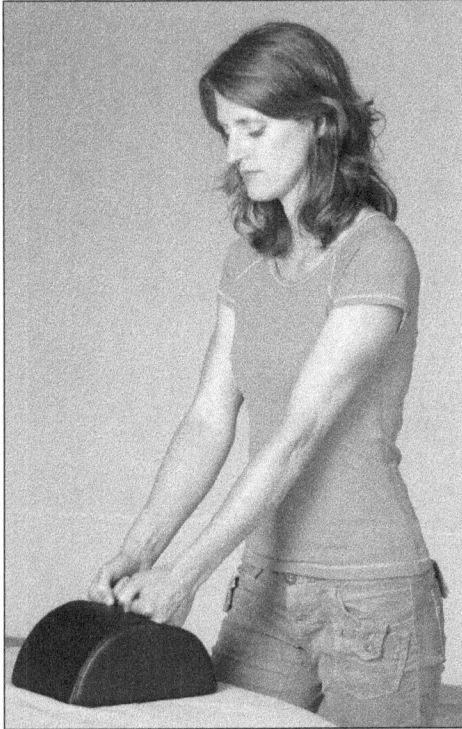

Practice applying pressure in neutral posture on a bolster until this motion feels comfortable and natural to you.

There should be three curves in your spine, an inward (lordotic) curve in your lumbar region, a slight outward (kyphotic) curve in the thoracic region where your ribs attach, and another lordotic curve in your cervical spine. Your head should be level, with your forehead and your chin perpendicular to the floor. Your shoulders should be relaxed, with your clavicle bones parallel to the floor. Your scapulae should be down and flat against your ribs to keep them stabilized. Your upper arms should hang down at your sides. To allow good blood flow between your upper arm and forearm, your elbows should be just slightly bent. Avoid locking your elbows in a completely straight or hyperextended position; even though this position will relax the muscles in your upper arms, it will transfer too much stress to your joints. Keep your wrists straight and your hands close to the "handshake" position, to avoid too much pronation or supination, which could stress muscles and tendons. To simulate the feeling of beginning to work in this posture with a client, put a bolster on your table and apply pressure to it in this posture.

To be able to maintain a neutral posture as you work while standing, you will need to adjust your table height according to the size of your client and the type of techniques you do. For work that requires a moderate amount of downward pressure but long strokes, such as relaxation massage of the torso and limbs, adjust your table so that the client is a few inches below your elbow level. This table height is low enough to allow you to use some of your body weight to apply pressure, without being so low that you will have to bend and stress your lower back. A "thicker" client or a client in side-lying position will require a correspondingly lower table height. Performing deep tissue techniques, passive stretching exercises, and other techniques requiring more force may require an even lower table setting. A lower setting allows you to use more of your body weight to apply pressure. While you will bend over more, you will be supporting your upper body weight with your arms as you are applying the pressure.

Seated Neutral Posture

Except for the position of your legs, seated neutral posture is basically the same as standing neutral posture. Since your legs are no longer weight-bearing, you can bend your knees as much as 90 degrees, or sit with your lower legs extended a bit in front of you, which will open up the angle at the back of your knees and improve circulation. Your hips should be higher than your knees, and there should be greater than a 90-degree angle between the tops of your thighs and your torso. Increasing this angle to 110 to 130 degrees will increase your circulation, and help the muscles in your torso to relax.

You may want to sit higher while you perform manual techniques than you would at a computer or at the dinner table. Place your feet flat on the floor for stability, so you can sit forward a bit more. In this position, your legs will be a little straighter and take up less room between you and the table. A higher position will also allow you to use more of the muscles in your torso and hips. It will also make the transition to standing easier, so you will be more likely to "pop up" for a quick

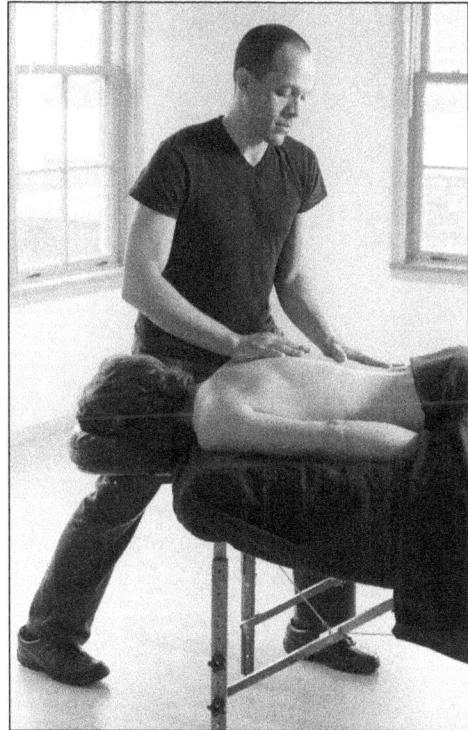

Work in standing neutral posture for work that requires moderate to deep pressure.

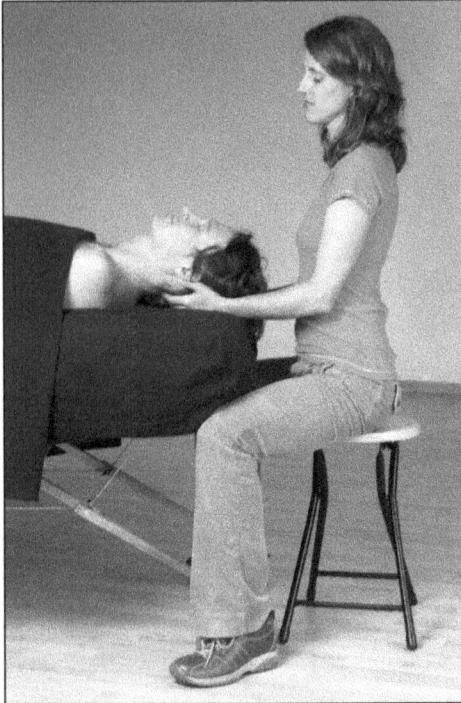

Work in seated neutral posture for light, precise or delicate work.

technique that is better done while standing. Options for sitting higher include a stool that adjusts higher than a typical chair height for you, a saddle chair or an exercise ball. Stools or chairs should have wide bases for stability and wheels for mobility, although they should not roll too easily or they will be unstable. For delicate work, such as treatment to the head and neck area, place the table at or just below seated elbow level. It may also help to have your elbows supported or resting on the table as you do these small motions.

Standing and seated neutral postures should feel comfortable. If you find these postures difficult to attain or maintain, it may be that your body has made adaptations over the years that have tightened or weakened your muscles. To restore neutral posture, you will need to stretch tight muscles and strengthen weak ones. Changing postural habits is a slow process; it takes at least several weeks of concerted effort to get back on the right track. Exercises designed to improve posture can be very helpful; you can find some exercise suggestions to get you started in Chapter 11. It may also help to receive some manual therapy yourself, if exercise and posture retraining is not enough. If you are not in the habit of working in a neutral posture, getting back into it may feel uncomfortable at first. If getting into a neutral posture causes pain, move out of that posture and recheck it against the descriptions above.

Working in Near-Neutral Postures

As you stand or sit in neutral posture, one thing will quickly become obvious: you are not going to get much work done in this posture. Even if you could maintain a totally neutral posture as you work, the lack of movement would cause static loading, a harmful risk factor. The goal of using good body mechanics is not to maintain perfect neutral posture, but rather to move through a range of near-neutral postures in order to minimize stress on your body. Good body mechanics are dynamic, with postures that are always changing.

As you start your day, arrange your table, your seating, and other elements of your workplace to enable you to begin your work in a neutral posture. You will not be able to stay in a neutral position at all times as you work, but you should at least start there. As you work, try to stay as close as possible to neutral posture, and come back to totally neutral posture as frequently as possible. If you get in the habit of working in this way, neutral posture will become a reference point for you, both intellectually and proprioceptively. Your body will eventually develop a memory for that position and will instinctively want to return to it.

> **Your goal is to move through a range of near-neutral postures that are dynamic and always changing.**

Positioning Your Client

We tend to think about positioning the client in ways that will make them feel the most comfortable. Of course, client comfort is a priority, but so is your comfort as a practitioner. It is nearly always possible to find a position that is comfortable for the client, and also allows you to maintain near-neutral postures as you work.

Position your client so that the part of their body you want to work on is directly in front of you, close to your body, and facing up toward you. A good rule of thumb is to work only on the parts of your client's body that you can access directly, both visually and manually. For example, with your client lying supine, you would work on the front of the quadriceps, but then move the client into a side-lying position to work on the iliotibial band.

You can ask your client to lie on your treatment table in one of three positions: prone, supine or side-lying. You can also work with your client seated; in this position, massage practitioners sometimes use an on-site massage chair. You will find that certain techniques are more effective and easier to perform in

> **To maintain a near-neutral posture, work only on the parts of your client's body that you can see. Reposition your client as necessary to make this possible.**

one position than in another. Each position places the therapist at a different angle relative to the client's body. Each provides unique opportunities to access parts of the client's body while allowing you to work comfortably. Take advantage of the opportunities each position affords you. Experiment by placing your clients in all four positions, and identify which of your techniques works best in each position. Learn to work with the position, not against it. By doing so, you will be able to lean in with body weight, and avoid awkward postures. Unfamiliar positions may take some time to get used to, so you may want to practice on a friend or fellow professional before using them with a client.

Working With the Client in Side-Lying Position

Of the four possible client positions, side-lying is the most often overlooked and underutilized. Those therapists who seldom use the side-lying position do themselves a disservice, since it is arguably the best position for the therapist for many techniques. It is also the most comfortable position for a large number of clients. With proper bolstering, most clients find a side-lying position more comfortable than a prone or supine position, particularly clients with large or sensitive breasts or those suffering from back pain.

In this position, one entire side of the client's body is turned toward you. Your client can easily move close to the edge of the table nearest you, so you can work without reaching out in front of you. You can remain upright nearly all of the time, maintain near-neutral posture, and keep your wrists straight, cutting down on stress to your arms and hands. Muscles located on the side of the body that would be difficult to work on with the client prone or supine are very accessible with the client

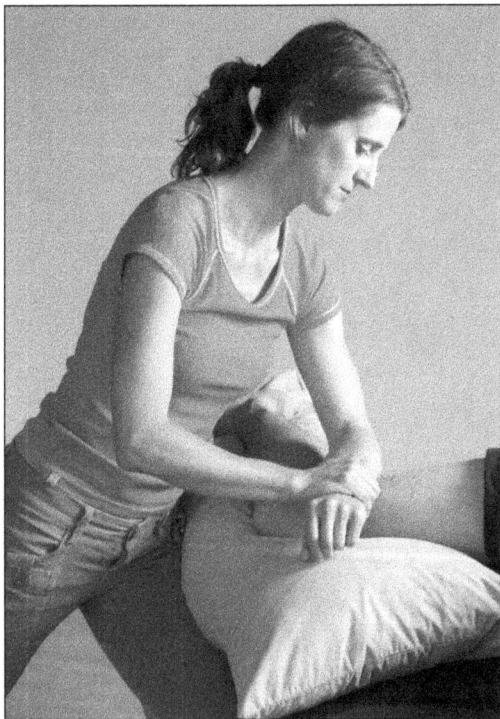

Use your forearm to apply broad, even pressure on a client who is in a side-lying position.

on their side. You can use your forearms extensively to work with these muscles in this position, to give your hands a rest, and to achieve a broad, even stroke.

Working With the Client Supine or Prone

To maintain near-neutral posture with the client in supine position, work only on the anterior aspect of the body. In prone position, concentrate on the posterior aspect of the body. Your client's back and the posterior aspect of the legs can be easily addressed in prone position, and you can use your forearms to give your hands a break.

Some therapists perform techniques that use the client's body weight to provide downward pressure on the therapist's hands. For example, with the client supine, they place their hands underneath the client's back and support the client's weight on their fingertips. This type of technique is very stressful for the practitioner's hands and arms. Instead, get the client into a prone, side-lying or seated position, where the back is stretched out in front of you and you can easily access the entire surface. If you choose to do this kind of work, keep it to a minimum, working at the edges of the body with very little of the client's weight on your hands.

Working With the Client Seated

A number of techniques can be performed with client sitting upright in a regular chair, backless stool or on the treatment table. Massage therapists use this client position for on-site massage using a specialized

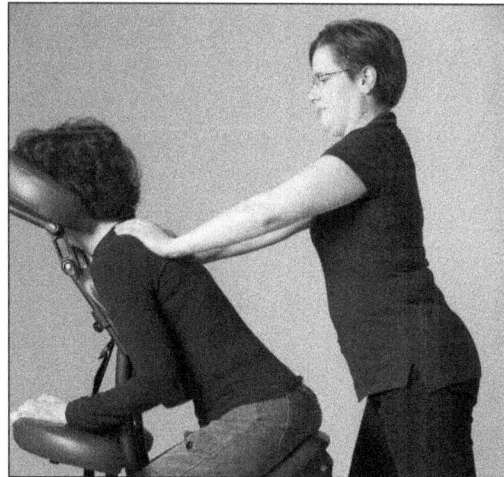

The client's position in an on-site massage chair may cause the therapist to adopt awkward wrist, shoulder and back positions such as wrist extension and shoulder flexion.

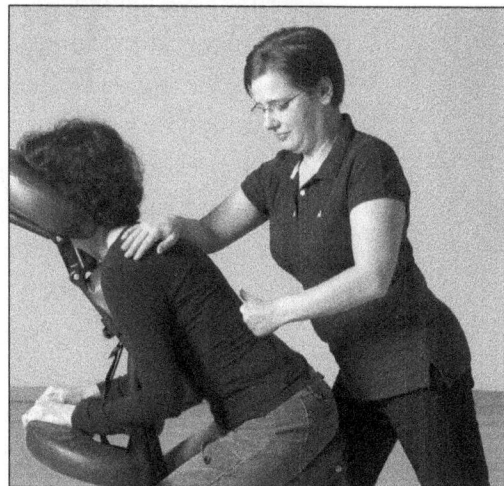

Support yourself with a forearm on your client, and use a loose fist to avoid bending your wrist.

massage chair. Working with the client seated is a good choice for treatments to the neck, shoulders, upper back and arms, which are often the focus of a typical 15- to 20-minute chair massage session. Many physical therapy examination tests and interventions for the shoulder and neck are also performed with the client in a seated position. If treatment is focused on the client's upper body, the seated client position typically allows the practitioner to remain upright and avoid stressful bending at the waist.

Working on a seated client also offers several challenges for the practitioner, particularly for massage therapists who do chair massage or rehabilitation therapists who work with clients seated on a non-adjustable treatment table. If you use your palms to apply compression across the client's shoulders or upper back, you can end up bending your wrists and elevating your shoulders. It is also easy to get into awkward postures when treating the lower back, legs and feet. There is a greater vertical area to cover when your client is seated than when the client is lying flat on a table, which encourages more bending, kneeling and squatting to address these lower areas.

In the course of a 15-minute chair massage, the time you spend in these awkward postures will be brief, and not likely harmful. These short periods do have a cumulative effect, though, so be careful about scheduling too many chair massages in one day. When the treatment time is extended to 30 minutes or more, or much of the treatment focuses on the lower body, you will need to pay particular attention to good body mechanics and the ergonomics of your workspace. To avoid wrist bending, use your elbows, forearms or fist when applying compression or making long strokes across the back. When treating the mid back, it may help to place one foot behind you and use some of the strength in your back and hips to generate more force. If you have to bend at the waist, rest one hand or forearm on the client or on part of the massage chair, to help hold up some of your upper body weight.

Spend as little time as possible bending at the waist, a position that is hard on the lower back. This awkward position also doesn't allow you to use the larger muscles of your upper back, along with your stance, to take some stress off of your upper extremities.

When squatting, keep your knees behind your toes as much as possible and limit the time you spend in a deep squat to protect your knees. It may also help to squat on one leg, while extending the other leg out to the side, and to alternate legs each time you squat. Use a foam pad to kneel on and limit the time you spend on your knees, as this position can create pressure behind the patella. Over time, that pressure can irritate bursae and damage cartilage. If you do a fair amount of chair massage in your practice, add some exercises into your workout routine to maintain strength and flexibility in your hips and legs, to better prepare you for the amount of squatting involved in this kind of work.

Working With the Client at Floor Level

Some modalities, including Thai massage, The Rossiter System® techniques, and some forms of Shiatsu, are done with the client lying on a mat on the floor. Many of the techniques for these modalities allow practitioners to use their feet to apply pressure, providing a good break for the upper extremity. These methods are not without their challenges, especially to the practitioner's balance. Awkward postures can arise, including extreme neck flexion if the practitioner is in the habit of looking down at the client continuously during treatment, as well as kneeling and squatting to get down to the client's level. Tractioning during mat work does allow use of the entire body to generate the pulling force, but practitioners must be careful to use both hands to grasp the part of the client's body they are tractioning. If you work with your client on the floor, be sure to use good body mechanics, and use leverage and your body weight effectively, just as you would with any other type of bodywork. Physical therapists that work with pediatric clients and have to stoop and bend to their level should also be aware of the particular challenges of working closer to floor level. Elevate your patients whenever possible by placing them in a chair or on the table, rather than bending or lowering yourself to their level.

Keeping the Client Close to You

Since the healthiest working position is one that allows you to remain upright with your arms at a comfortable distance in front of your body, position your clients close enough to you that you do not have to hold your arms far out in front of you or lean forward to reach them.

If you are standing at the side of the table, work only on the side of the client that is closest to you. Do not reach across the client to work on the other side; instead, walk over to that side and work there. If you are applying a particular technique, use the hand that is closest to the area you are treating to avoid reaching. There is nothing wrong with asking clients to move over to the side of the table closest to you. You may want to organize your work to address one side of the body at a time, so you and the client can stay on one side for a while and then switch to the other.

You can also position just the client's legs or arms for easier access. Abducting a client's leg or arm so it angles towards the side of the table will allow you to work on that body part without having to twist, bend or reach. By keeping your work close to you, you will be able to use good body mechanics no matter what technique you use, and lean in with body weight to apply pressure.

Using Positioning Aids

There are a number of products available to manual therapists that can help maximize your client's comfort and your own. These supports allow you to adjust the client's position to give you better access to the part of the body you want to work on. They also provide extra support and cushioning for clients with special needs, including pregnant women and people suffering from low back pain. Bolsters designed for manual treatment work are easiest to wipe down, but you can also use pillows and cushions with washable covers to position your clients. Use bolsters rather than your hands to hold a client's limb or head in place while you work, reducing static loading on you and allowing you to use both hands to perform techniques. Bolsters can also help you create slack in a muscle by shortening it slightly. For example, you can bolster the lateral part of the leg as you rotate it outward to work on the medial aspect. You will gain access to the adductors without placing them in a full stretch that would make them taut and more difficult to work on.

Movement

Now that you are aware of your breathing and posture, and your client is optimally positioned, it's time to start moving. Remember, to avoid static positions and remain dynamic as you work in order to increase circulation and use your larger muscles to generate force. As you move, use your breathing to counteract any tension that may develop so your movements remain fluid and relaxed.

Starting With a Solid Base of Support

To be able to use the force and momentum of your entire body as you work, you need a good, stable base of support. With your lower body stable, but flexible, the rest of your body can move fluidly, including your knees, hips and shoulder girdle. No part of your body should be "locked down" as you work. It is particularly important not to move the upper extremity independently from the rest of the body, as it is already overused in your work. The entire body should move as a unit.

To generate force as you work, start at the ground and work your way up. In general, keep your feet approximately shoulder width apart.

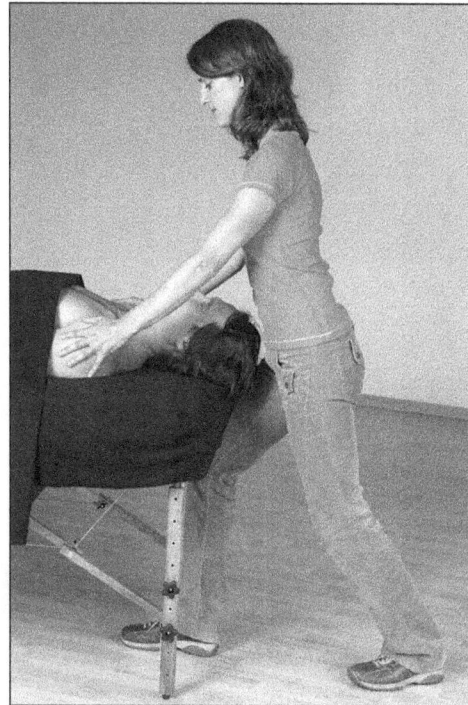

When working from the end of the table, keep your shoulders and hips in line with each other to avoid twisting your torso.

- **When you work at the head or foot of your table**, your feet should be directly under your shoulders, or place one foot a bit forward and one behind. Face the client squarely and avoid any twisting motions. This position will help you keep your hips and shoulders in line with the table as you work.
- **When you are working at either side of the table**, place your outside foot ahead of you and the foot closest to the table behind you. This position will turn your hips in towards the table while allowing you to shift your weight back and forth during longer strokes or movements.

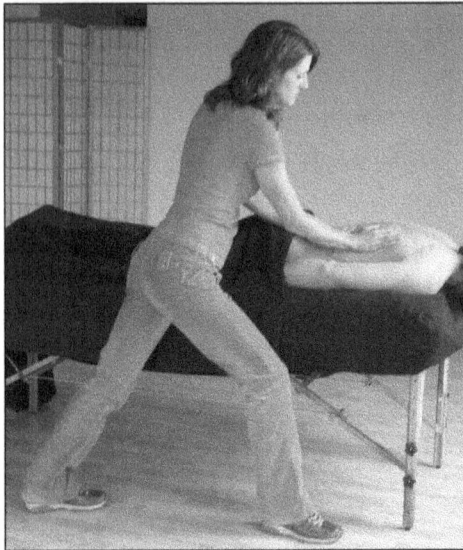

When working at the side of the table, place your outside foot in front of you and your inside foot behind you, to minimize twisting your torso.

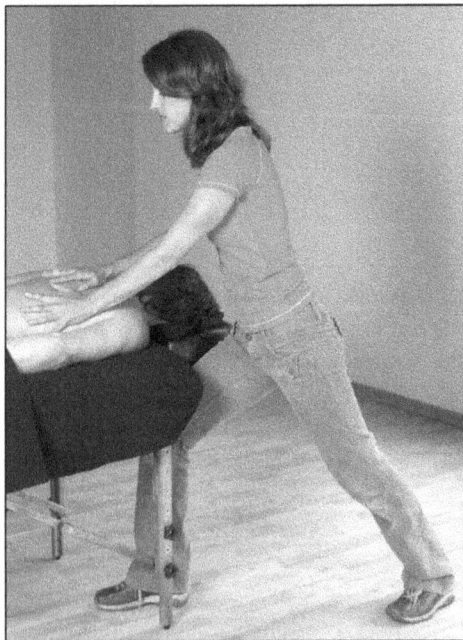

By adopting a lower stance with one leg well behind you, you can use your hip and leg muscles to generate force.

Keep your ankles, knees and hips loose and relaxed as you work. Be sure to maintain the natural curves of your spine as you work and avoid "rounding" your back, particularly in the lumbar spine. If you do not have a power-adjustable table and you need to work at a lower angle to the client, widen your stance and bend your knees a bit to get lower rather than bending at the back. Using a lower stance and standing behind your strokes, with your feet well back of where your hands are on your client, will allow you to more consistently use your legs and hips to create movement. This position has the added advantage of reducing the degree of extension at your wrist.

Avoid twisting at the knee, which can lead to knee injury. For the same reason, avoid flexing your knee past your toes. Focus on keeping your hips under your torso rather than letting your pelvis tilt back or forward. Tilting your pelvis backward can put you into a forward-leaning position and prevent you from using the strength of your lower body as you work. Tilting your pelvis in either direction could also affect your balance and generate static loading in the lower back. Review the photo on page 85 demonstrating standing neutral position and note the position of the hips directly under the upper body.

Movement of the Torso

As you work, pay particular attention to the way you move your lower back, neck and shoulder girdle. Many muscles run between the neck and shoulder, so movement (or lack thereof) in one of these areas will necessarily affect the other. The thoracic spine is relatively inflexible because the ribs attach to it, so the way you move your shoulders will directly affect your lower back and hips, and vice versa. Practicing movement patterns that protect all of these vulnerable areas will help you prevent injury to them.

Movement of the lower back: To protect your lower back, avoid bending forward more than 20 degrees or twisting at the waist, particularly while you are lifting or applying any amount of force. Instead of twisting, move your feet to bring your hips into alignment with your shoulders. Take the time to reposition your body as you work to ensure that you are squarely in front of the part of your client you want to work on, so that twisting is unnecessary. There will be situations where you will have to bend forward, but you can minimize strain on your lower back by maintaining a neutral spine, keeping the lordotic curve in your lumbar spine intact, and by supporting the weight of your upper body with your arms. A good example is working down your client's back from the head of the table. While you will be out of neutral posture, as long as you are applying downward pressure with your arms you will not be supporting your upper body weight solely with your back muscles. The tradeoff is that you will put pressure on your hands, though, so be sure to follow the guidelines for movement of the upper extremity that are explained later in this chapter. Be careful not to move too quickly as you straighten up again, especially if you have been in this position for more than a few seconds, since your muscles may have fatigued due to static loading. Reaching out and bending at the same time, without putting even a single hand down to support your weight, is very stressful to your lower back and should be avoided.

Movement of the neck: Try to maintain the inward (lordotic) curve in your cervical spine and keep your head in a neutral position: balanced squarely over your cervical spine rather than thrust forward, tipped downward, tilted or twisted to the side. While maintaining the lordotic curve is important, try not to hold your neck rigidly. A small amount of movement in the neck will prevent tension from building up in the neck muscles.

To protect your neck, it is important to recognize the essential role that your vision plays in the way you position your head and neck as you work. We take in most of our information through our eyes. For this reason, vision tends to dominate the other senses and dictate the postures we work in. We have a tendency to focus our vision on our work, even when it is not necessary to do so. When that work is a client lying on a table, the result is a forward tilted head posture that stresses the neck muscles. Visual assessment of the client is important prior to treatment, and so is periodic monitoring of the appearance of their skin, body position and facial expressions for reactions to the treatment. But it is not necessary to stare down at them during the entire treatment session. Peripheral vision is actually better attuned to small movements than foveal, or central, vision, so you may be more likely to pick up a small flinch or facial twitch if you keep a softer focus over your entire client rather than a more intense one. When you do need to look down, do so mostly by gazing downward with your eyes, tipping your head down as little as possible. Shift your gaze frequently to different areas on your client's body, which will change your head and neck position with each glance.

Movement of the shoulders: One of the most common postural problems for manual therapists and their clients is forward head and shoulder posture. Many people stand with their shoulders internally rotated, their chests caved in, and their heads jutted forward. This

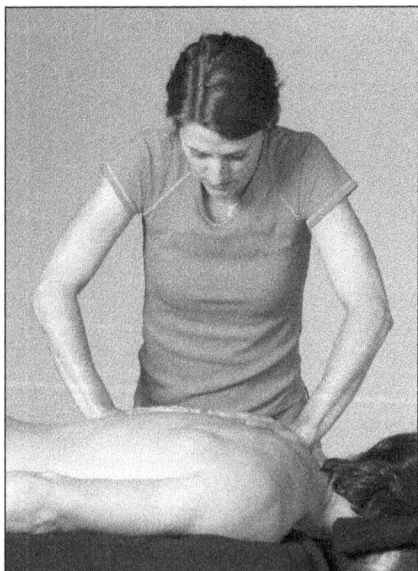

Fatigue may lead to poor postures, such as elevating your shoulders.

posture is encouraged by the fact that nearly everything we do in our daily lives, from cooking to writing to brushing our teeth, requires us to have our arms out in front of our bodies. As a manual therapist, you are also working in this position throughout your workday. Since so much of your time is spent with your arms extended in front of you, making even small, subtle changes to the way you use your body in this position can reduce your injury risk.

Working with your shoulders rounded forward or elevated (see photo, left) is one of the more awkward and potentially damaging positions you can get into as you work, because it:

■ overstretches the muscles in your back
■ shortens the muscles of your chest

- prevents the muscles in the shoulder from working effectively
- puts pressure on the thoracic outlet
- places tendons in positions where they can rub on bone, creating irritation and inflammation
- causes excessive friction on shoulder bursae, creating inflammation

Protect your shoulders by keeping them in a neutral position, keeping them down and back as much of the time as possible. If you tend to round your shoulders forward, doing backward circles with your shoulders can help you keep them in a more neutral position. You can also do a corner stretch (see Chapter 11 for a description of this stretch.). If you tend to hold your shoulders elevated, try exaggerating that movement, shrugging and holding it for a moment, and then letting your shoulders drop down to neutral. As you work, ask yourself periodically "where are my shoulders?" and consciously bring them back down if necessary. Bring your elbows in close to your sides and allow your shoulder blades to slide down your back. Squeeze your shoulder blades together a little using your rhomboid muscles to help stabilize them. Breathe deeply in and out to counteract tension that could be causing you to raise your shoulders as you work. Focus on keeping your sternum forward and lifted, to avoid rounding forward and caving in at the chest.

Avoid reaching your arms far out in front of you, out to the side past the width of your shoulders, or across the midline of your body. Applying pressure in any of these positions, particularly if one or both of your shoulders are internally rotated, will stress the structures of the shoulder, placing them at risk for injury. If you find yourself extending your arms too much, move in closer to your work.

Movement of the Upper Extremity

We naturally associate performing manual treatment with using the hands and arms to apply pressure or perform techniques. Much of the training manual therapists receive concentrates on these techniques. The term "manual therapist" literally means someone who uses her or his hands to do therapeutic work. It isn't hard to see why manual therapists get into the habit of using their hands and arms nearly exclusively to do their work.

Stabilizing Your Scapulae

The scapula is an important part of the kinematic chain of the upper body. Many muscles attach to it, and most of those muscles are brought into play when doing manual techniques. For the upper extremity to work efficiently, you need to stabilize the scapulae, placing them into a neutral position so that the stress coming through your arms can be distributed evenly between the larger muscles of your chest and upper back. By stabilizing your scapulae, you can avoid the tendency to move the upper extremity by itself, a habit that stresses the small arm muscles and increases your exposure to risk factors like repetitive movement and hand force.

To stabilize your scapulae, relax your shoulders and lift your chest slightly upward, just until your shoulders, rib cage and head line up with the rest of your body. Use a mirror to check your alignment. Lift just enough to get back into a comfortable, relaxed, neutral position—don't stick your chest out or push your shoulders back unnaturally. Use your breath to counteract any tension in your shoulders. Let your arms hang naturally by your sides.

Now that your scapulae are stabilized, your upper extremities can move in concert with the rest of your body. Try this simple exercise that illustrates the difference between working with scapular stabilization (with your scapulae engaged and neutral) and working without it:

Stand at the side of your treatment table with your feet a comfortable distance apart. Start out in a good standing neutral posture, then stabilize your scapulae by lifting your chest slightly upward and squeezing your scapulae slightly together while keeping your shoulders down and back. Make a loose fist with both hands. Keeping your arms straight, lean forward and rest the front of your fists on the table. The broad, flat surface of your fist creates greater stability, which will help distribute stress evenly. Check your scapulae to make sure they are still in neutral position. Keep breathing deeply and evenly to make sure tension doesn't creep in and distort your posture.

Bend your knees slightly and lean in to let your fists sink into the surface of the table or into a bolster (refer to photo on page 83). Be sure to keep your hands soft, but still in a fist. Don't push your fists into the table with your arms. Don't let your arms move independently from the rest of the body in any way. Allow your arms to stay firm but not locked to absorb movement generated by the upper body, and initiate your movement with your whole upper body rather than just your arms. If you know CPR, you will recognize this concept from the way chest compressions are performed. Let your body move as one unit, so your body weight moves through your arms from your upper back and shoulders to create the downward motion that increases the pressure. Experiment with applying different degrees of pressure using this technique, from very light to very deep.

Now try the same exercise without scapular stabilization. Allow your shoulders to internally rotate, and the chest to cave in slightly. You will notice that it is now difficult for the upper extremity to work in concert with the rest of the body. Without proximal support, the arm can easily become unstable, and the arm muscles have to work harder to control arm movements. You can see that scapular stabilization allows movement of the arm to be initiated and controlled by the muscles of the chest and back, reducing stress to the smaller, less powerful muscles of the arm as you create pressure.

Try not to think of your upper extremity as the main part of the body you use for your work. Although you may use your hands and arms to deliver treatment, they should be the last part of a chain of movement, rather than the initiators of the movement. Whenever possible, avoid moving your upper extremity independently from the rest of your body. Your power should come from your core muscles, chest, back, hips and legs, not just from your arms. The only exception to this rule will be small, precise techniques done with light pressure, for which you will necessarily use only the small muscles of your hands and arms. Be aware, though, that you may start by using light pressure, generated by the smaller muscles of the distal arm, and progress to using deeper pressure. As you increase the pressure you are using, you will need to consciously take the time to transition to using larger muscles that are better suited to this kind of work. If you are seated, you may need to move to a standing position to allow you to engage the rest of your body in your work.

Using your hands, fingers, and particularly your thumbs by themselves should be kept to a minimum in your work. Moving these small, vulnerable structures independently places them at too great of a risk of injuries like ligament tears and tendonosis. Restrict your use of these delicate structures to the work you do with little to no pressure: the more pressure you use, the greater your risk of injury. Keep your hands soft and relaxed as you work to avoid static loading of the intrinsic muscles of the hands.

As you lean in with body weight, keep your elbows fairly straight, but not locked, so you can actively use the muscles in your upper arms to protect your elbow joints. Avoid fully pronating or supinating your forearms, particularly when you apply pressure, since these positions stress the attachments of the flexor

The most important single piece of advice to follow to avoid hand and wrist injuries is to keep your wrists straight as you work.

and extensor muscles at the epicondyles of the elbow. Your flexor and extensor muscles have only so much stretch to them, and if they are pulled taut by forearm rotation, they will be more easily strained by finger movements or wrist bending.

Your lower arms are at their strongest, and under the least amount of stress, when they are in a "handshake" position with your wrists

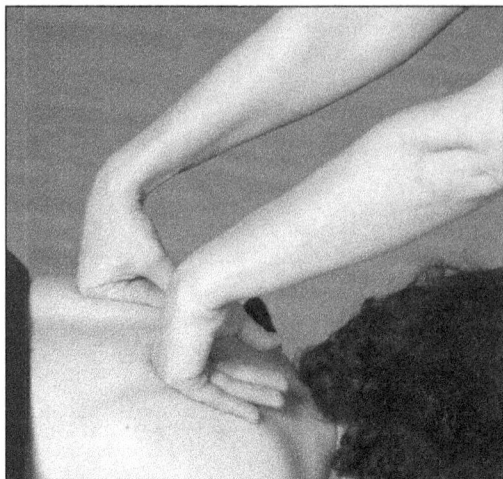

Hyperflexion of the wrists while applying downward pressure can put you at risk for wrist injury.

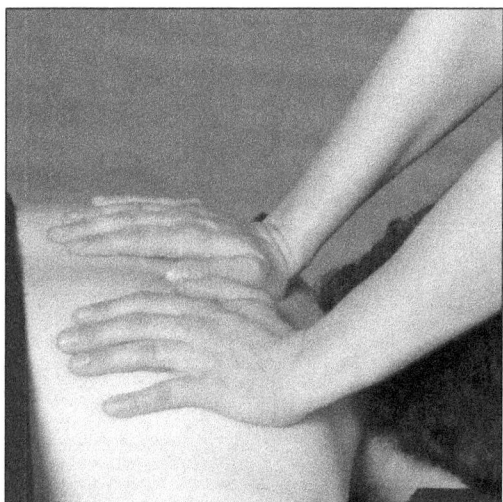

Hyperextension also increases the risk of injuring your wrists.

straight, mid-range between supination and pronation. The most important single piece of advice to follow to avoid hand and wrist injuries is to keep your wrists straight as you work. When using hand force, you should not only avoid flexion and extension, but also ulnar or radial deviation. By taking your wrists out of neutral as you apply pressure with your hands, you use your wrist flexors and extensors more than you do when your wrists are straight. This places more stress on their tendons, and increases the pressure within the carpal tunnels in your wrists, all of which can lead to injury.

There is a small range (10–15 degrees) of wrist bending or deviation from neutral position that is acceptable and will not add undue stress to the joints. Many manual techniques can lead to a considerable amount of ulnar deviation, hyperflexion or hyperextension if you don't pay enough attention to your body mechanics as you do them. These awkward positions make injury more likely, particularly when combined with hand force. A good visual indication that you are bending your wrists too much is the appearance of any wrinkles or folds in the skin on the side you are bending toward.

Varying Your Movements

Even if you are using good body mechanics, you can still overuse a part of your body. If you rely too heavily on using your hands, fingers and thumbs, even if you are using your larger muscles and stabilizing your scapulae at the same time, you can still injure yourself. For this reason, varying the parts of your upper extremity that you use to deliver treatment is essential in preventing upper extremity MSDs. The same holds true for your neck, back and lower extremities; you need to keep moving to avoid static loading or repetitively doing the same techniques in the same position. Practitioners who maintain a sense of fluidity and ease of motion as they work are generally more relaxed and less likely to get into potentially harmful static positions.

The human body develops "motor programs" as it moves, in a process known as neuromuscular facilitation. As you repeat a motion, the muscle recruitment and firing pattern involved in that motion is facilitated; the motion becomes fluid and easy for you, but you are constantly recruiting the same muscles, placing the same stress on the same tendons, and holding the joint in the same position. Making these motions over time in positions that are far from neutral can lead to injuries from repeated, cumulative trauma. Facilitated motions may become easier for you to perform, but make sure they are not the only motions you use. In addition to causing injury, they can lead you to repeat the same treatment sequence for nearly every client, whether it is appropriate to their condition or not.

Moving and changing your position help dispel muscular tension, and have the added benefit of increasing your general physical conditioning and circulation. The impact of your work is more evenly distributed to your body as a whole, rather than fatiguing just your upper extremities. Make it a goal to move frequently and fluidly around the table, repositioning yourself and your client as needed.

The best strategy for your long-term health is to develop multiple ways to treat any given part of the body or pathology. Using a variety of approaches is not only easier on your body; it also increases the likelihood that you will be able to find an appropriate approach to the myriad number of clients and conditions you will encounter in your practice. Some clients will respond better to some treatments than others; some respond better to lighter techniques than to deep tissue techniques, and the opposite can also be true.

In observing a number of very experienced manual therapists who have worked for years and reported no serious symptoms of injury, it is obvious that these practitioners have a very important point in common: they all vary their movements, techniques and positioning frequently as they work. They keep moving, never spending too much time in one position or posture: they walk around their client as they work, addressing the client's back one moment, then moving to the client's head, then walking over to work on the shoulder, etc. They are constantly adjusting their own or the client's position to achieve the optimum posture and leverage to do their techniques. They also change technique and hand/arm position frequently: first they may use a fist, and then change to an open hand, then to a few fingers together. Each hand position lasts no more than a few seconds, and then they move on to a new one to avoid too much repetitive motion.

Using a variety of motions and frequently changing the part of the hand or arm they employ allows these practitioners to use many different muscle groups without overusing or overstressing any single one. In so doing, they avoid static loading and turn their work into a kind of whole-body workout that encourages good circulation and regular breathing—all of the good things that keep us healthy. It may also be that their ability to vary their motions demonstrates the flexible approach they take to their work, another very healthy attribute.

Using a variety of motions during a hands-on treatment session can allow some muscles to rest as you use others. But even when you use a variety of motions, there may be some parts of your body, such as your arms and lower back, which are always in use. Variety by itself may not protect the parts of your body that are always engaged in those motions. True variety involves finding ways to completely rest a muscle group while you use others. For this reason, you still need to build in breaks where you do not use your arms at all, as you saw in Chapter 4.

Balancing Large Movements and Small Movements

Manual therapists often work on small areas where they find adhesions, trigger points, pain or injury. Too often, practitioners feel they have to do a lot of small, repetitive movements on a small area of a client's body, particularly if the treatment plan addresses just one area. Even if you are treating just one part of the body, there are many modalities and techniques that can be applied, including those that incorporate larger motions or are less repetitive. Continual, intensive treatment of small areas during a lengthy session is not a good idea for your musculoskeletal health, nor is it an effective treatment strategy for most clients.

In your treatments, try to balance periods of intense treatment with lighter treatment, interspersing large and small movements throughout your sessions. To reduce your risk of injury, keep the time you spend treating small areas with fine, intensive movements to a small percentage of the total treatment time for that client.

Striking a balance between small movements and techniques using broader, larger movements is important for all manual therapists, but it is particularly pertinent to the work that massage therapists do. Massage is a holistic method of healing; the most effective massage treatments address the entire body, not just a few spots. Addressing the whole body reminds your clients that they are more than just an injured shoulder or a sore back. This change in attitude can significantly affect how well they progress in their treatment.

Large, broad, gentle strokes also serve another important pur-

---

Five Reasons Not to Over-Treat Your Clients

1. Clients can only integrate so much work into their bodies in one session. For example, limiting your work to treating a half dozen major trigger points in one session will avoid overloading your clients' ability to adapt to the changes in their neuromuscular systems.

2. The stress of too much deep work can create new muscle guarding and considerable soreness over the next couple of days.

3. Some muscle guarding may be protective in nature, preventing greater damage and pain, for example, from a bulging disc in the spine. Releasing that muscle guarding too quickly might actually cause more harm than good.

4. Over-treatment can create nausea, dizziness and grogginess that can be unpleasant and counterproductive.

5. Too much pain as a result of treatment can create a fear/avoidance response that can cause a client to stop seeing you, and may even stop them from seeing any other manual therapist in the future.

pose: they aid in lymphatic drainage of the area. Part of the goal of massage is to help move accumulated metabolic byproducts and waste products out of the muscles. Broad, light strokes used every few minutes between treatment techniques gently sweep the lymph fluid away from the affected area, moving metabolic byproducts back toward the general circulation where they can be processed and flushed out. Larger strokes can also help your clients become calmer and more relaxed, which will aid in healing and promote general health and well-being. Breaking up your spot work with more general lymphatic drainage strokes is good for your client and easier on your hands. While large strokes are not without their own risks, combining small and large work in your sessions will help you avoid most of the risk that comes with doing any one type of technique for long periods of time.

How Good Body Mechanics Impact the Client's Experience

Using good body mechanics is not only better for your health; it also makes the work you do feel much better to your clients. Working with larger muscle groups and body weight will make your movements smoother and more flowing. Hands that are tense, stiff and unyielding because you are generating force using only the upper extremity will feel unpleasant to your client while causing stress and discomfort for you. You want to relax your clients, not transmit your tension to them. Let your hands relax so they can mold to the individual contours of your client's body. Lean in with your body weight to apply pressure rather than pushing with your arms, since that type of movement can feel stiff and aggressive to your clients. Keep your hips and knees "soft" so you can more easily use the strong muscles of your legs to create movement. When your clients perceive your touch as fluid, relaxed and assured, they will be more confident in your skill as a professional, and more open and responsive to the treatments you provide to them.

Mutual Observation

To reinforce your self-awareness, ask a colleague to watch you as you do manual techniques. Proprioception only goes so far; it is very helpful to have someone else observe your work and give you constructive feedback, or to videotape yourself working and analyze your body mechanics.

Find a colleague you trust, and schedule a mutual observation session. Plan on observing for at least a half hour for each of you, to give you time to get into your work and demonstrate a variety of techniques. After watching your colleague work, reinforce good habits and then point out some areas that could use improvement. Then switch and have your colleague do the same for you.

Top 10 things to observe as you watch each other work:

1. Do you stand for long periods in one place, or do you move around your client?

2. Do you use your body weight and your larger muscles to perform techniques, or are you mostly using your upper extremities to create and execute your techniques?

3. Do you use the same kind of stroke or technique for a long time before changing to a different stroke?

4. Do you keep your wrists straight?

5. Do you use your thumbs too much (i.e., more than 5 minutes total during the session)?

6. Are most of your techniques done with one part of your hand? For example, do you use your fingers 50 percent of the time, or do you use your flat palm to the exclusion of any other part of your hand?

7. Do you keep your shoulders relaxed and down, with your scapulae stabilized?

8. Do you lean forward too far (more than 20 degrees forward from vertical) or too often (more than 20 percent of the time), or do you remain upright most of the time?

9. Are you doing any lifting that could be avoided?

10. Are you breathing deeply, or are you breathing shallowly or holding your breath?

You might ask another colleague to videotape you as you work, or videotape yourself using a tripod. Then watch the tape and evaluate your work. As you develop awareness of the way you work, you can start incorporating more movement and variety into your sessions. Needless to say, it takes practice to develop the confidence and flexibility to work in this manner. It is definitely a model to emulate in your effort to stay injury-free.

Maintaining Awareness of Your Body Mechanics

Understanding the principles of good body mechanics does not necessarily mean that you will use them as you work. Even with the best of intentions, it can be difficult to practice good body mechanics consistently during your workday. It takes a good deal of effort to maintain awareness of your own sensations, breathing and movements as you work on someone else. It is easy to get distracted or lose yourself in your work. As your awareness slips, you can find yourself pushing your body past its limits or developing bad habits over time.

In healthcare professions, it is easy to focus so much on treating the client that you neglect to think about the physical process by which you are accomplishing the treatment. There is a tendency among healthcare workers to concentrate more on the intellectual process of treatment than on the physical work they are doing. Some practitioners may even feel guilty thinking of themselves rather than the client. But to avoid injury, it is necessary to pay close attention

Signs of Stress to Watch Out For

As you are performing your work, be on the lookout for the following warning signs:

- Your hands or arms are shaking

- Your fingertips are turning white

- You get a muscle spasm

- You are holding your breath or breathing shallowly

- Your legs, back, or upper extremity is feeling like the technique you're using is too tiring or taxing

- You feel discomfort or pain in any part of your body

- You feel you may lose your balance

to the way your body is responding to (or suffering from) the intense work you are doing. A happy medium does exist where your own needs and self-awareness are balanced with your concentration on your client's needs.

Awareness is an essential part of injury prevention. It helps you stay in tune with your body and respond promptly to symptoms. As you work, try to remain as attentive as possible to the signals your body is sending you. Fatigue, tension, discomfort, pain, and shallow or held breath are important indications that trouble is brewing. They can indicate that your body mechanics are less than ideal, that the techniques you are using are putting too much stress on your body, or simply that you are emotionally stressed or overworked. The faster you can react by identifying the cause of the problem and doing whatever is necessary to correct it, the better you will be able to protect yourself from injury. See Appendix C for a simple practice that can help raise your body awareness and gauge and reduce your level of stress or tension, before and/or during your sessions.

---

1. Rajeev Kaushik, Reshma Kaushik, Sukhdev Mahajan, Vemreddi Rajesh, "Effects of mental relaxation and slow breathing in essential hypertension," Complementary Therapies in Medicine, 2006; 14 (2): 120-126.

6

Modifying Your Techniques

Applying the general principles of ergonomics and good body mechanics to your work is the first step on the road to career longevity and musculoskeletal health. The next step is to examine specific techniques you use, and identify those that are stressful to your body and can lead to injury. When evaluating your techniques, keep in mind one primary rule: *if it hurts, don't do it*. If any of the techniques you use cause you pain or discomfort, even if it is only for a brief time, you could be damaging your tissues. You will need to find alternate techniques that allow you to remain comfortable and symptom-free as you work. Until you stop doing techniques that cause musculoskeletal symptoms, you will continue to injure yourself, and your symptoms will not go away. Techniques that do not cause pain but feel uncomfortable or awkward should also be avoided or adapted. Those feelings of discomfort are often the first indication that the techniques you are using may eventually cause pain and injury. Changing your techniques before your body sends you the pain signal can stop the injury process before it gets started.

The primary injury prevention rule for specific treatment techniques: if it hurts, don't do it.

Reducing Stress to the Fingers and Thumbs

Among the most overused parts of the manual therapist's body are the fingers and thumbs. These small, sensitive parts of the body are perfectly adapted for precise, intricate work and for providing tactile feedback. Manual therapists tend to use them extensively as pressure tools, a use for which they are not well suited. Because these structures are easily injured, it is important to find alternative techniques that allow you to minimize the time you use your fingers and thumbs in your work.

Fingers and thumbs are frequently used for techniques such as cross-fiber and other types of friction, breaking up adhesions, performing light effleurage on delicate areas, and working through deep layers of muscle and fascia in small or very specific areas. Using the tips of the fingers and thumbs to apply pressure is a common technique for releasing trigger points and myofascia. Many techniques used in manual therapy, like reflexology, treatment massage, and PT techniques like applying pressure to the occipital area, extensively use the thumbs in a repetitive manner. Fingers are relatively long levers with very little supporting musculature to stabilize them. You must use your forearm muscles to move or apply pressure with the fingers. By doing so, you can increase pressure in the carpal tunnel. With the addition of force or awkward positioning, this can elevate the risk of tendinopathy and carpal tunnel syndrome. Sustained pressure applied with your fingertips can cause them to lose sensitivity. That sustained pressure can also increase joint laxity and damage the cartilage between the joints. All techniques that use the fingers and thumbs to apply pressure are inherently risky, and the repetitive nature of these techniques, when combined with force, can result in injury.

You may feel that a few of the techniques you do with your fingers and thumbs are so effective that you are not willing to give them up, especially if you cannot find

Reducing Effort in Your Sessions

Manual treatment work can be fatiguing. When you are working near your maximum level of effort with muscles that are fatigued, injury is likely to occur. It helps to know your maximum level of effort, and then consciously work at a much lower percentage of that maximum. Everyone has a different maximum level of effort. You can identify your maximum level by your perception of the effort you use in your work.

Think about grading your techniques according to the effort you use to perform them. Use a scale of 1 to 10, where 1 is practically no effort and 10 is the most effort you could possibly exert. To be safe, stop using any technique you rated 6 or more; limit techniques with a 3–5 rating to no more than once or twice per session; and any techniques that you do repetitively should not have a rating of more than 2.

adequate alternatives for them. There may be some areas of the body that you feel are too small or delicate and would be endangered or unreachable with any other part of your body or technique. Certainly there are some muscles, such as the subscapularis, that would be hard to work on with any other part of the body. Muscles in sites of potential endangerment, such as the scalenes, require both the precision and sensitivity that the fingertips provide. Using a tool designed for treating small areas may help (of course, keep endangerments in mind). You can certainly continue to use your fingers and thumbs in these cases. The goal is to stop overusing them in your treatments, not to stop using them altogether.

It is particularly important to limit the time you use your easily injured thumbs. Think about setting a limit, before you start working, for how much time you will use your thumbs in any one session, and use them only in those instances when you feel you have no other good choice. Keep your effort down to a "light" or "easy" level when using your thumbs repetitively. To keep your thumbs healthy, use them as little as possible in each session, and even then for only brief periods before switching to a different part of your hand, or a different technique altogether. The idea is to stop using your thumbs *before* the muscles that support them become fatigued, so your thumbs remain in proper alignment when you use them.

Applying and Maintaining Pressure with the Fingertips or Thumb Tips

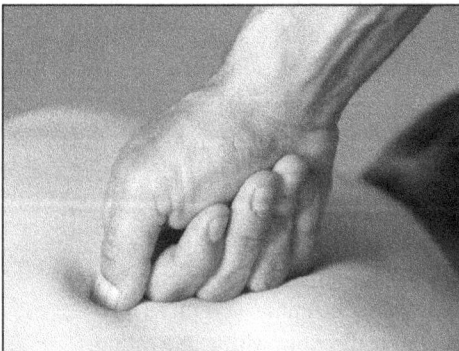

Keep your thumb straight, not flexed or extended, to protect it when applying downward pressure.

If you use your thumb to apply downward pressure, the healthiest method is to keep the thumb supported and in line with the rest of your hand and arm, with a "power hand" over it to help provide the force. Keep the joints of the thumb essentially straight with just a slight amount of flexion, avoiding both hyperflexion and hyperextension. In this position, you can use the fist and fingers to support the thumb. To work on trigger points, try first palpating with the thumb, then laying your forearm on top of the thumb to apply pressure. In this way, you avoid stressing the CMC joint by using the delicate muscles of the thumb to apply pressure. An alternative would be to palpate the tissue with the thumb first, to find the right spot, then using the elbow to carefully apply the pressure. If you are using gliding pressure with the thumb along the length of a muscle, ensure that the base of the thumb (the thenar eminence) stays in contact with the client's body so that pressure is not applied exclusively with the tip of the thumb and it remains relaxed as you glide.

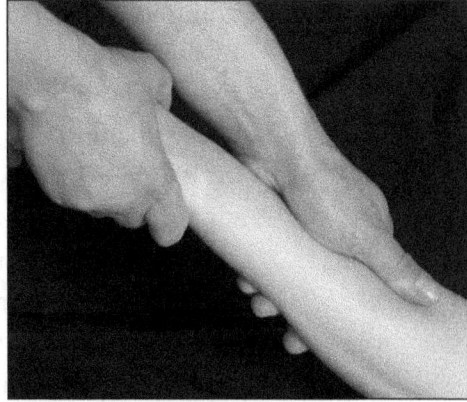

Keep the entire thumb, including the thenar eminence, in contact with your client when applying gliding pressure.

Avoid applying pressure with just one finger or thumb by itself, which places too much stress on that one digit. It also forces you to hold your other fingers out of the way, creating an awkward position that increases stress on the hand and wrist. Try to use several of your fingertips together as a unit if you use them in your work. In situations where you need to apply pressure in a tight space—when working around the neck, for example—use your index and middle fingers together, since these are your strongest digits. If you can, brace them with your other hand by laying it across the back of your knuckles.

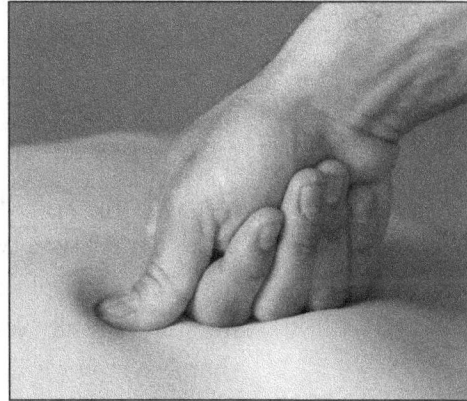

Any combination of hyperextension and flexion in the IP and MCP joints of the thumb will increase the force concentrated in the CMC joint, and should be avoided.

When applying pressure with the fingertips or thumbs, take steps to protect your hands and wrists at the same time. Keep your wrists straight, and allow the rest of your hand, including the thumb, to relax as much as possible as you apply pressure, to avoid any unnecessary effort or static loading. Keep your fingers evenly flexed at each joint as you work. Don't let any joint bend back into extension, since this position will transfer stress up to the next more proximal joint. It is particularly important to keep the thumb in a good position, since applying pressure with either the interphalangeal (IP) or metacarpophalangeal (MCP) joint in hyperflexion or hyperextension will transfer stress to the carpometacarpal (CMC) joint. The position of your thumbs determines where the forces are concentrated, whether they are born by the muscles or shifted to more delicate, easily damaged structures like ligaments and cartilage.

If you cannot avoid hyperextension or more than slight flexion in all of the joints of your fingers and thumbs as you work, then you are applying more pressure than your muscles can sustain. The stress in this case will be transferred to tendons, ligaments and joint cartilage, which can lead to injury. Too much pressure on the thumb and fingers also creates ischemia, cutting off circulation there and increasing your risk of injury. You can support one hand with the other to help maintain a good hand position, but you still need to be careful about applying too much pressure. Much of the force you apply with the supporting hand will still be transferred to the fingers of the treating hand, and can damage the cartilage in your IP joints.

For all of these reasons, it is best to use the thumb as little as possible for direct pressure. Remember that manual therapists have a very high incidence of thumb injury as a result of their work. If you are already experiencing pain or other symptoms of injury or impending injury in your thumbs, you will need to stop using them completely until they have healed. Explore other options for creating direct pressure, including using the elbow or using hand tools, even if you are not having any thumb symptoms as a preventive measure. The process of discovery can be very creative and fun!

Supporting the Client's Weight on Your Fingertips

Some manual therapists do techniques that use the weight of their client's body on the therapist's fingertips to generate pressure or apply manual traction. For example, when performing suboccipital release, they place their hands, palms up and fingers extended, underneath their client's occiput, so that the weight of the head on their fingertips provides the force necessary to release tight suboccipital muscles. Practitioners use similar techniques to work on trigger points in the erector spinae or rhomboids, or to apply traction to the scapula. It is not unusual to see the practitioner's hands or arms shaking with effort as they perform this type of technique. While these techniques can be very effective for the client, they need to be approached with caution. Some parts of clients' bodies can be quite heavy (see Table 5 on page 129), and place a great deal of stress on your hands, wrists and forearms.

It is actually more stressful to support weight on your fingertips or hands in this way than to apply downward pressure. This kind of technique isolates your upper extremity, stressing the small muscles of the shoulder, arm and hand. Over time, the pressure on the joints, particularly the interphalangeal joints, can damage the cartilage and cause osteoarthritis. When a technique carries so much risk, and so many alternatives exist that accomplish the same goals as well or better,

---

Trigger Points: Work Smarter, Not Harder

- Part of the reason for using ischemic compression on trigger points is to suffuse the area with blood to help restore a biochemical balance in the tissues. Ensure an adequate supply of blood in the area by first warming the tissues with moist heat before you work on trigger points, and releasing any adhesions that may be restricting circulation.

- Use a hand tool instead of your fingers or thumbs whenever appropriate.

- Don't hold pressure for long periods of time. If the trigger point does not begin to react after a few seconds, you may not be directly on it (some trigger points are very small and hard to locate). It may also be a tender point that is better treated with techniques like Strain-Counterstrain or positional release. Reposition your pressure, or try a different technique.

- If an area has a series of trigger points, work on the most tender one first. If all are similar in tenderness, work on the most proximal or medial one first. These points are more likely to be the original trigger points, while the others in the area may be secondary or satellite trigger points. Treating the primary point may make the secondary points release by themselves.

- Use passive and active stretching of the muscles you have treated to help your clients integrate the work you have done.

- Limit the number of primary trigger points you treat in one session to avoid overworking your clients.

it is best to simply stop using the technique. The client's back and neck muscles can be addressed easily in prone, seated or side-lying positions, using your body weight as well as your hands, forearms and elbows to create the pressure.

Alternatives to Using the Fingers and Thumbs to Create Pressure

You will be less likely to injure your thumbs and fingers if you learn to use other parts of your hand or arm to accomplish the same treatment goals. Use the sensitive tips of the thumb and fingers to palpate tissue before applying pressure. Palpation should be done lightly; if you apply too much pressure, your thumb or fingers will lose sensitivity. Once you have found the spot you want to treat, mark it with your thumb or fingers, and then apply pressure with another part of your hand or arm. Vary the part of the hand or arm you use to apply pressure, so you don't use one part exclusively or repetitively.

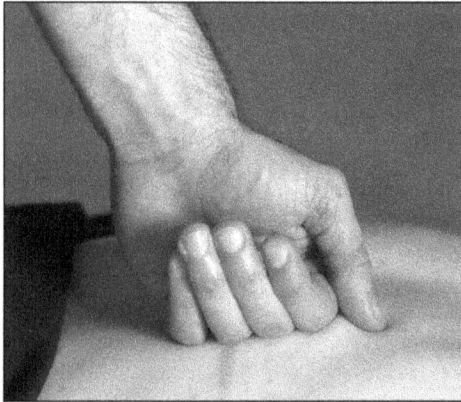

Using your knuckles gives your fingers a break and allows you to keep your wrists straight.

Instead of using your thumbs or fingers, try using your knuckles (you can alternate using the proximal and middle phalanges) or the edge of the hypothenar area (the edge of the palm between the pinky finger and the styloid process of the ulna). If you want to use just one knuckle, it is best to use the middle knuckle on your middle finger, since it naturally sticks out more and you can use the fingers on either side for lateral support. Use less pressure when you use your knuckle, to protect both yourself and your client. You have less sensation in your knuckles than in your fingers or palm. Knuckles are also unyielding, and you can damage delicate tissues in your client's body by trapping them between your hard knuckles and one of the client's bones. Too much pressure on your knuckles could

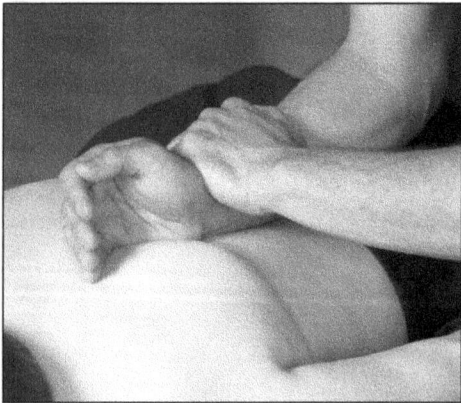

Use your hypothenar eminence and styloid process to apply more concentrated pressure, while supporting your wrist with your other hand.

also damage the ligaments and cartilage that support and cushion them. Avoid overusing your knuckles for the same reasons discussed above for the fingers and thumbs. If you have any form of arthritis or a family history of arthritis, you should be particularly careful about using your knuckles to apply pressure, as you could cause additional damage to the joints.

Elbows are another alternative for working on larger muscles that are not close to potential endangerment sites. If you use your elbow, be sure to keep the hand of the same arm relaxed and loose as you apply pressure. Keep your upper arm in close to your ribs, stabilize your scapulae and keep your shoulder down, to avoid placing stress on your shoulder muscles. Take a deep breath to release any tension if you're not used to this position. When applying deep pressure, avoid using the point of the olecranon process, which may provide pressure that is too focused. Try using the part of the elbow just distal or just proximal to the olecranon process itself to provide a broader pressure. Using your elbow, knuckles or the side of your hand will allow you to use your stronger proximal muscles to create force, so you can apply the same amount of pressure with less effort than you would use with your fingertips or thumb.

As you saw in Chapter 4, hand tools are another alternative to using the fingers and thumbs. They exist in varying sizes, shapes and hardness, depending on the use you have in mind. Although you will still need to use some hand force, gripping and repetitive motions when using hand tools for tasks like trigger point treatment, cross-fiber friction or muscle stripping, you will be

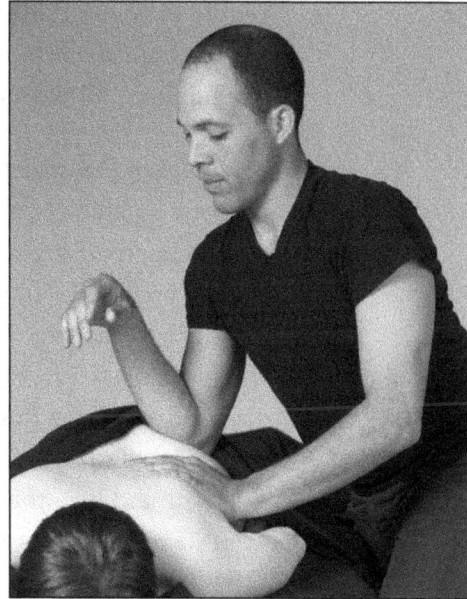

Stabilize your scapula and keep your wrist relaxed when using your elbow or forearm.

Reducing the Use of Your Fingers and Thumbs

Avoid overuse of your fingers and thumbs by using the following to perform techniques and apply pressure:

- Forearms
- Elbows (with caution)
- Knuckles
- Backs of middle phalanges
- Ulnar stylus
- Ulnar edge of palms
- Hand tools

able to create those motions using much larger muscles. Your fingers and thumbs are best used as diagnostic tools to find trigger points or adhesions, for example, so keep them in good shape for that purpose.

Applying Pressure to Bony Surfaces

Some techniques, such as releasing trigger points on the suboccipital muscles, require placing pressure on thin sheets of muscle that lay over hard bone. The pressure is a form of contact stress for the therapist, which can damage the small blood vessels and nerves of the fingertips. This damage can cause inflammation of the nerves, which will reduce sensitivity in the fingertips until it subsides. Contact stress at the palm, particularly the base of the palm where the medial portions of the thenar and hypothenar eminences meet the carpal bones, can result in an increase in pressure in the carpal tunnel, potentially damaging the median nerve there.

Broad pressure can be applied to larger bony areas, such as the infraspinatus, by using the forearm or knuckles. Using the flexor muscles in your forearm to apply pressure over the scapula can avoid the potential for bone-on-bone contact between your ulna and the spine of the scapula. At the same time, you'll get a massage for your own flexors. Smaller muscles in bony areas, for example the supraspinatus, may be better treated with a hand tool to avoid contact stress to your fingertips. Using one that has a rubber tip will allow you to create a more focused pressure while maintaining comfort for your client.

Grasping Tissues Between the Fingertips and Thumb

Manual therapists sometimes use techniques that involve grasping a small amount of tissue between the tips of the fingers and thumbs. They use these techniques when working on muscles such as the upper trapezius, the sternocleidomastoid, the thumb adductors, and the pectoralis major, or to lift superficial fascia.

When you grasp tissues in this manner, you use the smaller, weaker muscles in the hand and around the thumb, rather than the larger, stronger muscles of the forearm. This grip is inherently weak as a result. The internal force created by this type of pinch grip (known as a tip pinch grip) also increases pressure in the carpal tunnel. The

Figure 4. Relative Strength of Grips

Grips that allow you to use the larger muscles in your forearms, such as a power grip or hook grip, are much stronger than grips that primarily use the intrinsic muscles of the hand, such as pinch grips.

Optimal power grip (e.g., grasping a client's wrist with your entire hand)

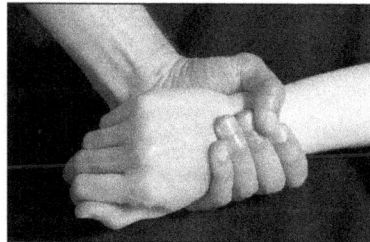

100%

Hook grip (e.g., grasping a client's upper trapezius between the fingers and palm)

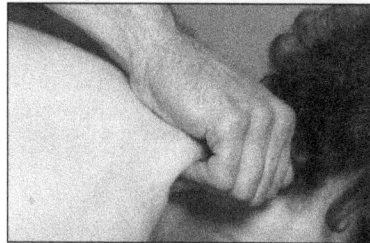

Power grip, too wide or narrow (e.g., grasping a client's entire ankle, or a single finger)

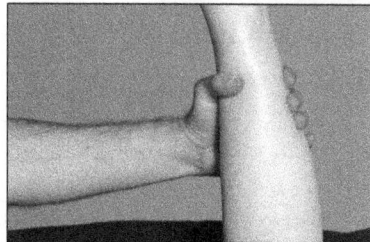

Lateral or key pinch grip (e.g., squeezing tissues between the thumb and side of index finger during petrissage)

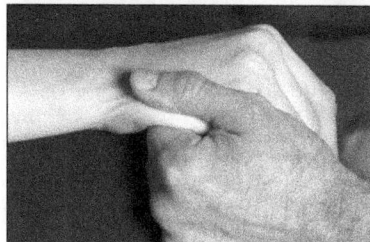

Tip pinch grip (e.g., lifting the client's skin between the fingertips and the tip of the thumb)

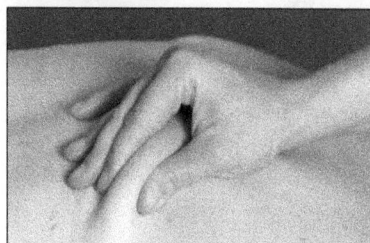

15%

repeated use of pinch grips can cause hand and wrist injuries such as tendinopathy and carpal tunnel syndrome. To make things worse, therapists often bend their wrists when using the tip pinch grip, further increasing the risk of injury.

Your strongest grip uses your entire hand to grasp the tissues, with your fingertips coming close to your thumb, such as when grasping a client's wrist. Your grip will be slightly weaker if you cannot bring your finger and thumb close together because the part of the client's body you are gripping is too wide (like their calf), or when your fingers and thumb overlap too much because the body part is too narrow (like their thumb).

Another way to achieve a stronger grip is to alter your position (or your client's) so you can grip these tissues with your fingers pressing toward your palm, keeping your wrists straight. This "hook" grip is the one you use when you grasp a client's upper trapezius between the fingers and palm, or when you carry a portable treatment table by the

Ergonomics Principle—Avoid Pinch Grips

Gripping between the fingers and thumbs is one of the greatest risk factors for thumb, hand and wrist MSDs. Pinching can increase pressure in the carpal tunnel while fatiguing muscles around the thumb and placing stress on the CMC joint surfaces. Because pinch grips involve such small muscles, using even a small amount of force can increase your risk of injury. Just 2 pounds (0.9 KG) of pinch force, about the amount required to open a clothespin, can result in microtrauma and eventual injury if that force is sustained or repeated often enough.

Several petrissage techniques call for gripping between the thumb and the fingers or palm, and should therefore be used sparingly. Whenever possible, grasp tissues between the base of the index finger and the first phalange of the thumb, rather than the tip of the thumb.

Compression of thinner sheets of muscle, such as the upper trapezius or external obliques, is sometimes performed using a pinch grip. Instead, grasp the tissue between the palm and fingers. You may need to reposition yourself in relation to your client to keep your wrist straight as you do this technique.

handle. Another option is to grasp tissue between the side of the index finger and the IP joint of the thumb in a lateral or "key" pinch grip.

In general, limit the duration that you hold a grip at any one time in the course of a session and during a workday. Even your strongest grips should be used sparingly. If you are using this kind of technique to release trigger points, let go after several seconds if you do not sense a change in the tissues, and try another approach. See the boxed section on treating trigger points on page 113 for more information.

Increasing Hand and Arm Stability

Techniques become harmful when they overuse the hand, elbow or arm, or when they use one of those parts of the upper limb in an unstable position. Instability can lead to unnatural positioning, one of the main factors that contributes to work-related injury. Instability is inherent in some structures, like the CMC and shoulder joints, but you can also create instability by damaging the ligaments around a joint through overuse. For these reasons, avoid using any technique that puts the arms and/or hands in positions that are hard to control, or causes them to wobble. Using broad, flat areas, like the forearm or front of the fist or knuckles, will give you the most stability. The thumb and the fingers are the most unstable parts to use, since they tend to buckle and wobble when pressure is applied.

You can enhance stability by reinforcing your hands, wrists and fingers. The more stable the wrist or finger joints are, the less the muscles have to work to keep the joints in alignment. The added stability distributes stress more evenly, and allows the muscles to relax, since they no longer have to work so hard to maintain stable positioning (the photo on the bottom of page 114 provides a good example). For example, using a "hand-on-hand" position is a technique familiar to chiropractors during an adjustment.

There are many simple techniques for reinforcing your hands and fingers. Use your free hand to enhance stability at the wrist. When using your fingers, create stability by using at least two fingers at a time: never use just one finger to apply pressure. When using a flat palm, place the other palm on top of it. Keep the bottom hand soft and relaxed, so it can palpate properly and retain its sensitivity. Think of the bottom hand as the "palpating hand," and the upper one as the "power hand," the one that propels and creates the pressure of the stroke. This same technique can be used when you apply pressure with your fingertips.

Reducing Stress to the Hands and Arms

Manual therapists use their hands as their main working tools, and perform a great variety of treatments with their hands and arms. While the hands are versatile and flexible instruments for delivering treatment, repetitively using them in your work, especially when force is involved, places the weak links at the thumb and wrist at risk. There are several good alternatives to using the hands that lower injury risk for the practitioner without reducing the effectiveness of treatment.

Grasping and Lifting Tissues (Petrissage)

Petrissage techniques like skin rolling or kneading typically involve grasping and lifting tissues between the fingers and thumb, or the fingers and palm. Sometimes both hands are used in a wringing motion to lift the tissue between them. These repetitive gripping and squeezing motions are stressful to the thumbs, hands and forearm flexors.

If you do this type of technique, be sure to use the larger muscles of your upper torso to initiate the motion that creates the stroke, to lessen the stress on your upper extremity. For some practitioners, though, these techniques may still be too uncomfortable or painful. If that is the case, stop doing them altogether. Remember that there are other ways of lifting tissue. Using your forearms in a forward circling motion (a technique used in Lomi Lomi massage) lifts tissue while also increasing circulation to the area. You can also try "cupping," a traditional Chinese medicine technique that can be used in massage treatments. Cups are applied to specific areas to lift the skin and underlying fascia and pull blood into the tissues. While traditional cupping used a small flame to heat the air in a glass cup to create a vacuum, newer forms of cupping use a hand pump to create the suction in

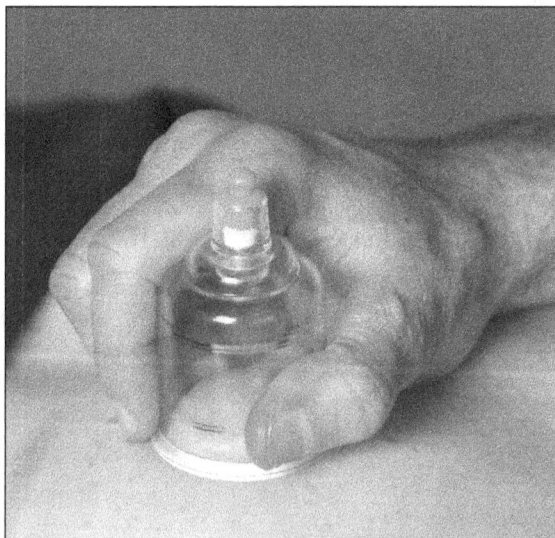

Cupping can be used to lift tissues without the need for pinch grips or repetitive motions.

either glass or plastic cups, a safer and more practical alternative. Cups can be used in one location, or they can be moved about to treat a broad area with the use of massage oil or a similar lubricant. Care must be taken not to create too much suction, which can break blood vessels and cause significant bruising. With practice, cupping can be used in place of techniques such as petrissage and skin rolling, accomplishing the same results with much less stress to the practitioner's hands and wrists. Grip the cup with a relaxed hand as you place it and/or move it over the tissues. Be sure to check the scope of practice rules in your jurisdiction, and the coverage provided by your professional liability insurance, before using cupping techniques on your clients.

Working on Large, Hypertonic or Guarded Muscles

The larger muscles of your clients' lower extremities, such as the gluteals, quadriceps and hamstrings, are very strong, particularly when compared with the muscles of the upper extremities. Yet many manual therapists work extensively on large muscles by applying pressure with their palms or grasping the tissues with their open hands. If your client has significant muscle guarding or very hypertonic muscles, and you attempt to overcome this resistance using your hands, this is a battle you are likely to lose. Your hands stand at least a fighting chance to get through the small muscles of your client's neck or upper extremity, but you should not wear them out on large, guarded or hard muscles. When working on large muscles, use your knuckles, fists, forearms and elbows rather than your fingers or thumbs, and avoid using your hands to apply pressure or grasp large muscles.

One of the more physically demanding aspects of doing manual treatment is working on hypertonic muscles, particularly when a client has significant guarding in the area, has been doing a lot of strength

An Opportunity for Self-Massage While You Work

Working on bony surfaces on your client's body can provide you with an opportunity to massage a part of your own hand or arm. For example, you can drag your thenar eminence (the fleshy part of your palm at the base of your thumb) across the edge of your client's patella, scapula, malleolus, etc. For larger bony parts, such as the iliac crest, you can run the flexor (volar) side of your forearm across them. Your clients will appreciate the use of these softer parts of your hands and arms on sensitive bony areas, and you will get the benefits of flushing out metabolic by-products and increasing circulation to these heavily used parts of your own body.

training, or is involved in athletic activities. Working too aggressively on guarded muscles with either pressure or stretching can damage muscle fibers (both your client's and your own) and cause more muscle guarding.

You can work on these muscles through sheer repetition, warming them with lots of broad strokes, and then working layer by layer through the guarding to get to the trigger point or adhesion at the root of the problem. This approach can be taxing for you if you're able to do it (not everyone has the physical fitness to do long stretches of kneading hypertonic muscles). It would be easier to try an alternate approach that takes advantage of human physiology to make your work easier. The technique of reciprocal inhibition is based on the concept that contracting an antagonist to the muscle you want to work on will, in most cases, cause the muscle to relax to some degree, allowing you to work deeper. If you are trying to work on trigger points in a deep muscle in the triceps, asking the client to flex their arm to engage the biceps may give you better access. You can also ask your client to make small, slow movements that recruit the muscle you are working on, stopping them once you have reached the depth you want.

There are other techniques that can also be effective in this situation. Ask your client to focus on moving an entirely different body part, using a fairly complex movement that will distract them from the muscle you are targeting. A good portion of muscle guarding is related to non-specific pain, so if you can change your client's focus for a while, they may relax enough for you to take care of trigger points that are the underlying cause of the guarding. You can also try using positional release to shorten a muscle and relax it enough to work through it.

You may be able to access some parts of the body more easily by having the client perform specific movements or get into specific positions. To better access the vertebral border of the scapula, for example, you can have your client place their hand palm up in the small of their back while they are lying face down or on their side, causing the scapula to lift off the ribs. If your client is face up, you can have them reach across and place their hand palm down on their opposite shoulder. This will not only lift the vertebral border slightly, but it will also bring it toward you so you don't have to reach as far.

Keep in mind that it may be easier to loosen tight or guarded muscles with heat, ultrasound or a vibrating massager (depending on the situation and the scope of your practice) before going in with your hands. Asking the client to take several slow, deep breaths with you can also reduce tension in tight muscles and reduce muscle guarding.

If you work with athletes, you will likely find they have large, hypertonic muscles. Don't try to get those muscles to relax by using brute force. You may lack the necessary strength, and you may cause muscle guarding with these clients. If you want to work on athletes, it's best to pursue specialized training in sports massage or athletic training.

Keeping Your Wrists Straight When Applying Pressure

Bending your wrist slightly as you work is not a bad thing, as long as you use little to no force while doing it (for example, when you are applying oil or making light strokes). When you apply force at the same time, it is imperative to keep your wrists as straight as possible. Once you begin applying force with the hands, the tendons in and around your wrist come under tension, and pressure begins to build in the wrist. Bending or deviating your wrists only increases the tension and pressure, making microtrauma to the tendons, inflammation, fibrosis or damage to the median nerve more likely. Movements near the end range of motion also place stress on the ligaments in a joint, increasing the likelihood of damage and subsequent joint laxity. The additional tension on muscles and tendons caused by wrist bending also affects the more proximal attachments at the elbows, increasing the likelihood of conditions such as epicondylitis or epicondylosis.

It is easy to start bending or deviating your wrists as you do compression or effleurage (stroking) techniques with a flat palm. Wrist hyperextension is especially common when using the flat palm to apply pressure while working close in to your body. An alternate technique you can use sparingly when working on thicker muscles is to make a loose fist and use the flat part of the backs of your fingers to apply pressure. This technique must be used with caution as well, since it can lead to wrist hyperflexion when working farther from your body (see top photo on page 100). Another option is to use the forearm, which works well for larger surfaces and allows you to relax your wrists as you work. Manual therapists tend to take their wrists into ulnar or radial deviation when working on parts of the body that are hard to access, or when performing percussion (tapotement) techniques. You have less range of motion in ulnar/radial deviation than you do in flexion/extension, so it is more likely for you to get into the end range of motion without noticing it.

Use these techniques to help you keep your wrists straight when applying pressure with your hands:

- Instead of using your flat palm to apply compression when working directly over your client, use the back of a loose fist (proximal phalanges) or your forearm.
- When using your forearm to apply pressure, support your wrist by grasping it loosely with your other hand, just proximal to the wrist.
- When using the palms of your hands, stand well behind your strokes so that your arms are at a shallow angle relative to your client, to keep wrist extension to a minimum.
- Adjust your position by using a lower stance or adjusting your table height if you notice that you are bending your wrist when applying pressure. You can also try sitting down to adjust your position if you are applying light pressure.

Keeping your wrists straight as you work is the single most important postural point to keep in mind for avoiding hand, wrist and elbow injuries. This advice also applies to anything you do outside of work, such as typing at the computer, playing a musical instrument, holding the steering wheel while driving, or cleaning up around the house. Pay careful attention to your wrist posture as you work, and over time you will develop the beneficial habit of keeping your wrists straight during any exertion, whether during a treatment session or outside of work. For more tips on injury prevention outside of work, see Chapter 9.

Using Your Forearms and Elbows Instead of Your Hands

The best way to save your hands is to avoid using them whenever possible. Your forearms and elbows can be very effective tools for soft tissue work, and can replace your hands for many techniques requiring broader pressure or less precision. Lomi Lomi techniques use the forearms and elbows extensively to apply pressure. The basic Lomi Lomi techniques can be easily adapted for use as an alternative to techniques that use the hands.

The fundamental Lomi Lomi stroke uses the forearm to compress and lengthen a broad area of tissue. Supporting the wrist with your opposite hand provides support, and leaning in with the elbow can provide some specific linear pressure as you move along (for example, to the erector spinae—see photo on next page). In addition to providing an alternative to using the hands for petrissage, Lomi Lomi strokes are very effective for addressing broad areas like the back, the gluteals, the anterior or posterior thigh, the posterior calf, and the bottom of the foot. You can apply pressure either with the ulnar side of the forearm (for more specific pressure) or the flexor muscles on the volar side of the forearm (for softer, more general pressure). Be aware of the tendency to clench your fist in response to tension, especially when you are new to these forearm techniques. If your hand becomes tense, relax it consciously and with your breathing.

You may find that forearm techniques are too rough for thin clients who have prominent bones. Experiment with using the forearm on different parts of the body in different ways to see what works best for you and your client. Be sure to use sufficient lubrication for forearm techniques, and maintain communication with your client about pressure and comfort.

If more focused pressure is required, your elbows can be wonderful tools if they are used carefully. Refer to page 115 for guidelines on the safe use of the elbow with your clients.

Reducing Stress to the Shoulders and Lower back

Saving your shoulders and back is just as important as saving your hands. As you saw in Chapters 2 and 3, these areas are also at risk for injury from the work you do. The arms and the torso are fairly long lever arms, so forces tend to concentrate in the shoulder joint and at L4/L5/S1 in the lumbar spine. It is important to find ways to adapt techniques that stress the shoulder and lower back, to avoid the injuries that are common in these areas.

Reaching and Bending Forward for Long Strokes

Long, fluid strokes work well for spreading oils, warming tissues, and relaxing a client before and after deeper treatments. You may wish to address a large area of tissue, like the entire length of the back, in one long stroke. Long strokes also give you an opportunity to stretch and break up the repetitiveness of short strokes. Unfortunately, long strokes are the most likely to take you far out of neutral posture, causing you to reach out from the shoulders and bend at the lower back. You can reduce stress on your lower back when bending forward in your work by maintaining a neutral spine and supporting your weight with your arms. A good rule to follow is to extend a long stroke as long as you can comfortably support your weight, and end the stroke as soon as you begin to feel any strain in your lower back, arms or shoulders from reaching out.

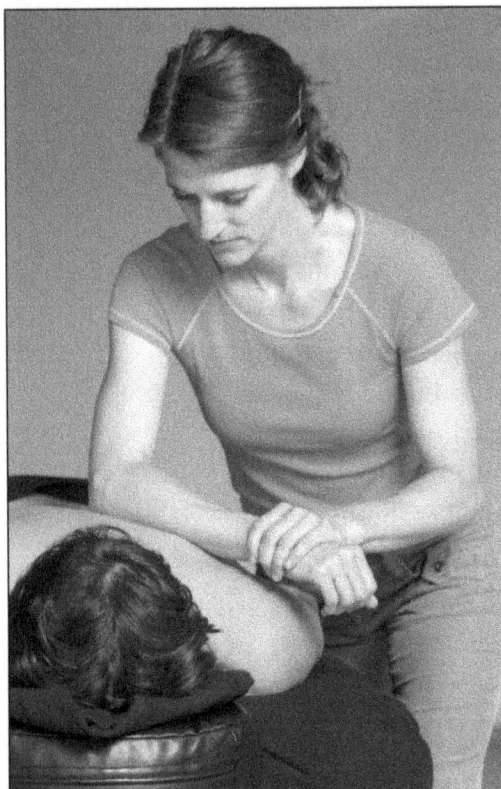

When using your forearm, lean in toward your elbow to create more focused pressure.

If you are a shorter person, you may want to do long strokes from the side of the table instead of the head or foot of the table. Standing at the side of the table, remain upright and walk along with your stroke, taking small steps along the side of the table so that your body propels the stroke forward. Avoid reaching to the end of the range of motion of your arms and back, as it will be that much harder to get yourself back up. After bending over for a while, bend your knees and flex your hips a little as you stand up straight again. This movement will get some of your upper body weight back over your hips so you can use your legs, not just the muscles of your lower back, to help you straighten up again.

Leaning Over the Table Without Support

When you lean over your client without applying downward pressure, the muscles in your lower back have to support the entire weight of your upper body. That weight can be over half your total body weight. If you have ever worked for a long period of time while bent over, and then felt soreness, weakness or pain in your lower back when you straightened up, you have experienced the fatigue that this static loading can cause.

Physical therapists, osteopaths and chiropractors often bend over their clients while mobilizing or adjusting the spine or torso. These practitioners may bend and twist their own bodies while at the same time holding and lowering their clients into the proper position before applying downward pressure. These awkward working positions, along with the physical stress of supporting part of the client's weight, contribute to the high rate of low back symptoms among these practitioners.

To avoid back injuries caused by leaning over, raise your table so you can work in a more upright position. A power-adjustable table allows you to easily raise and lower your client whenever you find yourself leaning over without support. Asking your client to move closer to the edge of the table can also reduce the need to lean forward. In some situations it may help to put your knee up on the table or even to sit on the edge of the table to get closer to the client, rather than leaning forward. If you do need to lean forward, look for opportunities to place a hand or forearm down on the table or client to support yourself. Avoid placing your palm down flat on the table with your wrist in extension, which would create too much pressure on the hand and wrist.

Lifting

Lifting is one of the most common causes of occupational injury in any profession. Among healthcare workers, the incidence of lifting-related injury is particularly high. Back and shoulder injuries are very common, particularly among nurses, who have to frequently lift and reposition patients in bed. The worldwide shortage of nurses can be partially attributed to this high injury rate. Lifting all or part of a client's weight was listed as one of the primary causes of injury in surveys of physical therapists, physical therapist assistants, chiropractors and, to a lesser extent, massage practitioners.

Manual therapists may find themselves lifting and transferring clients on and off the treatment table if the clients are in a wheelchair or other mobility aid and are not able to transfer themselves. This particularly awkward type of lifting causes considerable stress on your spine and the muscles of your lower back. One thing is very clear from reading the injury statistics and studies of the effects of lifting on the body: there is simply no safe way for one person to manually lift the entire weight of an adult human being. Even with two practitioners lifting together, the forces on the body exceed recommended occupational limits. This fact remains true even with clients who can provide some limited assistance during the move. If a client reacts unexpectedly during a move, the risk to the practitioner is even higher. If anything goes wrong while manually transferring a client, both the practitioner and the client can be injured. For all of these reasons, if you have not been specially trained in lifting techniques, do not have the appropriate equipment or assistance available, or do not feel prepared to lift people, then you should not do so.

In hospitals and other treatment settings, specialized equipment and training are available to help healthcare workers lift and move patients. If you are a practitioner working alone or in a clinic without this equipment or training, you should not transfer clients who need anything more than minimal assistance. For your clients' safety and your own, refer any clients who need more substantial assistance to a rehabilitation clinic or other facility that has the proper equipment and trained personnel.

Lifting Specific Body Parts

Manual therapists perform many techniques that require the practitioner to lift a part of the client's body. While this type of lifting may not seem difficult at first, you may quickly find yourself straining to sustain the weight if you are not truly strong enough to lift it. Before you lift any weight, whether it is at the gym, in your home, or in your practice, stop and consider whether you really have the strength to lift it before doing so. Consider the possible weight of the body part, and whether you will be lifting momentarily or holding the body part suspended for

Table 5. Approximate Weights of Parts of the Body[1]

Part of the body	Percentage of total body weight	150-pound client (68 KG)	200-pound client (90.9 KG)	250-pound client (113.6 KG)
Head and neck	8%	12 pounds (5.5 KG)	16 pounds (7.3 KG)	20 pounds (9.1 KG)
Head, neck and trunk	60%	90 pounds (40.9 KG)	120 pounds (54.5 KG)	150 pounds (68.2 KG)
Forearm and hand	2%	3 pounds (1.4 KG)	4 pounds (1.8 KG)	5 pounds (2.3 KG)
Entire arm	5%	7.5 pounds (3.4 KG)	10 pounds (4.5 KG)	12.5 pounds (5.7 KG)
Lower leg and foot	6%	9 pounds (4.1 KG)	12 pounds (5.5 KG)	15 pounds (6.8 KG)
Entire leg	15%	22.5 pounds (10.2 KG)	30 pounds (13.6 KG)	37.5 pounds (17 KG)

any amount of time. If you are not absolutely sure you have the necessary strength, don't take the chance. If you start to lift the body part and find yourself straining or wondering how you will be able to hold that weight for any length of time, lower it back down again as quickly as you can while taking care not to hurt the client. If your hands start to shake, or you find yourself holding your breath or excessively tensing your shoulders or neck, you are lifting beyond your strength capacity. Even if you have the strength to initially lift the body part, you may not have the strength to hold it for very long. Bear in mind that physical conditioning, including endurance, is more important than strength alone in preventing injuries due to lifting.

Table 5 shows the average weight of different parts of the body, to help you judge your ability to lift them. Not everyone has the strength to lift and hold a 12-pound (5.5 KG) weight for several minutes with just their hands, and yet many manual therapists will lift a client's head and hold it suspended in one hand for 5 to 10 minutes at a time. The more you are aware of the real weight of the different body parts, and the more honest you are with yourself about your own strength, the better you will be able to avoid injury from lifting on the job.

In addition to taking into account the weight of the body part you are lifting, you will also need to consider your posture while lifting. You may be strong enough to lift a 30-pound (13.6 KG) leg, but if you do it while bending and reaching out, you will be adding over 300 pounds (136.4 KG) of additional stress to your lower back. It will be much better for your back if you lift that same 30-pound leg while in an appropriate posture, holding the leg close to your torso while maintaining a neutral spine and using the muscles of the hips and legs to assist you.

Even if you are strong enough to lift a body part, doing so places stress on your already heavily used upper extremities. Holding a client's head with one hand, for example, creates pressure in the carpal tunnel and stresses the forearm flexor muscles. That's another good reason to keep lifting to a strict minimum in your work.

Fortunately, there are many alternatives to lifting heavy body parts. Manual therapists can avoid lifting body parts by changing the client's position, using a bolster, or, when possible, simply asking the client to lift the body part themselves. Here are several examples:

The Torso: Since the head, neck and trunk represent well over half of the client's weight, lifting (or lowering) the weight of the torso can be almost as risky as lifting the entire client. To return clients to a seated position, have them assist in lifting their own torsos using their arms and core. Ask them to roll onto their side and swing their legs off the edge of the table. If possible, have them use the arm on that side to push down on the table to help lift the torso. The weight of the legs will act as a counterweight, so it will be easier for you to assist them (NOT lift them) up to a seated position.

The Shoulder: With the client prone, therapists will often lift the shoulder, either to access the anterior aspect, to manipulate the shoulder joint, or to make the scapula "wing out" to access its medial border. It is not uncommon to see a therapist's hands shaking as they strain to hold the weight of the shoulder as they work. Again, unless you are very strong, do not lift the shoulder or hold it up for any amount of time. Shoulder massage and mobilization can be done quite easily in supine, seated or side-lying positions. If you want to work on the shoulder with your client prone, take a bolster or small pillow and place it under the client's shoulder to support it as you work. Ask the client to roll slightly to the other side to allow you to position the pillow (again, avoid lifting the shoulder if your clients can do so themselves). Using a bolster or pillow can often take the place of lifting and suspending parts of the body. The medial border of the scapula can be made more prominent by placing the client's hand behind the lower back instead of lifting the shoulder.

The Arm: Most clients' arms will not be very heavy, but larger clients' upper limbs may be heavy enough to require particular care when lifting and holding them. With the client supine, take hold of the wrist and fold the hand up towards their shoulder by flexing the client's elbow. You can then lift at the elbow to access the upper arm and lateral aspect of the shoulder. In this position, you can hold the arm up more easily, since most of the weight of the arm will be directed straight down toward the shoulder. From this position, you can more easily pull the arm up over the client's head or across their body to the opposite shoulder if you wish.

The Leg: There are times when you may want to lift one or both of a client's legs, whether to place a bolster under them or to perform a treatment. Keep in mind that a single leg can weigh as much as 15 percent of the client's total body weight. If you lift the entire leg at

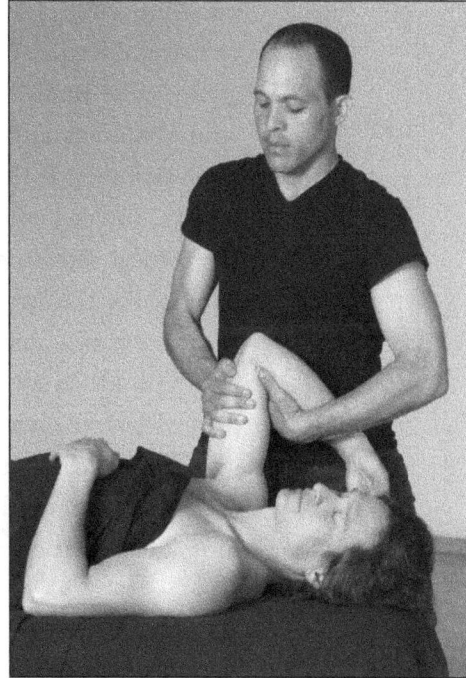

Fold the lower arm up toward the shoulder before lifting the upper arm, rather than lifting the entire weight of the arm at once.

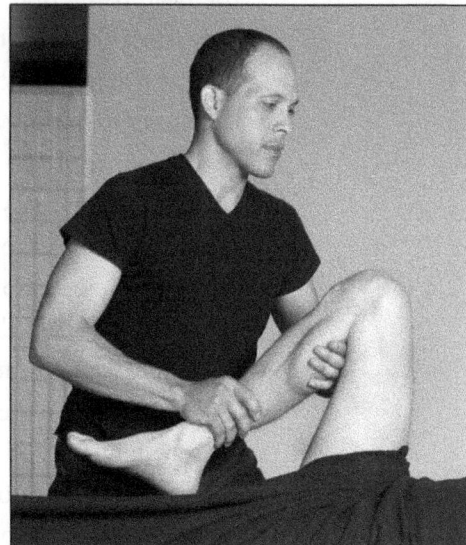

Slide the foot along the table to flex the knee, then push the leg up and over the hip joint rather than lifting the entire leg at once.

one time while it is straight, you could be lifting 25 pounds (11.4 KG) or more, since you will also be lifting a good deal of the hip musculature at the same time. Lifting the leg in this position is not only hard on your shoulders and back; it can also injure your client's knee if not done properly. If the treatment does not require your client to remain passive, you can enlist their help in lifting their own leg or legs. If your client must remain passive, have them relax their knee, then place one hand under the knee and slide the foot along the treatment table with the other hand. Once the leg is flexed, you can then lift the leg by pushing the ankle and knee up toward the client's head, keeping the weight of the leg over their hip joint. In the same way, you can slide both legs up with the feet on the table in order to slide a bolster under the knees. Again, bear in mind that you can simply reposition the client to access muscles and structures, rather than lifting for that purpose.

The Head: Taking into account the musculature of the neck, the head can weigh 12 pounds (5.5 KG) to 20 pounds (9.1 KG). That would not be a lot of weight to lift for a short amount of time while standing upright and using both hands, while being sure to also use your leg and back muscles to support the weight. But manual therapists often lift the head using one hand, and then hold it for long periods of time as they work on the neck with the other hand. Many practitioners also do this treatment while they are seated, using only the small muscles of the upper extremity to do the lifting.

If you must lift the head, do so with both hands, while standing. Instead of holding your client's head while you work on the posterior neck, lift it for a moment and then place a folded towel under the top of the head, just above the occiput, to keep it elevated. To avoid lifting the head at all, roll the client's head to one side and place a small folded towel underneath the top of the head. Roll the head to the other side so it rolls onto the towel. The top of the head will now be supported and a space will be created for your hands to slip under the neck. You can also choose not to work on the neck at all when the client is supine. Instead, do this work with the client seated, prone or in a side-lying position.

Suboccipital release is a popular technique done with the client lying supine. It involves lifting the head, and then placing it on the therapist's flexed fingertips. The weight of the head creates the direct pressure on the suboccipital muscles. It also stresses the therapist's forearm flexor muscles and increases pressure in the carpal tunnel. The suboccipital muscles can be accessed without lifting the head (for example, with the head elevated on a towel as discussed above), or fully accessed with the client side-lying, seated or prone. Another way to work on these muscles with the client supine, instead of using the fingertips, is to make a loose fist with both hands, roll the client's head to the side, and then roll the client's head onto your MCP knuckles. Do not press upward with your hands. Encourage the client to breathe deeply, and then on the exhale let the head sink down onto your knuckles, and allow the weight of the head to provide the pressure. There are also small supports available that are designed specifically to place pressure in this area, simulating the practitioner's hands.

Stretching and Tractioning

Tractioning a client's arm, leg or head brings several risk factors into play that increase the possibility of injury for the manual therapist. Pulling motions tend to require a considerable amount of back muscle contraction to stabilize the practitioner's torso. Overexerting the back muscles in this way can lead to low back injuries in much the same way that lifting does. In general, pulling motions use weaker muscles than pushing motions, and it is more difficult to use body weight to provide the necessary force. The grip you use on the client's body while providing traction is also an important factor. Maintaining a strenuous grip while providing traction can place a great deal of stress on your hands, wrists and elbows. Tractioning can also result in static loading if it is held for 30 seconds or more.

On the positive side, the pulling motion of tractioning uses a different set of muscles than the pushing motions that are much more common during most treatments. Varying the muscles you use in your work avoids overuse and fatigue, and contributes to good whole-body conditioning. The key is to find ways to use large muscles and body weight to provide the tractioning force, and to use good body mechanics during the movement.

If you have applied a lubricant to the client's skin, wipe off as much

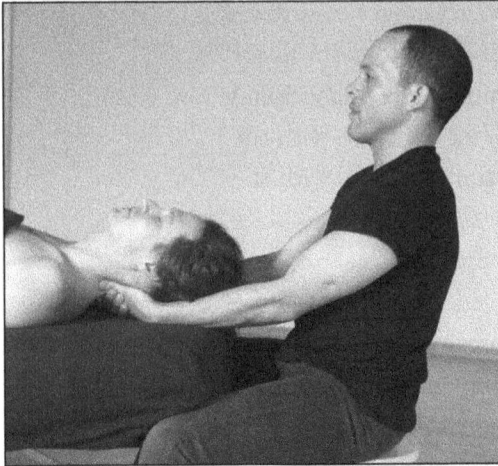

Cross one hand over the other with your palms facing you and hook the sides of your hands into the occiput and mastoid processes to get a better grip when applying traction to the head and neck.

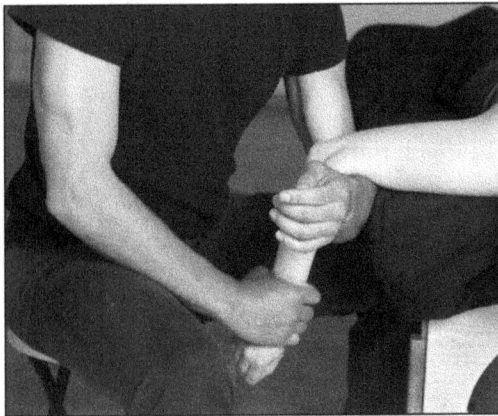

Hook your forearm around the client's elbow to traction the upper arm and shoulder without having to grip the arm tightly.

as you can from the client, and from your own hands, before attempting to grip and traction that part of the body. When tractioning, try to grip with your whole hand, with the thumb wrapping around to meet the fingers, as if you were starting to make a fist. This power grip is easiest to achieve around the client's wrist, since most wrists are small enough that you can wrap your hand around them fairly comfortably. You may also find it easier to hold the wrist just proximal to the hand, where the broader structures of the palm will keep your hand from sliding distally as you pull. Position your grip carefully to avoid putting pressure on the client's carpal tunnel.

It may be more difficult to get a comfortable grip on the client's leg, and even more difficult to get a comfortable grip on their head. To safely provide traction to the leg, grasp the client's ankle and heel with both hands, keeping your wrists straight. Stabilize your scapulae, keep your arms straight, and lean back with one foot behind the other, to allow your body weight to create the traction and maintain your balance. You can also traction the leg while seated, as long as the table is low enough to allow you to pull back with your arms between mid-sternum and waist level. Do not lift the client's leg—just let it slide along the table as you lean back. If you have a power-assisted table, raise the table to the height of your hands, so you can stay upright as you traction.

The client's head or arm can be put into traction in the same manner, using your body weight to create the traction. You may find it easier to grip the head by forming your hands into a loose 'U' shape, overlapping them a little, and hooking in at the base of the head using the mastoid processes and occiput as gripping points. Stop applying traction at the first signs of fatigue in the muscles of your back, shoulders or arms. Fatigue is a sign that you have put too much stress on your muscles, and it can also be an indication that you are being too forceful with your client. Traction should provide a gentle stretch that your client can relax into, not a force that they will resist.

There are ways to traction limbs without gripping. For example, with the client lying prone, abduct the arm to 90 degrees and let the forearm hang off the edge of the table. Lower yourself by sitting on a stool or squatting, so your shoulders are level with the top of the table. Hook your forearm into the flexor side of the client's forearm just below the elbow and hold the client's wrist with your other hand. Lean back while stabilizing your scapulae to traction the upper arm and the muscles that attach to the scapula. Move your client's arm into different angles of shoulder adduction to stretch all of the muscles in the shoulder and upper back. You can traction the upper leg in the same way, with the client prone, by flexing the client's knee and hooking your forearm around their calf while the other hand continues to hold the ankle loosely.

Some of these same techniques can be used to reduce the demands on your body when you do passive stretching or resisted exercises with your clients. Find ways to grip the clients' limbs at their smallest diameter, so you can use a good power grip. Grasp parts of the body that give you a good handhold, such as the top of the foot, or the wrist just proximal to the carpal bones. With proper positioning, you can even use your forearms to hold parts of the body, and then use your body weight to provide the force of the stretch. To stretch the calf using this technique, for example, have your client lie supine, then cup your hand under the heel, and lay your forearm across the sole of the foot. Raise the

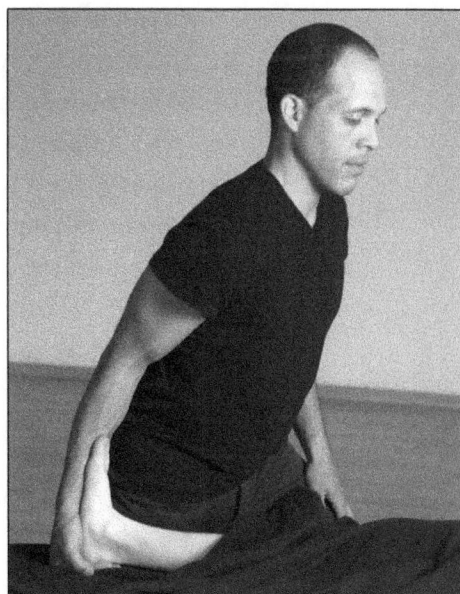

Cup the heel in your hand, line your forearm up with the sole of the foot, and lean in using body weight to stretch the calf.

table height, if you can, to allow you to remain upright. Place one of your feet slightly behind your other foot. Then bring your body weight over your forward leg, gradually adding pressure to the sole of the client's foot with your forearm until a stretch is achieved. It will be relatively easy to hold this position since the necessary force is provided primarily by your larger postural muscles.

Being Creative with Your Techniques

There are so many techniques that are used in the different modalities that it is impossible to present an exhaustive or complete list of alternative techniques here. The possibilities are nearly endless, and depend on the type of work you do, your own body type, the needs of your client, and many other variables. Combine the principles you have learned in this chapter with your own experience and creativity to find techniques that are safer and more comfortable for you. As time goes on, you will become more aware of feelings of stress or discomfort as they occur, and learn to adapt your technique accordingly in your work.

Continue to experiment with modifying your technique and finding alternative approaches that can reduce stress to your body. If some of the alternate techniques suggested here do not feel comfortable for you, try a different approach. The process of experimentation can be as important as the new techniques you discover or invent. Every time you work on modifying your technique, you will develop greater awareness of your capabilities and limitations. After a while, you will know your body and how it responds to your work so thoroughly that adapting your techniques to lower your injury risk will become second nature.

---

1. Tarek M. Khalil, Elsayed M. Abdel-Moty, Renee S. Rosomoff and Hubert L. Rosomoff, Ergonomics in *Back Pain: A Guide to Prevention and Rehabilitation* (New York: Van Nostrand Reinhold, 1993; 217).

7

Looking at Your Emotions and Your Work

Your emotions play an important role in the way you approach your work. Feelings, attitudes and beliefs about your clients and your professional life or work environment can affect you in a positive way or a negative way. They can either reinforce or undermine your ability to integrate principles of ergonomics, good body mechanics, and technique modification into your daily work life. If that happens, you can find yourself making choices or putting yourself in situations that can increase your risk of injury.

It is very important to recognize negative or counterproductive feelings, attitudes and beliefs that may come up for you when you are with clients. Becoming aware of the role your emotions play in your work will allow you to lessen their impact on your ability to protect yourself from work-related injury.

Manual treatment work, like all healthcare professions, brings with it a number of emotional challenges for the practitioner. Some of these are specific to the nature of the work, and others are common issues that many workers experience and which can increase the anxiety and distress that are risk factors for injury. Whether you identify with the following examples, or experience different emotional issues in your work than these, this discussion will hopefully get you thinking about how your emotions influence your work in ways that could contribute to your risk of injury on the job.

Difficulty Setting Limits with Clients

Most people find that setting boundaries with others is challenging. For manual therapists, whose work involves helping people who are often in pain and feeling needy, it can be particularly difficult to set limits with clients. Practitioners who are just starting out are particularly vulnerable. They may not have the confidence yet as professionals to feel justified setting limits, nor the experience to know how to do it gracefully. They may hesitate to limit the types of work they will and won't do, or possibly turn clients away, for fear of losing income or damaging their reputation.

At some point, all health professionals are faced with clients who have needs or demands that the practitioner cannot, and should not, try to meet. You may have a client who needs or requests numerous sessions of very intensive manual therapy that you would find too physically stressful. You may be asked to work with a disabled client who requires a considerable amount of assistance getting on and off the treatment table, which would increase your risk of back or shoulder injury. A client who is particularly large or has very developed or hypertonic muscles may demand very deep work that you do not feel capable of providing.

If you come in contact with these clients, you may feel compelled to comply with their demands. It is normal to want to please your clients. You likely decided to enter your profession because you have a real desire to help your clients and make them feel better. The fact that they are paying you for their treatment creates additional pressure. For all of these reasons, you can end up feeling obliged to provide the treatment these clients request, even if it places your own body at risk of injury.

A good number of these clients or patients don't realize that there are other ways to achieve the same results. Some clients who say they want deep work would in fact not benefit at a particular time from deep tissue treatment or heavy manipulation. Take the time to do a thorough intake with them, to get a full picture of why they are experiencing the symptoms they came to you to treat. You may need to educate your client on other approaches to their treatment. For example, sometimes it's more beneficial to point out things they may be doing (e.g., lifting heavy objects, using poor ergonomics at work) that could be contributing to their symptoms. Changing those factors could alleviate their discomfort or pain. Inform them that this is a part of your job as much as the manual work you do and can be quite beneficial to them. Or you may want to point out to them that the type of work they're asking for would not have the effect they're hoping for at this time in their injury or recovery, and lighter work would be more beneficial.

If you need to, there is nothing wrong with referring these clients to other healthcare practitioners. Not only will you be saving your own body so you can continue to treat those clients you are able to help, you will also be ensuring that the clients you refer out get the treatment they need. It may be helpful to network with practitioners of different healthcare professions in your area, or those who do different modalities than you do, so you feel comfortable making referrals to them. While you may be giving up the occasional client, if you build the right referral network, you should get plenty of new clients in return.

It is contrary to the therapeutic process to hurt oneself in order to help someone else.

Another option is to politely say "no" to the type of treatment you do not want to give, for whatever reason, and offer an alternative that you feel will be just as effective. For example, some of your clients may be under the impression that deep, intensive techniques are the only truly effective kind of treatment. Why not educate them about the value of other treatments that involve lighter touch or movement to accomplish the same treatment goals? They may be more open to change and experimentation than you think, and will appreciate your expertise and guidance.

Don't fall into the trap of fearing that your clients will never come back to you if you refuse to do that certain technique they always ask for, but that you feel is unsafe for you to do. Having a strong sense of personal boundaries and limits is healthy in any relationship, and an important element of professionalism. It is contrary to the therapeutic process to hurt oneself in order to help someone else. Doing so will set up a kind of martyr dynamic between you and your client that will ultimately make both of you uncomfortable. Realize that your clients do not come to you because you do that one technique with your thumb that they just love. Most clients use a number of different criteria to choose a manual therapist; the particular manual techniques the therapist uses is just one of those criteria. You are more than the sum total of all your techniques. Your clients come to you because you are YOU, because you are professional and competent, and because they are comfortable with you and trust you. Being clear, firm and consistent about your personal and professional limits will help deepen that trust. A client who does not respond to that level of honesty and integrity probably would be better off with a different therapist.

Inflexibility about Treatment Methods

You can end up creating extra work and physical stress for yourself by making assumptions about the kind of treatment your clients want. You may assume that your client wants deep work or extensive treatment when all the client really wants is a relaxation massage, some assisted stretching, or some help with their exercises. Simply checking in with your clients and asking them what they want and don't want eliminates the guesswork that can needlessly overload you during your sessions.

On the flip side, you may be the one who believes that deep, intensive or extensive work is necessary in every session. You may have fallen into a routine of treating all your clients in this manner, even though this kind of work is not appropriate for all clients. It is important to assess each client's needs individually and treat them accordingly. Certainly, if you specialize in a particular form of deep bodywork, then it is certain that your clients come to you for that modality. But for many practitioners, it is better to learn several ways to address any one condition, including some that are easier on your body. Lighter, more general massage can be more effective in treating some kinds of pain syndromes or injuries than more specific or deeper techniques. Other times, your client may benefit as much from a discussion of aggravating factors in their work and home life and how to reduce or eliminate them than from any hands-on treatment you can offer. Remember to remain responsive to the client and try to discover and understand what they really want and need.

Unrealistic Expectations of Yourself

For some manual practitioners, the title of "therapist" brings to mind an image of someone who is perfect, never makes mistakes, and can fix all problems. The title and the image that goes with it can be burdensome to these practitioners. The pressure of living up to this ideal can make them self-conscious, self-doubting and self-critical. When they bring the stress and tension of this attitude to their work, they can lose the objectivity and flexibility necessary to remain self-aware and protect their own health.

Unreasonable expectations can lead to a fear of not doing their work the "right way." This fear can make new students or graduates feel that they must incorporate every technique they have learned into their work, even those that both the practitioner and the client find uncomfortable or painful. They may feel that this is the right way to work, and any other way is wrong. Manual therapists who are anxious about being wrong and overly concerned about doing a good job tend to exhaust themselves in every treatment session, trying to give every client the best treatment of their life. These therapists often have difficulty keeping to a schedule and finishing their treatment sessions on time. This anxiety often causes static tension in the therapist's own muscles, a risk factor for injury. In addition to increasing their risk of injury, their perfectionism also stifles their creativity, preventing them from growing in their profession and finding pleasure in their work.

There really is no one right way of doing your work. There are many ways to go about treating any condition, and many modalities and techniques can be used to reach the same treatment goal. What you learn in school is a good basis from which to develop your own approach to your work. Throughout your career, you will need to experiment and find the techniques you like best, adapt others as needed, and abandon any that don't suit you or cause you discomfort or pain. With more realistic expectations of yourself, you will be able stop doing any techniques that overstress or hurt your body.

Some manual practitioners also come to view themselves as "healers," a perception that can be reinforced by teachers or fellow practitioners, and then by clients who look to them for help. In reality, your clients heal themselves, and you can only help facilitate that healing process. If you begin to believe that you are responsible for your clients' healing, you run the risk of becoming more of a caretaker than a care provider. This attitude can create an unhealthy relationship between you and your clients. Your clients are responsible for their own well-being; you need to avoid taking on that responsibility so you can be free to take on the one that does belong to you—your own well-being.

Therapists, whether manual or psychological, are only human beings. There are limits to what you can do for your clients, no matter how perfect you try to be. It really is enough to do what you can for them, and let them take the rest of the responsibility. Accepting the limitations of what you can do for others is another part of the awareness and mindset that can keep you from getting injured.

Dropping unreasonable expectations of yourself will allow you to relax and regain some perspective on your work. You will be better able to accept the information and suggestions in this book and let them become part of the way you live and work. You will become more flexible and more willing to try different ways of working that may be more comfortable for you and ultimately allow you to protect your own health. As you develop your own individual style of working, you will be better able to set yourself apart from other practitioners and attract the type of clients who will benefit from the type of treatment you provide.

It's also vitally important to schedule time off from work in your weekly, monthly and yearly schedule. In a physically demanding profession like yours, time off not only gives your body a break from the stress of your work. It also gives you time to mentally and emotionally recharge and gain valuable perspective on your career. If you truly go easy on yourself during your time off, you'll come back to your work feeling refreshed and ready to treat yourself as well as you treat your clients.

Inaccurate Beliefs about Work-Related Pain and Injury

Manual therapists have traditionally suffered silently with pain and injury. Some practitioners may be convinced that this suffering is a normal part of their profession and must simply be tolerated. If you are not as stoic as they are, they may have a hard time understanding why you are "making such a big deal" about being in pain. Unfortunately, there can be a certain pride and feeling of superiority among practitioners who have not been injured, and that can cause others who are injured to feel ashamed or "less than." They may look down on those who complain as "wimps" or "amateurs." If these practitioners are teachers, they pass this unhealthy attitude on to their students. If you work for an employer, you may also fear that the employer does not want to know that you're in pain and may suspend or fire you if you become injured.

This can become a vicious circle. You're afraid your employer will let you go if you are injured, so you continue to work despite your pain. In time, your symptoms turn into a full-fledged injury that ultimately interrupts your job. If pain or discomfort arise, use the information in this book to see if adjusting your technique, posture, or work schedule helps.

If that doesn't work, speak with your employer. A smart employer will want to work with you to find a solution that works for both of you: perhaps a shorter schedule for a few weeks, or taking some time off to see a doctor and get a treatment plan.

If your employer is indifferent or annoyed, it may be a sign that you're not going to be able to properly safeguard your health with this employer. In that case, it may be best to part ways amicably. Attitudes about potential injury and how a prospective employer deals with it may be wise to ask about in your job interview. It is certainly a good way to judge whether this workplace supports their employees' health or not, and that may affect your feelings about taking this job or not.

We now know that the old "no pain, no gain" attitude is counterproductive. New or acute pain should not be thought of as a normal by-product of your work as a manual therapist. If pain is severe and/or lasts more than a week or two, it should not be ignored. It would be a mistake to think that you can just "work through the pain" and everything will be alright. It is wiser to see a healthcare professional to figure out why the pain is occurring and make the changes necessary to resolve it, or start developing a treatment plan together. One can only wonder how many of those practitioners who learned to live with pain ended up having to stop working because of injury.

Listen to and trust your instincts. When that voice in your head says something isn't right, it is important to pay attention to it. With increased awareness, you will start to hear and heed that voice early on, while there is still plenty of time to keep pain from turning into chronic injury.

8

Special Considerations and Tips

In previous chapters, you learned about injury prevention issues and considerations that are common to all manual therapists. There are also specific challenges and vulnerabilities that practitioners in certain sectors of the manual therapist population face. These challenges can occur at different stages of a practitioner's life or career, in certain work situations, as a result of their gender, or due to any number of other circumstances or characteristics too numerous to mention here. You may belong to one or several of the following sectors of the manual therapist community. The tips and suggestions provided here will help you avoid the risks associated with the particular circumstances you face in your life as a manual therapist.

Students

School is an exciting time, but it is also a time when musculoskeletal issues can arise. Students are constantly faced with new physical and intellectual challenges. They are usually anxious to do their best, and in a hurry to become professionals. When students are first learning techniques, they tend to use less than optimal body mechanics and more effort than is necessary. Reconciling school time constraints with stress outside of school can cause a great deal of pressure and anxiety. As a result of all of these factors, school is a place where people can get injured.

It is common for students in physically demanding professions to experience injury during their training. In sports, overtraining injuries are common among young athletes, and in music, where schooling involves a great deal of practice as well as performance, injury is quite common. Several studies have shown a significant rate of injury in training programs for manual therapists. The Canadian study (cited in Chapter 1) indicated that inexperienced massage therapists (those in their first five years on the job), like inexperienced workers in all industries, report a higher rate of injury than those with more experience. An Australian study revealed an increasing prevalence of low back pain among PT students in their second, third and fourth years of schooling.[1] The survey found that close to two-thirds of the students had experienced low back pain within the previous year. The findings of these studies indicate that inexperience in performing physically demanding work is an additional risk factor for injury among students. The authors' personal experiences as students, as well as observing students while teaching workshops at schools, provide additional anecdotal evidence that students in the manual healthcare professions have an increased risk of developing symptoms and injury during their training. Schools that train manual therapists obviously agree, since an increasing number of them now teach injury prevention courses for their students (some of them using *Save Your Hands!* as a textbook). These schools are dedicated to protecting their students from injury from the start, while they are still in training.

Paying attention to injury prevention from the very beginning of your training will get you into good habits that can keep you healthy throughout your career. Here are some suggestions and tips to start applying now if you are already a student, or if you are getting ready to start a training program:

- **Get in shape:** Make sure you are in good overall physical condition before you begin your training. If you are already in school, start getting into shape now. See Chapter 11 for a conditioning program designed specifically for manual therapists, including special tips for students and prospective students. Be honest with yourself about your physical abilities, and set your goals accordingly. Build strength and endurance in the muscles you will use most in your work by gradually increasing the amount of exercise you do with those muscles.

- **Don't start school when you are injured:** It is best to be free of acute or subacute musculoskeletal injury at the time you begin your training. Even low-level, chronic conditions can flare up under the unfamiliar stress of learning hands-on techniques. If you are experiencing musculoskeletal pain or injury, see an appropriate healthcare provider as soon as possible and make sure you start treating the problem. Wait to begin school until your injury has healed and your symptoms have subsided.

- **Reduce stress outside of school:** When you are in school, your body has to adapt to new physical challenges, and your mind to the pressures and challenges of dealing with new situations and new information. To prepare yourself for these challenges, try to resolve or postpone any stressful or difficult situations in your personal life. Since the physical and emotional stress of going to school is already a risk factor for injury, adding any other stress to it will increase your chances of becoming injured.

- **Pay attention to symptoms:** Students can think that early symptoms like muscle fatigue, discomfort and pain are normal parts of their training that they can work through. They may not have the information or experience to recognize the warning signs of injury. Be sure to read Part Three of this book for important information on injury physiology and symptoms of injury, so you can recognize and take action on any symptoms that may occur while you are in school.

- **Build work endurance slowly:** Gradually increase the number of practice treatment sessions you do during your training.

Don't get too enthusiastic and carried away when you are first in school and try to work on everyone you know. Allow the endurance and strength to develop gradually as you practice new techniques. Learn to pace yourself, so you don't exhaust yourself in every session.

- **Avoid taking on additional hand-intensive work:** If you are doing a good deal of hands-on practice as part of your training, avoid also taking on multiple hands-on continuing education workshops or volunteering at sporting events. The combination of a sudden increase in work hours and learning new techniques can bring on symptoms. At home, don't spend your weekends doing hand-intensive chores around the house. If you do participate in additional manual work, plan on taking it easy in your school-related manual workload the following week, and be on the lookout for any symptoms that may indicate that you have overstressed your body.

- **Ask for feedback on techniques:** It is common for students to use poor body mechanics or too much force as they learn the manual techniques they will use in their careers. Don't hesitate to ask your instructors to comment on your technique and help you make the necessary adjustments.

- **Be flexible about techniques:** If you start experimenting early on with different ways of doing the same treatment, you will more quickly develop the flexibility that will help keep you healthy throughout your career. If you are learning a technique that is done with a flat palm, try it also with your knuckles or forearm. If the technique is taught with the client prone, try it with the client lying on their side. If you are unsure about an alternative technique, ask your instructor for advice. The first time you learn a new technique is also the best time to practice doing the technique with either hand. Since the new technique probably feels a little awkward to you anyway, it may not seem awkward when you perform it with your non-dominant hand.

- **Create an optimal work environment:** Follow good ergonomic guidelines in setting up your workspace, as discussed in Chapter 4. While you are a student, it is particularly important that your workspace fits you properly. If your student clinic or classroom workspace is not set up to allow you to work safely, speak with your instructor and work with them to modify it so you and your fellow students can adequately protect yourselves from injury. School is the best time to develop good body mechanics, and it will be difficult to do so if your workspace does not fit you well.

- **Develop Your Self-Awareness and Self-Care Mindset.** It's never too early to develop a proactive self-care mindset about how you will safeguard your health in the context of your work. You know after reading this far that a large number of manual therapists become injured as a result of their work. Take the recommendations here to heart from the beginning, and start incorporating them into your work. It's much easier to start out on the right foot than to wait to get injured before you make the necessary changes to have a long, healthy career. Developing self-awareness is a vital part of staying healthy. From the first treatments you give, keep your own comfort and ease in mind instead of only concentrating on your client or patient. You can take better care of them if you're taking care of yourself. Check in with yourself every day before you start work to ensure that your mindset is clear and focused on your self-care. Even better, check in with yourself before each treatment. Make a plan for how you'll react if you're starting to feel tired, or uncomfortable, or tense. The more awareness you can have from the very beginning, the less likely it will be that you become injured as a result of your work. See Appendix C for more information and techniques to help you develop greater awareness and a healthy self-care mindset.

- **Don't give in to peer pressure:** If you are experiencing pain or discomfort doing techniques that others are comfortable doing, you may be afraid to say anything for fear that the other students will put you down. Competitive feelings can run high among students, and other students may make you feel inadequate or imply that you cannot keep up with them. While in the short term, saying nothing may spare you the potential criticism of your fellow students; in the long term, it can get you injured. Your health is much more important than proving something to others. Tune them out, and do whatever is necessary to protect yourself from injury.

- **Be communicative with instructors and administrators:** It is very important to speak up and let your instructors know if you feel any discomfort or pain during your training. Your instructors cannot help you unless they know that something is wrong. Remember that there is no shame in admitting you're having some difficulty. It's perfectly normal to need some extra help at times, particularly while you're a student. Alert your teachers when you first start feeling symptoms, and discuss with them the steps you need to take to keep your symptoms from turning into an injury. Your instructors should help you find alternate ways of working that will be more comfortable for you, and, if necessary, refer you to an appropriate healthcare professional for evaluation. In the unlikely event that an instructor is not receptive to your needs, you can always ask another instructor or a school administrator to intervene and address your concerns.

Remember that the ultimate responsibility for your health rests with you. You must be your own advocate while you are in school. Have the courage to do whatever it takes to stay healthy, even if that means taking some time off from school if you need to. Interrupting your schooling may be upsetting and frustrating, but it is better than developing an injury that can shorten, limit or end your career. It is usually possible to negotiate some time off from school that will enable you to heal, and then pick up where you left off. Injuries that start in school can continue and worsen as you progress through your training, and after graduation with the demands of professional employment. Protect your investment in your training, your new career, and your quality of life by dealing with injury swiftly, responsibly, and completely.

School administrators and instructors can help students protect themselves from injury by following a number of guidelines and instituting some simple practices in their programs. Massage schools will find recommendations for methods to reduce the risk of students developing MSDs in Appendix D.

New Professional Practitioners

Studies have shown that the most injuries happen in the first five years of practice.[2] It takes time to develop mastery and ease in the very physically demanding work you do. New practitioners are very susceptible to comparing themselves and competing with colleagues, and to meeting the demands of employers. These pressures can reduce their self-awareness and cause them to push themselves beyond the limits of their physical abilities.

New practitioners need to have a heightened awareness of injury risk and be particularly on the lookout for the very beginning of any symptoms that may arise. They also need to be very communicative with employers about scheduling and the types of techniques they may need further training to master.

Make sure you have support from a group of fellow therapists and hopefully a mentor who can help you surmount the demands that come with starting a career. Ideally, you would start out with just a few clients at first (whether you are self-employed or work for someone else) and slowly work your way into a busier schedule. Many of the recommendations for students are applicable to new practitioners as well, so be sure to carefully read that section, above.

Chair and On-site Massage

As you saw in the discussion of body mechanics in Chapter 5, practitioners who do chair massage can end up working in awkward postures such as bending at the wrist or back, kneeling and squatting. You will be more likely to get into awkward postures if you spend a significant amount of time treating the client's lower body. Since on-site massage sessions tend to be brief (15 to 30 minutes), massage therapists may feel that they can schedule many more sessions in a day than they would if they were doing hour-long sessions. Bear in mind, though, that encountering risk factors like repetitive motions or awkward postures without adequate recovery time is still a concern, even for brief sessions. Scheduling numerous brief sessions in your workday will increase your injury risk, particularly if you do not leave much time between the sessions.

Use these tips to help address the following postural and scheduling issues:

- Limit the length of seated massage sessions to 30 minutes or less; longer sessions should be done with the client on a table or mat.
- Avoid the temptation to schedule even 15-minute sessions one after another. Leave adequate recovery time, at least 10 minutes, between sessions, and take longer breaks every couple of hours to sit, stretch, eat and hydrate.
- Instead of using your flat palm to apply compression, use your knuckles, loose fists, forearms and elbows, to avoid wrist bending.
- Change your posture and position frequently as you work; try sitting on a low stool to help you minimize time spent bending at the waist, kneeling and squatting.
- Use kneeling pads to avoid some of the compression on your knees that can come from kneeling on hard surfaces.

If you use your massage chair or table for on-site massage, take a look at these tips for massage therapists who have a mobile practice:

- Buy the lightest table or massage chair you can find.
- Use a cart or wheeled carrying case for transporting the table or chair. If you prefer to use a carry strap, realize that you'll be carrying most of the weight of the table or chair on one side of your body. At the least, place the strap across your body to spread out the weight. See if you can get a second strap to put across your body and on the opposite shoulder, to balance out the weight.

- Consider the type of vehicle you drive to clients' homes. Look for one that gives you good access to the table or chair without having to reach or bend to lift it out of a trunk or cargo space.

- Check out the path to the client's home and the area where you will be setting up your table before carrying it in, to make sure there are no obstacles or impediments that could make the lifting and carrying awkward or more difficult.

- Avoid being put in a position where you are expected to help the client move heavy furniture to make room for your table. When you schedule appointments, give clients guidelines for the amount of working space you will need, so they can find an appropriate space for you to work in their home or office. Inform them that you cannot help them move furniture or heavy objects. If they still ask you to help move things, be firm and remind them this is not part of the service you provide, as you explained in advance, and they will have to find someone else to help them.

A Note to Massage Therapists

There are so many different types of treatments and modalities that fall under the larger heading of massage therapy and bodywork that it would be impossible to address them all here. These include treatments that do not involve using the hands with any pressure at all, like breathwork and Reiki, or small amounts of pressure like lymphatic drainage.

However, nearly all of these modalities include some risk factors. A reflexologist who works only on the feet still needs to maintain near-neutral postures and be aware of risk factors to their upper extremity, neck and back. If you use only your feet and legs to do massage, like Ashiatsu massage, you'll need excellent balance and strength in your core, legs and feet to prevent injury. These therapists also tend to look down at their clients most of the time and can develop neck injuries as a result of that static loading. Unless you do not touch the client at all (for example, when doing some types of breathwork with them), you must stay aware of your body mechanics, the ergonomics of the treatment space, getting into awkward postures and other risk factors.

Spa Practitioners

An increasing number of massage therapists are now working in spas. In fact, spas are now one of the biggest employers of massage therapists in the United States. The spa environment presents special challenges and considerations for practitioners, including working on wet floors, lifting heavy linens, and performing highly focused treatments such as facial massage. While some treatments such as body wraps may not require much forceful exertion or repetitive motions, spas may expect practitioners to follow set protocols, so practitioners may have less control over the work they do. Treatment tables designed for lighter spa work may not adjust low enough for deep tissue work, even though this kind of work may be offered as an option for clients.

Therapists working in a spa, as well as estheticians who do some massage with clients, face the challenge of sharing the responsibility for safe work practices with the spa's management. The management is primarily responsible for ergonomic changes to the physical workspace, equipment, scheduling and breaks; practitioners are responsible for adjusting treatment tables when necessary, using good body mechanics, and communicating concerns promptly with management. The following information is intended to help both parties deal with these issues:

- Practitioners and spa managers should work together to review the physical layout of treatment rooms and equipment, and to establish schedules that balance the workload among the practitioners. While some practitioners may be particularly proficient with certain techniques, over-specialization often leads to overuse. At the same time, some practitioners may not be adequately trained or conditioned for deep tissue work, and doing too much of this work would greatly increase their injury risk.

- Using a variety of motions is one of the better ways to prevent musculoskeletal disorders, and providing that variety is more easily accomplished in spas that offer a number of different services. Treatments such as body wraps or hot stone therapy can be fairly easy on the practitioner's hands compared to deep tissue massage, for example. Massage done on the client while they are wrapped is typically light in pressure, which is appropriate to this type of treatment. Some of this massage can be done while seated to provide a short break from standing.

- Lifting is one of the most frequent causes of injury in any profession. Large or heavy pieces of equipment, stones for hot stone massage, and bundles of wet linens should not be placed on the floor or in a high location where awkward lifting postures could increase the likelihood of back and shoulder injury. Place heavy objects at mid-thigh to waist level, where they can be lifted close to the body in an upright posture, or, better yet, slid onto a rolling cart and wheeled to their destination.

- Bending over for long periods of time is another frequent cause of low back injury. Performing hydrotub treatments, for example, often requires the spa practitioner to bend over to actively participate in the treatment, either by using a hydro wand or performing manual massage as the client soaks. Depending on the design of the hydrotub, the practitioner may do a considerable amount of bending and twisting at the waist. Minimizing time spent in any one posture, or spending some of the time sitting, squatting or kneeling on a folded towel or a cushion can help in this situation (with mats on the floor, see next bulleted point). Placing one hand on the edge of the tub to hold some of the weight of the upper body, or placing a folded towel against the side of the tub to use as a chest support may also help to reduce stress on the therapist's lower back when leaning forward. In any situation that involves water, be particularly careful about the possibility of slipping and falling. Speak to your manager if you feel that the floor is too slippery or there are trip hazards, in which case adjustments should be made to ensure your safety.

Appendix E provides recommendations to help spas reduce injury risk for massage therapists working at their facilities.

- Floor mats can benefit the practitioner by reducing fatigue from standing on hard surfaces, and by helping to prevent slips due to wet floors. A good mat will be at least half an inch thick, and allow some give without making you feel like you are "sinking in." Tiled mats, each about one foot (30 cm) square, are lighter in weight than full size mats, which makes them easier to move for cleaning. Beveled edges on mats help prevent tripping, and can make it easier for carts or other wheeled objects to move over them. Avoid mats with an overly-aggressive tread pattern, as the treads can grip the soles of the therapist's shoes and make it difficult to reposition their feet. Massage therapists even outside of the spa environment can benefit from having good mats alongside their tables, to ease the stress of standing.

- If mats are not feasible, impact-absorbing shoe insoles are the next best thing. Wearable outsoles that provide cushioning similar to anti-fatigue mats are also available. Footwear should also include a good EVA (ethylene vinyl acetate) or similar midsole to provide cushioning, and should have a non-slip sole. In fact, any manual therapist in any setting should wear supportive footwear.

Older Practitioners

Many manual therapists continue to work well into their 50s, 60s and even beyond. In earlier generations, it was generally accepted that aging brought with it an inevitable decline in physical capacity. While some amount of decline does occur, we now realize that it is possible to maintain a good level of physical condition by staying active and exercising regularly. Manual therapists who are still practicing past middle age have typically arrived at that stage because they have learned to work in ways that place less stress on their bodies. As a result, they tend to get injured less frequently than their younger, less experienced colleagues. However, older practitioners generally do not heal as quickly, so it is important for older therapists to be even more aware of symptoms and even more cautious and quick to seek treatment so they can avoid full-blown or chronic injury. It is also wise for younger practitioners to start preparing now for the physical changes that occur later in life.

Good habits and good planning for the future can keep you healthy throughout a long career. Here are some to tips to consider:

- Plan ahead for the decrease in strength, flexibility, balance and work capacity that usually comes with age. Learn modalities that are less stressful on your body, and that take advantage of your years of experience.

- Include weight-bearing exercise in your conditioning program to maintain muscle strength and slow the possible loss of bone density.

- Balance tends to become less steady with age, so avoid any techniques that involve reaching out without support. Be particularly careful to keep your weight centered over your feet as much as possible. Do exercises to work on your balance, and do them in a safe environment so you don't fall.

- Cartilage tends to thin with age, so limit the amount of time you spend leaning in with your body weight, which places a good deal of pressure on your IP joints, wrists and other upper-extremity joints and can lead to osteoarthritis.

- Connective tissue loses elasticity with age, so you may not be able to do some of the techniques that were easier when you were more flexible. Be prepared to walk around the table more and work closer to your neutral posture.

- With the decrease in muscle mass that is common as we age, your maximum strength will also decline, so the effort you put into any of your techniques should be reduced accordingly. Usually, the decline in strength will be very gradual, so you should be able to adjust your work methods gradually as well.

- Put a savings plan into effect that will allow you to gradually scale down your practice and reduce the number of treatment sessions you do per day as you near retirement.

- Know when it's time to "fold up your table" for good and enjoy your retirement.

On the positive side, with age comes experience. You have most likely learned many ways to work with clients, so you have more skills to bring to your treatment sessions.

There is no specific age at which a manual therapist should retire. Listen to your body and your heart, but remember that you want to spend your time relaxing and enjoying life when you retire, not recovering from a chronic musculoskeletal injury.

Female Practitioners

Some studies have shown a higher rate of MSDs among women than men. While female manual therapists share the same injury concerns as male manual therapists, they have a few additional challenges due to their gender:

Pregnancy: During pregnancy, women may have temporary symptoms of carpal tunnel syndrome, since the increase in hormone levels can cause fluid retention and edema in the wrists.[2] The symptoms can very often be corrected by wearing wrist splints at night, and they typically resolve completely following birth. If repetitive motions and wrist bending while pregnant aggravate these symptoms, these temporary CTS symptoms can become more long lasting. For this reason, pregnant women need to exercise caution and not overuse their hands and wrists during this time. Low back pain is also common in pregnancy, and is likely due to a combination of additional stress on the musculoskeletal system from weight gain and joint laxity caused by an increased secretion of hormones.[3]

Other hormonal changes: Women who have hormonal changes due to gynecological surgery or oral contraceptive use also tend to report higher levels of MSDs. Peri- and post-menopausal women seem to be particularly at risk for MSDs.

Strength: Women generally have about two-thirds the strength that men do. This lower level of strength is not necessarily a risk factor, as long as female practitioners take advantage of the strength of the rest of their bodies to do their work.

Women may also have certain physical advantages over men. They generally have a lower center of gravity, which gives them better balance. For women, leaning over can be less of a strain on the lower back because they generally have less upper body weight to support. Women are generally smaller and shorter than men, which has several benefits. Smaller hands allow women to apply more concentrated pressure requiring less force than a person with a larger hand would tend to apply. Shorter limbs can mean more reaching, but with shorter lever arms, that reaching will generate less stress on the shoulders.

Working During Pregnancy

If you continue to work during your pregnancy, keep these tips in mind:

- As your belly grows, it will push you further away from the table and keep you from using good body mechanics. Position your clients so they are closer to you as you work, and experiment with different client positions that allow you to keep reaching to a minimum.

- If you find that your belly truly prevents you from using good body mechanics, it may be time to take a break from work until after the baby is born.

- Many women start to develop low back pain during pregnancy, particularly during the final months when the weight of the belly pulls them forward. Sitting more of the time that you are working can help alleviate pressure and pain on the lower back, and the fatigue that can come from standing for long periods while carrying this extra weight.[4]

- To avoid additional strain on your already overtaxed back, avoid any movements or activities that could increase stress on the lower back, like lifting, bending or twisting.

- If you start experiencing symptoms of carpal tunnel syndrome, ease up on any repetitive motions you do with your hands and be particularly vigilant about keeping your wrists straight as you work. Wearing wrist splints at night may reduce symptoms. Talk to your physician or obstetrician about your work and follow their advice, particularly if you begin to develop symptoms. See Chapter 14 for more details on CTS symptoms.

- Be careful as you return to work after taking time off. Women are still often largely responsible for taking care of children and the home, so balancing those physically demanding activities with your work should be taken into consideration. If this is your first child, or you are adding to a growing family, the additional responsibilities and physical demands of childcare can combine with the physical demands of your work on your body and increase your overall risk of injury.

- Staying active is important during pregnancy, but be aware that your changing body makes the ergonomics and body mechanics issues involved in your work even more complex.

Male Practitioners

In general, men tend to be stronger than women, but don't let that fool you into thinking they can't get injured. Overall conditioning, including endurance and flexibility, are more important than strength alone in determining your risk of injury. While studies show that men are less likely to have MSDs than women, they are nearly as likely to have low back injuries as women are. Men generally have greater grip strength, so they are more likely to have injuries at the base of the thumb, possibly from overusing their strength. To avoid injury, keep these principles in mind:

- **Don't rely on upper body strength alone:** If you are very strong, your muscles may not be in danger of injury, but your joints, ligaments and tendons are still vulnerable. It is just as important for men to use their entire body to generate force as it is for women.

▪ **Avoid leaning over without support:** A large proportion of a man's weight is in his upper body, which is one of the reasons that taller men are prone to back injury. Whenever you lean forward without supporting yourself by putting a hand down, the muscles in your lower back have to hold up a great deal of your weight.

▪ **Don't get stuck with all the deep work:** There is a common misconception that male practitioners are best suited to doing deep tissue or sports massage work, because of their size and strength. Clients may come to you looking for deep work with a lot of pressure, and other manual therapists may refer clients in need of intensive work to you. Either way, you may find yourself being assigned more deep tissue or sports massage work than your female counterparts. Be aware that the high forces required to do deep tissue work may increase your risk of injury. Be careful to limit the number of deep tissue sessions you schedule in a day or week. Give yourself plenty of time to recover from a difficult session, as it can take up to 48 hours for muscles and tendons to heal after a significant exertion.

▪ **Be careful with off-work labor:** As a man, you may also be asked to do more of the heavy physical labor around the house, or at a second job. Heavy lifting, gripping and repetitive motions from using hand tools, and vibration from power tools, are just some of the risk factors that you can be exposed to at home. Be as careful about overloading yourself in your off-work time as you are during your workday.

1. Leah J. Nyland and Karen A. Grimmer, Is Undergraduate Physiotherapy Study a Risk Factor for Low Back Pain? A Prevalence Study of LBP in Physiotherapy Students, *BMC Musculoskeletal Disorders*, 4:22 doi:10.1186/1471-2474-4-22, 2003.
2. Mary Beth Braun and Stephanie J. Simonson, *Introduction to Massage Therapy* (Philadelphia: Lippincott Williams & Wilkins, 2007; 26).
3. Andrus J. Voitk, John C. Mueller, Diane E. Farlinger and Richard U. Johnston, "Carpal tunnel syndrome in pregnancy," *Canadian Medical Association Journal*, 1983; 128(3): 277–281.
4. Darryl B. Sneag and John A. Bendo, "Pregnancy-related Low Back Pain," *Orthopedics*, 2007; 30: 839.

9

Injury Prevention Outside of Work

Everything you have read so far in this book about your work—ergonomics, body mechanics, overall awareness—is equally applicable to your life outside of work. Many aspects of your day-to-day life affect your ability to prevent injury. You use your upper extremities almost constantly every day. Even in your sleep, the position in which you hold your hands and arms can contribute to injury. You may subject your shoulders and back to the insults of lifting and bending as much at home as you do at work. To stay healthy, you must try to incorporate injury awareness into all areas of your life.

This task is actually easier than it sounds. Once you become more aware of injury risk factors and prevention methods, you will find that this consciousness becomes an integral part of the way you live your life. You will begin to notice potentially harmful activities that you used to do without thinking, and start adapting them (or avoiding them) to be easier on your body.

Protecting Your Hands Every Day

There is an old story about a famous violinist who was so protective of his hands that he never used them in his daily life. Other people fed him, opened doors for him, and chauffeured him, all to save his precious hands and fingers for the more important work of playing the violin. Of course, never using your hands is a rather extreme and impractical method of injury prevention. Most manual therapists have no choice but to use their hands and arms in their daily lives in addition to their work. But it is possible to pay more attention to the way you use your hands to reduce or eliminate some everyday stresses that could increase your chance of injury. Reducing the amount of manual labor you do outside of work and avoiding using your hands in an unnecessarily stressful manner can greatly reduce your risk of developing an MSD.

In fact, the violinist was not completely wrong in his approach to injury prevention. It is reasonable to ask others in your life to do some things for you that might be overly stressful to your hands. If you live with a spouse, roommate or family member, you can certainly ask them to occasionally open stuck jar tops or stiff faucets for you. Part of injury prevention is acknowledging your limitations as well as your strengths, and asking for help when necessary. The people you live with know that you need to save your hands for your work as much as possible, and will likely be happy to help out with small tasks that are easy for them but could be too stressful for you.

A number of day-to-day activities commonly done with the hands can be done with other parts of the body. For example, most people open even heavy doors with their hands. Unless a door has a knob that must be turned, you can push it open with your shoulder or your foot. You may be able to find electric devices to do some work that you currently do with your hands, such as electric can openers and power scrubbers. Stop using your bare hands to do tasks that could be done with a tool designed for that purpose. There are many tools now available to help make common but stressful household tasks, like opening cans or jars, easier on your hands. Many of these tools were designed for people with arthritis or other limitations to hand strength, but the tools also reduce stress to healthy hands. Turning, twisting or wrenching things open with your hands may prove how strong you are, but it is also unnecessary and potentially harmful. Place objects or tools you use often at waist level or a bit above, so you can avoid reaching for objects that are not easily accessible. If you must reach for something low down or high up, consider purchasing a long-handled reaching device, easy to find and inexpensive to buy online.

Carrying heavy objects can also be stressful to your arms and hands. Carrying a pot of cold water to the stove by its long handle can put a tremendous strain on the forearm of the person carrying it. Supporting some of the weight by placing the other hand underneath the pot at the same time will distribute the weight between the two arms. If the pot is cold, hold it as close to your body as you can, to allow you to use larger muscles to carry the weight. If the pot is hot, either use a potholder to support the bottom, or let it stay on the stove and empty the contents into a serving bowl or your plate. When you carry packages, distribute the weight between both arms. If your package has long enough handles, carry it on your forearm or your shoulder to avoid gripping the handles with your hands. These may seem like very small points, but the cumulative effect of this extra manual activity can be substantial.

Repetitive activities that cause sharp impact to the hands, like hammering nails and stapling papers, should be avoided or reduced as much as possible. Your hands are your livelihood; avoid anything that bangs, hits, pinches, vibrates or traumatizes them in any way. Choose your pastimes and hobbies carefully. Joining the bowling team, building furniture, or doing needlepoint may not be the best choices of pastimes for a manual practitioner. If you already participate in a hand-intensive pastime and really don't want to give it up, look for ways to apply the principles of ergonomics and body mechanics to your hobbies as you would to your work. Take frequent breaks and try to avoid doing those activities on days when you have had a particularly heavy schedule at work. Activities you do in your free time are a modifiable risk factor you can control, so do your best to optimize the circumstances under which you do these activities to lower the additional risk they represent.

Reducing Stress to Your Musculoskeletal System in Daily Activities

There are many ways to reduce possible causes of stress in all aspects of your daily life. Incorporating these tips can help you avoid additional exposure to risk factors on top of the physical demands of your work as a manual therapist.

Writing:

- Use pens with a larger diameter barrel and a cushioned grip.
- Use rollerball or gel ink pens that do not require as much downward pressure to write.
- Type into a computer instead of writing by hand.
- Avoid excessive cell phone texting, which has led to cases of "de Quervaine's Thumb" injury. Raise the phone up so you are not using it with your head bent down (remember that the head weighs as much as a bowling ball).

In the kitchen:

- Avoid lifting heavy frying pans or pots with one hand.
- Use electric can openers and a jar and bottle opener designed to reduce force and stress on the hand.
- Use an ulu knife (knife with handle directly over the blade), mandoline or food processor for chopping, or buy pre-chopped foods.
- Avoid carrying heavy bags of groceries—use a rolling cart instead.
- Buy products in smaller containers, or portion them out into smaller containers once you get them home, to avoid lifting heavy contents.
- Avoid working at counters that are too high or too low. If necessary, buy a kitchen work cart with a top surface that is a couple of inches below the height of your elbows.
- Use a paper towel instead of a sponge for clean up, to reduce wringing and squeezing motions. For the same reason, avoid using mops that must be wrung out manually.

Cleaning:

- Use long-handled cleaning tools to avoid bending, and padded, angled hand tools to reduce grip force and keep your wrists straight.
- Use furniture glides to more easily move furniture around the house.
- Try to push objects you need to move in your home, rather than pulling them, which is more stressful.
- Use lightweight or self-propelled vacuum cleaners.
- Lift only a small amount of laundry at a time, especially when transferring wet clothes from the washer to the dryer. Place the hamper on a chair to avoid bending over each time you pull clothes out. If a couple of articles of clothing are tangled in the washer, don't tug at them to free them. Pull out other items first to free some room to untangle them.
- Never wring out wet clothes with your hands. Roll them up in a dry towel instead.

Using tools:

- Wear anti-vibration gloves, and limit the amount of time you use vibrating power tools.
- Never use your hand as a hammer; use a rubber mallet instead.
- Use spring-loaded scissors with handles that can be gripped with the whole hand.
- Use pliers or locking pliers instead of your hands and fingers for anything that requires force.

Driving:

- Adjust your tilt steering wheel to allow you to keep your wrists straight.
- Don't hold your hands too high on the steering wheel, which may reduce circulation.
- Change hand positions frequently to help keep your grip loose.
- Keep your wheels balanced and aligned to avoid excessive vibration.
- Adjust the backrest so that you are reclining slightly on longer drives.
- Use a lumbar support if your current seats do not provide good lower back support.

General:

- Use a hands-free book holder or place books or laptops in your lap on a firm pillow to raise them closer to eye level, or on a table, so you don't need to bend your neck to read them.
- Avoid cradling a phone device between your shoulder and ear. Use a headset or speakerphone if possible, or hold the phone in one hand, high enough that you don't have to bend your neck more than 20 degrees, ideally, to look at it.
- Lift thin objects from underneath using your whole hand rather than with a pinch grip from above.
- Lift larger objects with both hands and hold them close to your body.
- Buy a hand truck (a two-wheeled dolly) and use it to move everything you can.
- Use a stable step stool to access higher shelves instead of reaching. Have someone with you to hand objects down to.
- Set up your computer workstation to allow you to work comfortably. See Appendix B for a detailed description of computer workstation ergonomics.

Protecting Your Joints

These tips have been developed to help people suffering from arthritis to avoid further pain or damage. Some of them are similar to the ergonomics tips for work and home that you have seen above, but they bear repeating from the point of view of protecting your joints. Following this advice as much as possible in your daily life, even while your joints are still healthy, can help prevent damage to joint cartilage that could lead to osteoarthritis.

- Avoid placing pressure on your bent fingers, for example, when leaning your chin on your fist or using your knuckles to push yourself out of a chair.
- Avoid holding small objects with a tight pinch grip. For example, type at a computer instead of writing with a pen or pencil (see Appendix B for computer workstation recommendations).

- Avoid motions of the hand into ulnar deviation, for example, when opening jars or faucets.
- Use assistive devices to make manual tasks easier, such as key holders that give you more leverage when turning a key, or extended door-knob turners.
- Use good body mechanics when lifting.
- Use both hands to carry objects, and grip them from underneath, or add handles.
- Lighten the load when carrying. Better yet, use a cart or hand truck.
- Use larger and stronger muscles to do the work whenever possible.
- Arrange your work and storage around the house to eliminate unnecessary bending and reaching.
- Avoid holding static positions for long periods of time, such as holding and squeezing the pump handle when pumping gas (use the handle lock to keep the gas pumping).
- Use good posture and lumbar support when seated.
- Stop performing any motion or activity immediately if you begin to feel pain.

10

Your General Health and Wellness

The musculoskeletal system works in concert with the other systems of the body. Whatever happens in the other body systems, whether positive or negative, will impact your musculoskeletal health. Recommendations like eating well, getting enough sleep, and avoiding unhealthy habits like smoking or excessive drinking are more than just good advice you get from your doctor. They can have a direct effect on your ability to withstand the rigors of your work and heal tissue damage before it progresses to the point of injury.

Eat Well

Your diet affects more than just your overall health. It can also have direct and indirect effects on your musculoskeletal system. A poor diet can slow down your body's ability to heal, and contribute to conditions like diabetes that are risk factors for MSDs. The good news is that certain foods can actually help you maintain good musculoskeletal health while also benefiting your overall health. A complete description of proper nutrition would take up a whole book by itself, but the following general guidelines are a good starting point for manual therapists:

Eat whole foods with minimal processing: There are good reasons that whole foods are widely recommended. Vitamins and minerals are best taken in from food sources, rather than from supplements, and whole foods have more of them. Foods in their natural state contain beneficial elements—antioxidants, vitamins, minerals and fiber—which balance out the oxidizing elements that can cause cell damage. In highly processed and modified foods, such as trans fats and high-fructose corn syrup, these beneficial elements have been stripped away. The oxidizing elements in processed foods can cause cell damage in connective tissues, joints and even the brain.

Replace pro-inflammatory foods with anti-inflammatory foods: Some foods, such as fried foods, can cause inflammation in the body tissues. In addition to avoiding processed or modified foods that can directly damage tissues, try to reduce or eliminate foods that can create an inflammatory response. Replacing these pro-inflammatory foods with their anti-inflammatory counterparts will be healthier for your musculoskeletal system, and for your entire body.

Eat to sustain energy and repair tissues: Eat every 3 to 4 hours during your workday to keep your energy level up and replace essential nutrients. Keep healthy snacks such as fruits, vegetables and nuts at work. Have your last meal about 3 to 4 hours before bedtime, and avoid unhealthy snacks at night, particularly those with a high glycemic index.

You also need to take in the nutrients necessary to help repair minor tissue damage. Make sure you eat enough protein from lean meats (poultry, seafood), eggs and non-animal sources (whole grains, beans, lentils, nuts, soy) to help repair muscle tissue. Eat foods rich in calcium and vitamin D to help strengthen bones, and other minerals such as magnesium and potassium to help maintain the electrolyte balance in muscles. Vitamin C is an important component in tissue repair, another good reason to eat lots of fresh fruits and vegetables.

Reduce your calorie count: The one lifestyle change that has been consistently shown to help people live longer, healthier lives has been caloric restriction. Eating fewer calories not only helps keep your weight at a healthy level, it also allows you to take in fewer potentially tissue-damaging components often found in high-calorie foods. Look for nutrient-dense foods, many of which also have anti-inflammatory properties, to give your body the essential nutrients it craves without loading up on unnecessary calories. However, don't neglect any food group from your diet, since you need a balance of your total calories from proteins, carbohydrates and fats.

Hydrate: Dehydration can cause a 20–30 percent decline in muscle function, leaving you fatigued and more vulnerable to injury. By the time you feel thirsty, you may already be slightly dehydrated. Try to drink water frequently during the day, whether you feel thirsty or not. Most people need somewhere between 2 and 3 liters (8 to 13 cups) of water or other beverages per day, but individual daily hydration requirements can vary greatly. You may need to drink more water if, for example, you live in a hot climate, are pregnant or nursing, have certain health conditions, or exercise vigorously. Generally speaking,

Pro-inflammatory foods	Anti-inflammatory foods
Trans fats: Baked goods, margarine, fried foods, vegetable shortening, fast foods **Saturated fats:** Red meat, butter, whole milk and whole milk products **Omega-6 fats:** Oils made from corn, cottonseed, safflower and sunflower; processed foods **High Glycemic Index:** Potatoes, white rice, sugar, highly processed cereals, soda/pop **Nitrites:** Hot dogs, lunch meats, sausage	**Omega-3 fats:** Cold water fish—salmon, herring, anchovies (best if wild caught) Flaxseed Walnuts Pumpkin seeds Omega-3 enriched eggs Olive oil **Whole grains:** Buckwheat Oatmeal **Colorful fruits and vegetables:** Leafy greens (spinach, kale) Berries (blueberries, strawberries) Sweet potatoes Broccoli Avocados **Spices and herbs:** Ginger Garlic Chili peppers Turmeric **Green or Black Tea, caffeinated or not**

A Simple Formula for Good Hydration

Drink at least 4 cups (1 quart or 1 liter) of water per 50 pounds (23 kg.) of body weight. A person who weighs 125 pounds (57 kg.) should therefore drink about 10 cups (2.5 liters) of water per day.

you are staying adequately hydrated if you rarely feel thirsty and your urine is abundant and very pale yellow.

Discuss your nutritional needs with your healthcare provider: The food and hydration guidelines mentioned here should be reviewed with a qualified healthcare practitioner, as some people may be allergic to certain foods or have medical conditions that could require a specific diet or level of hydration.[1]

Get Plenty of Sleep

A good night's sleep allows you to rest and recover from the stresses you put on your body and mind during the day. It is a time for you to give up some of the control you maintain over your muscles and tendons, allowing them to relax and repair themselves.

Sleep is more than just rest. While you sleep, the force of gravity on your joints is diminished, and fluids containing important nutrients flow back into your intervertebral discs. During deep sleep, also known as delta or Stage 4 sleep, the body's repair and regulation processes are the most active. Human growth hormone (HGH), a primary regulator of cellular repair, is secreted at its highest level during deep sleep. At the same time, your body is rebalancing its chemistry, particularly the neurotransmitters. REM stage sleep, when we dream, brings with it a complete relaxation of the muscles. Healthy sleep patterns in which all stages of sleep are normal and uninterrupted is often referred to as "restorative sleep," because it has all of these healing attributes.

You will often hear people who have chronic pain complain of sleeping poorly. Pain or discomfort can interrupt the sleep cycle, and slow the body's healing process. Sufferers of chronic fatigue syndrome or fibromyalgia, for example, tend to have their deep sleep cycles interrupted by periods of wakefulness. This disrupted sleeping pattern contributes to the chronic nature of their conditions.

Sleeping in a poor position, or on a bad mattress, can also cause discomfort and pain, especially to the back and neck. Many people are under the impression that a very firm mattress is best for preventing back pain. A number of research studies have found that this is not the case. Most people sleep better, and feel less discomfort upon awakening, on a moderately firm mattress that has enough give to prevent pressure points from forming. While no one type of mattress is best for everyone, high-quality traditional mattresses, memory foam mattresses, and mattresses with adjustable firmness are typically rated the best. While a good mattress is important for everyone, preventing pressure points is particularly important for anyone with an injury or a chronic condition like fibromyalgia. Pillow-top beds, feather beds, and memory foam mattress toppers can all be used to reduce pressure points.

Another important consideration when sleeping is the position of your hands and wrists. Many people clench their fists and flex their wrists as they sleep. This position increases pressure in the structures

Tips for Avoiding Insomnia

- Avoid stimulants like caffeine or nicotine in the afternoon and evening.

- Avoid using bright, artificial or "blue" light, like cell phones or a TV, in the evening, which can trick your brain into thinking it is still day.

- Keep to a consistent sleep schedule; go to bed and get up at the same time, even on the weekends.

- Practice meditation and relaxation techniques, such as deep breathing, just before bed, to help you let go of stressful thoughts and feelings.

- Play relaxing music or nature sounds, such as ocean surf, to mask any outside noises that might prevent drifting off to sleep.

- Take a warm bath to relax your muscles, but avoid hot baths, which can raise your body temperature and have a stimulating effect.

- Avoid exercise within a few hours of bedtime.

- Avoid heavy meals in the evening, but don't go to bed on an empty stomach, either; eat light, healthy snacks that are easy to digest.

and nerves of the wrists, which can impinge the nerves and cause numbness in the hands.

Try to get in the habit of consciously placing your hands in a good position before you go to sleep. If you start out in a good position every night, you will be more likely to stay in that position as you sleep. Try holding a small, thin pillow or cushion between flat palms as you fall asleep. If you sleep on your side, you can slide your hands under your pillow, in front of your head, to help keep them flat and in a neutral position as you sleep. If you know that you have a habit of clenching and flexing as you sleep, you can try stretching, massaging, and consciously relaxing your hands before you go to sleep. If you are experiencing symptoms in the hands or wrists, you may want to talk to an appropriate health-care professional about using night splints. These wrist/hand braces

Tips for a Healthy Sleeping Position

A good sleeping posture helps you get a more restful sleep, and may keep you out of positions that can stress connective tissue or compress nerves and blood vessels while you sleep. The best sleeping positions are on your back or your side. Avoid sleeping on your stomach, which forces you to turn your head to one side, shortening muscles on that side and overstretching them on the other.

If you sleep on your back:

- Use a thin pillow underneath your head, to avoid sleeping with your neck in flexion.

- If you sleep propped up on many pillows, make sure that all of the normal curves in your spine are maintained.

- Place a pillow under your knees, to reduce stress to your lower back.

- Avoid folding your arms across your chest, which can place pressure on nerves and blood vessels around the elbow. Train yourself to hold your hands low across your stomach or at your sides.

If you sleep on your side:

- You may need a thicker pillow for your head than back sleepers. Look for one that keeps your head level with the rest of your body, not flexed to the side.

- Place a pillow between your knees to keep your legs more in line with your hips.

- Avoid curling up in "foetal position," as this position eliminates the natural lordotic curve in your lumbar and cervical spine.

- It may help to gently hug a pillow as you drift off. The pillow will keep your arms out in front of you and not twisted into awkward positions.

are comfortable enough for a short time (long-term use can cause muscle atrophy). to sleep in, and can help you develop the habit of keeping your wrists straight and your palms open.

Don't Smoke

In addition to all of the other negative health effects it causes, smoking can also reduce circulation, which is critical to maintaining a healthy musculoskeletal system. Smoking robs the body of vitamin C, an important component in connective tissue repair. The intervertebral discs are particularly vulnerable, and smokers have a greater risk of disc bulges and herniations. The nicotine in cigarette smoke slows all of the body's healing processes, so microtrauma to tendons, ligaments, cartilage and other tissues will take longer to repair. Nicotine is also a stimulant, so smoking can contribute to insomnia and keep you from getting a good night's sleep.

How Sleeping Affects Your Intervertebral Discs

During the day, gravity takes a toll on your spine, compressing the vertebrae and slowly forcing fluid out of your intervertebral discs. Your discs end up quite a bit thinner at the end of the day than they were at the beginning; you can lose half an inch or more of height after a long day of standing upright. As you sleep, fluids, and the nutrition that they carry, re-enter your discs and bring them back to full height. While this is a beneficial process, it does raise one caution. When you first get out of bed and your discs are filled with fluid, your spine will be less flexible. For this reason, you should avoid any heavy lifting or prolonged periods of bending or twisting of your spine for the first few hours after you arise.

Limit Caffeine Consumption

In small doses, caffeine is a performance-enhancing drug. Caffeine acts as a stimulant by blocking the absorption of adenosine, a neurotransmitter that helps to slow nerve function in the brain. Adenosine is an important biochemical that allows your body to enter a deeper sleep. Too much caffeine can disrupt sleep patterns, causing more fatigue, which can make you reach for more caffeine to keep you awake! Caffeine also reduces blood flow to the extremities; without proper circulation, your hands will be cold and tissue repair will be diminished. It also increases muscle tension and can cause muscle twitches and jitteriness. In larger doses, the drug can increase feelings of anxiety. Frequent caffeine consumption can create a physical dependence, and withdrawal symptoms can include headaches, muscle pain, fatigue and depression.

Caffeine typically has a 3 to 4 hour half-life in the body, which means that only half of the drug's effects remain after just a few hours. However, the rate of metabolism of caffeine varies among individuals, so you may want to avoid taking in any caffeine after the morning hours, since it may interfere with your ability to enter a deep, restorative sleep.

The bottom line is that small doses of caffeine may help reduce feelings of pain and fatigue, but too much has negative effects, including increased muscle tension, loss of fine motor control, and higher blood pressure.

Limit Alcohol Consumption

Unlike caffeine, the consumption of alcohol will detract from your performance. The media and medical community used to talk about the potential benefits of drinking in moderation. More recent research has revealed that drinking alcohol in any amount can negatively affect your health.

The downsides of alcohol consumption can be serious. Even though drinking alcohol may relax you and help you fall asleep more easily, it can also disrupt sleep patterns. Alcohol can make you more susceptible to depression, liver disease and some types of cancer (by robbing your body of folic acid). Alcohol can also create potentially dangerous interactions with acetaminophen and other pain killers, antidepressants, sedatives, and other medications that are frequently prescribed to deal with MSDs.

Maintain Regular Social Connections

Pain and dysfunction, if they occur, can lead us to isolate ourselves and cut down on our social outings and connections with other people. Isolation tends to feed on itself, and can amplify the feeling that we are no longer capable of functioning normally in society. To counteract this effect, be sure to maintain your relationships with friends and family and continue to enjoy social functions to the best of your ability. The feeling of continued connection to your social circle and life in general will provide much-needed perspective and remind you that you can still enjoy all life has to offer, even if you are injured at the moment.

Receive Massage and Other Modalities Regularly

Although manual therapists certainly know the benefits of regularly receiving massage and other manual treatments, many of them do not take the time to receive these treatments themselves. As you know, massage is very effective as a preventive measure to reduce your risk of injury. Given the physical demands of manual treatment work, it may help to receive bodywork more often than the generally recommended once per month. Exchanging treatments with colleagues at least every 2 weeks can help you eliminate accumulated muscle tension and any incipient symptoms before they can impact you further. Try to avoid giving your half of an exchange on a day when you have already done a number of treatment sessions, particularly if they involve deep tissue work. Practitioners in the other manual therapies should also make sure they receive treatment themselves, as an injury prevention tactic.

Massage Your Own Muscles

Between exchanges, you may get some benefit from self massage. Remember, though, that use of your hands to massage yourself will add to your overall exposure to risk factors such as repetitive motions, gripping and awkward postures. In fact, self massage can result in more awkward postures and issues with grip force than massaging someone else, for example, if you reach across your body and bend your wrists in an attempt to massage your opposite shoulder and arm. If you massage one hand and arm with the other, you obviously will not be able to use the idle hand to support the one doing the work. You also may not be able to use your body weight to apply pressure in self massage. Keep in mind that self massage is often not as effective as receiving massage from someone else, since you are splitting your focus between applying the massage and relaxing the muscles you are working on.

In addition to paying attention to good body mechanics, limit self massage sessions to brief periods of time. A quick warm-up massage, similar to a pre-event sports massage, may be helpful before you do your first treatment session of the day. Briefly massaging your hands and forearms between treatment sessions may help flush out metabolites and improve circulation.

The best strategy for self massage is to avoid using your hands as much as possible. Here are some self-massage techniques that are not hand intensive:

- Use tools to reach trigger points, being careful to not assume awkward postures while you do so.
- Lay one forearm flat on a treatment table, and use the other forearm to apply effleurage and compression to the flexors and extensors.
- Place a tennis ball or racquetball on the floor and lie down on top of it to massage the superficial muscles in your back, especially your erector spinae, infraspinatus and rhomboids. A firmer ball, such as a handball or high bounce ball, will even allow you to work out some trigger points.
- Massage the flexors in your forearms by placing a small ball on a counter or other hard surface and rolling your forearms across it.
- Use a long, hooked tool to massage your shoulders, back, gluteals and legs. This type of tool allows you to do compression and work on trigger points in areas that would otherwise require you to get into awkward postures to reach. Try to avoid pressing so hard that you must hold the tool with great tension or apply a lot of pressure with your hands and arms.
- Borrow a rolling pin from your kitchen to massage a number of the muscles in your legs. With some creativity, you can find ways to use your body weight to massage most of your superficial muscles, while giving your hands and arms a break. Keep a loose grip on the handles of the rolling pin.
- Use cupping techniques to lift the tissues in your forearms, upper arms and shoulders, releasing adhesions in the superficial fascia.

Maintain Regular Physical Activity

In the next chapter, you'll find a physical conditioning program designed specifically for manual therapists by a doctor of physical therapy. Try to do these exercises and stretches on a regular basis (ideally, several times a week) to help you prevent MSDs. You can "sneak" some of them in at work between sessions, or at home as you wash the dishes, do chores or during your free time.

Practice Relaxation and Stress Reduction Techniques

Massage is a proven method for reducing stress and anxiety, but it is not the only one. Exercise, yoga, meditation and mindfulness, listening to music, engaging in hobbies, and spending time with loved ones or

---

Therapeutic Baths

"Detox" Relaxation Bath

In a warm to hot bath, dissolve the following:

> ½ cup (150 g.) Epsom salt
>
> ½ cup (150 g.) sea salt (*not* table salt)
>
> ½ cup (150 g.) baking soda
>
> Soak for 10–15 minutes, then rinse thoroughly.

The hot water opens your pores, allowing minerals from the salts to be absorbed through your skin, while the baking soda helps soothe your skin. The primary mineral absorbed will be magnesium from the Epsom salt. Magnesium, balanced with calcium, is an important mineral for muscle relaxation, nerve conduction, and the production of energy. It also acts as an anti-inflammatory.

Note: hot mineral baths are not appropriate for everyone. Consult your physician if you have any health issues before using this bath recipe.

---

a pet are all good ways of relaxing. By invoking your body's relaxation response, you will experience a number of health benefits, including reduced muscle tension, lowered blood pressure, and improved immune system functioning. All of these will help your body's ability to heal while at the same time improving your emotional well-being.

A valuable practice you can learn more about, in this book and elsewhere, is Mindfulness Based Stress Reduction (MBSR). MBSR is a proven technique that encourages relaxation, focus, staying in the present moment, good breathing patterns, and overall well-being. Regularly practicing MBSR is highly recommended to help enhance body awareness and prevent injury for hands-on health practitioners. It's also a valuable practice to recommend to your clients or patients. You'll find more information on MBSR, as well as an MBSR-based morning routine to prepare you for work, in Appendix C.[2]

1. Based on information provided by George Piligian, MD, MPH and Elizabeth Vucovik Gartlan, MS, RD. See Bibliography for a complete reference.
2. Courtney E. Ackerman, M.A., Feb. 19, 2017, "Mindfulness Based Stress Reduction: The Ultimate MBSR Guide," https://positivepsychology.com/mindfulness-based-stress-reduction-mbsr/

11

Physical Conditioning

To have a long, healthy career as a manual therapist, you must have the necessary physical condition to keep up with the physical demands of your work. We have already seen that lack of physical condition is a risk factor for MSDs. Staying in good condition not only gives you the necessary physical capacity to do your work; it also helps you maintain a good level of circulation to help your body more quickly heal microtrauma to your tissues, and prevent cumulative trauma from turning into injury.

> This chapter was developed by Janet M. Peterson, PT, DPT, to address the specific conditioning needs of manual therapists who are not experiencing any symptom of injury. If you are already experiencing any symptom of injury, do NOT do the exercises or stretches recommended without first consulting a qualified healthcare professional. If you have previously been symptom-free, and doing any of the exercises or stretches in this chapter provokes symptoms, do not continue doing the exercises and stretches in this chapter without first consulting a qualified healthcare professional. In either of those cases, ask a healthcare practitioner trained in rehabilitation to prescribe a conditioning program for you, designed to address your specific symptoms and diagnosis. Once you are feeling better, you can review the activities listed in this chapter with the practitioner you have been seeing to determine whether they are appropriate for you to start doing. Consult your physician before beginning any exercise program.

If you are in school or just starting to practice, it is important to begin a conditioning program that will get your body ready for the physical work you are going to be doing. Start early in your career, and staying in shape will become a normal part of your routine. You will need to maintain your physical conditioning throughout your career to help protect yourself from injury.

To maintain optimal conditioning for your work, you need to develop activity-specific endurance, strength and flexibility. Depending on the level of conditioning you already have, you may need to concentrate on one of these components more than another. But an effective training program must include all three components.

There is a common misconception among manual therapists that their work provides all the exercise they need, because it is physically demanding. While it is true that your hands-on work can help build strength and endurance in the muscle groups you use frequently, it can also result in overuse and tightening of some of those muscles and disuse and overstretching of others. It also tends to be fatiguing without providing much of a cardiovascular benefit. Many practitioners work every weekday, and may not have enough time between sessions for muscles and tendons to recover and repair themselves.

A well-designed conditioning program will reinforce the aspects of your work that benefit your conditioning, and make up for those aspects that negatively impact your physical condition. Keeping in shape will not prevent injury in and of itself, but it is an essential component of a holistic approach to injury prevention.

Note that many of these same concepts apply to your clients or patients. You can suggest that they do any of the following exercises and stretches you feel are appropriate for them.

A Multifaceted Approach to Conditioning

A complete conditioning program for manual therapists should incorporate all of the following elements:

- Endurance/Cardiovascular (Aerobic) fitness
- Flexibility/Stability/Balance
- Body awareness/Proprioception/Good movement patterns

- Strength
- Good circulation
- Lack of adhesions
- Breathing

Endurance/Cardiovascular Fitness

Building muscle endurance helps prevent muscle fatigue. When muscles "give out" from fatigue, they can no longer properly support your joints. If this happens, all of the force of the technique you are applying at that point will be transferred to your tendons, ligaments and cartilage, potentially causing damage.

Most of the exercises you do should focus on building endurance rather than just strength. By developing good overall cardiovascular (aerobic) condition, your heart and lungs will be able to provide the oxygen and nutrients to support the muscular endurance you have developed in your individual muscle groups. People who have both aerobic fitness and endurance in individual muscle groups tend to have fewer MSDs.

Flexibility and Stability

To prevent injury, you need to find a balance between flexibility of your muscles and stability of your joints. Manual therapists spend a great deal of their time doing strenuous work with their arms in front of their bodies. As a result, the front of the body gets overworked and tight, while the back gets overstretched and weak. You can resolve this imbalance by stretching the front of the body, which is tight from overuse, and strengthening the back of the body, which is weak from underuse. The idea is to counteract the forces that are creating the problem.

While maintaining a normal level of flexibility is a goal, too much flexibility, or hypermobility, can make your joints unstable. When your joints are not adequately supported, particularly the weak links in your hand and wrist, you risk injuring those structures. Strong muscles are the "first line of defense" for joint protection, so strengthening the muscles around the joints in your weak links can reduce your risk of injury.

Body Awareness, Proprioception and Good Movement Patterns

As you saw in Chapter 5, you can reduce your risk of injury by using good body mechanics and working in near-neutral postures. The goal is to learn what it feels like to be in a neutral posture, where your joints are aligned, your muscles are in their strongest positions, and there is the least amount of stress on nerves, blood vessels and connective tissues. Developing your proprioception will enhance your awareness of your body and the positions of your various joints relative to each other. Once you have a good sense of what a neutral posture feels like, you can practice movement patterns that keep you within a comfortable range of motion around neutral and allow you to use your strongest muscle groups to perform a task. A good movement pattern is one that allows you to use the least amount of effort and stress to your body to accomplish a physical task. Ask a fellow student or colleague to watch you as you work and let you know when you are straying from neutral postures.

Strength

Strength plays a role in conditioning, but it is not the most important part of staying in shape. If you worked at or near 100 percent of your body's strength capacity for an extended period of time, you would likely injure yourself. Your muscles would not be able to sustain that level of effort without either tearing or transferring the stress to your ligaments, bones and joints.

To avoid injury, anything you do repetitively should not require more than one-third of your available strength. For most practitioners, the focus should really be on strengthening postural stability muscles (also referred to as core muscles) and underused muscles that are antagonists to the muscles you use the most often. Again, the idea is to balance the muscle forces on either side of the joint to create and maintain stability.

At the same time, you do need a certain amount of distal arm and hand strength to perform intensive manual techniques. It's best to start doing upper extremity strengthening exercises before you begin your training as a manual therapist, before starting a new job, or after a period of inactivity, to increase your overall strength capacity.

Good Circulation

Your muscles need the nutrients, electrolytes and oxygen in your blood to function properly. Sustained muscular contractions, especially in awkward postures and with poor breathing patterns, can reduce local blood flow to your tissues. Without good circulation, it's as if your muscles "run out of gas." Manual therapists tend to hold the lower body and trunk in one position as they work, and perform most of their techniques with the upper body alone. Work performed in a static standing position, particularly on hard surfaces, can lead to venous pooling in the legs and a reduction in overall circulation. Doing some form of aerobic conditioning will help you maintain good circulation. Prior to starting your workday, even 10 minutes of brisk walking can improve the blood circulation to your muscles to prepare your body for the day's work.

Lack of Adhesions

Minor injuries can cause scar tissue to build up over time. This tissue is prone to further damage for a number of reasons. It is more fragile and less functional than the connective tissue it replaces. It is not as flexible as the original tissue, so scar tissue that forms in the muscle body will not be able to contract. Scar tissue is laid down in a random pattern that is not always in alignment with the direction in which muscle fibers and connective tissue run. As a result, it tends to adhere to fascia and other tissues, which can further reduce circulation and range of motion. Cross-fiber friction may be able to break up scar tissue, which could then be realigned with linear friction. As part of a conditioning program, stretching and rhythmic movement of the body part can also realign scar tissue fibers.

Creating Your Comprehensive Conditioning Program

Incorporating all of these important components of conditioning into a simple workout routine is really quite easy. You only need to do enough exercise to rebalance your body; increase endurance, strength and stability in underused muscles; and improve flexibility in muscles that have become tight from overuse and adhesions. Add in some aerobic exercise to further increase endurance and circulation or as a warm-up, and some postural and balance exercises to improve proprioception and movement patterns, and you will have a complete program that will fit easily into your free time.

The exercises in the following sections have been designed to address the specific conditioning needs of manual therapists. They will help you improve and maintain your strength, flexibility, endurance and balance; keep tension at bay; and develop your proprioception and awareness of your movement patterns. Creating and following a routine chosen from these exercises will help you develop the physical conditioning necessary to help minimize your risk of injury from your work. If you are already physically active, use these exercises to fill in the gaps of your current regime.

Mix and match exercises from the different categories above to create a balanced, multifaceted conditioning program. As a general guideline, you can start each session with a warm up, then do either aerobic conditioning or strengthening or balance activities, and end with at least two stretches. If you prefer, you can start with a warm-up, then move on to stretches, then strengthening and balance exercises. Later in the chapter, you will find several sample routines to use as a guide to get you started.

Breathing Exercises

Learning to breathe deeply and regularly will help you counteract tension as you work. Your clients will also benefit, as they are likely to unconsciously start breathing deeply with you. Maintaining steady, even, deep breathing is very important both when you exercise and when you work, to ensure that your muscles get sufficient oxygen. Between clients, try to combine at least one of the following breathing exercises with one of the arm or neck stretches to help you relax and prepare for your next client. Doing even one breathing exercise and one stretch will help you reduce stress and increase your energy during your workday. Taking several such breaks each workday is a good goal to keep you healthy in your work.

Finding the Bottom of the Breath

The point of this exercise is to notice how your breathing works when tension is removed, so you can develop a natural, conscious way of breathing fully and deeply. Think about letting the breath happen naturally instead of forcing yourself to breathe in any special way.

Sit in a chair, close your eyes, and relax. Take a breath and exhale naturally through your mouth. Don't force the breath out. Keep exhaling until your breath is used up.

Relax, and wait. If you think of the breath as a long, vertical oval, this is the "bottom" of your breath. Wait until you distinctly feel the impulse to breathe. It is not necessary to wait until you are desperate for air, just until you can identify that your body wants to breathe in. Try to notice where in your body the impulse to breathe originates (most people feel the impulse originating in the abdomen or below the rib cage). Then take a normal breath in through your nose. If you cannot breathe normally through your nose due to allergies or other issues, inhale and exhale through your mouth. Concentrate on keeping your jaw and lips relaxed as you practice.

Notice when your breath crests at the "top" and turns into an exhale. Exhale through your mouth again. Keep exhaling until your breath is used up, and wait again at the bottom. Repeat as many times as is comfortable. If you do this exercise correctly, you should not hyperventilate or feel at all dizzy.

Lateral Rib Expansion

When you breathe shallowly, the diaphragm cannot do as much of the work of breathing as it should. Underutilizing the diaphragm causes you to overuse the secondary muscles of respiration, including the scalenes, the upper trapezii, and the intrinsic neck muscles. These muscles can become hypertonic from overuse, making you more susceptible to thoracic outlet and tension neck syndromes. The diaphragm can become weak from underuse.

Expanding the ribs laterally as you breath develops and strengthens the diaphragm. A stronger diaphragm will participate more fully in breathing.

Starting Position: Stand in front of a full-length mirror.

Action: As you breathe in deeply, concentrate on expanding your rib cage laterally. You should be able to see the ribs clearly expand out to the sides. Exhale. It may take some practice before you can isolate your breathing in this way. Try resting a hand on the side of your ribcage as you perform this exercise in order to feel the expansion. Your goal is make the rib cage expand laterally by 2 to 3 inches.

Aerobic Conditioning

To keep your heart healthy, experts now recommend at least 30 minutes of moderate cardiovascular exercise at least 5 days a week. These 30 minutes do not have to be consecutive; for example, you could take three, 10-minute brisk walks at different times of the day. "Moderate" means that you are breathing hard but still able to talk.

The best aerobic activities for manual therapists are those that do not tax the arms in any significant way. Walking, hiking, dancing and low-impact aerobics classes are good, safe choices. Walking is particularly good if you have not previously been physically active; running is great as long as you do not have any back or lower extremity conditions. Swimming and outdoor bicycling may need to be slightly modified to reduce arm stress; for example, you may need to use an anti-vibration wrap and raise the height of bicycle handlebars. If you use a stationary bicycle, use only light pressure on the handles. Use a kickboard for a portion of your swimming workout. Playing sports that use the hands intensively, like tennis, squash, racquetball, golf and volleyball should be kept to a minimum. Use common sense in your aerobic activities to avoid further trauma to your already heavily-used hands.

Strengthening Exercises

These exercises concentrate on strengthening the large core muscles of the back, trunk, glutes and abdomen. Strengthening core muscles will help you counteract the forward shoulder and head posture that manual therapists tend to get into as they work. It will also help prevent back injuries by strengthening the muscles surrounding the spine and strengthening your thigh muscles so they can do most of the work when you perform lifting activities. Strong core muscles will also help prevent stress on the knees.

Because your arms are anchored to your trunk through the muscles around your shoulder and scapula and you depend on your arms to perform your work, it is especially important to strengthen the muscles that hold your shoulder and scapula to your trunk.

When you do strengthening exercises with weights, be sure to leave at least a day between workouts on the same part of the body. Your muscles need 36 to 48 hours to recover and heal from weight training. Stretching and cardiovascular exercises can be done daily.

The number of repetitions you do and the amount of weight you use for these strengthening exercises will vary, depending on your starting, or baseline, physical condition. To avoid injury, it is better to start with lighter weights and more repetitions than heavier weights. Feel free to substitute stretchy bands for the hand-held weights. Placing the end of a band around your wrist rather than holding it with your hand can reduce the hand effort needed for these exercises.

It is very important to perform these strengthening exercises at a smooth pace: each repetition should take 2 to 5 seconds to complete. To build endurance, perform two or three sets of exercises, each set with 8 to 12 repetitions. If you cannot complete 8 repetitions before tiring, then the weight you are using is probably too heavy; if you can easily perform 12 repetitions and not tire, then the weight you're using is probably too light. Some of these strengthening exercises use your own body weight as the resistance, so the number of repetitions will vary for those exercises.

You may add to this basic program any exercises that address the back, the abdominals/core muscles or the legs. Do not add hand or arm exercises that are repetitive in nature. See the Frequently Asked Questions section at the end of this chapter if you are just starting out and want to strengthen your arm muscles before you start learning manual techniques.

Warm Up First

Remember to warm up with general body exercise like brisk walking or pedaling a stationary bicycle for 5 or 10 minutes before your strength-training session. If you feel pain as you perform any of these exercises, you may be injured. Discontinue exercising until you have been evaluated for a possible injury.

Core Strengthening

You won't need any particular equipment to do the exercises and stretches noted here. Using the weight of your own body will suffice. However, if you wish to further challenge your balance and build your core muscles, using certain pieces of equipment can be helpful once your core muscles start getting stronger. For example:

- Stability ball
- Bosu
- A sturdy chair
- An exercise cushion to practice balance

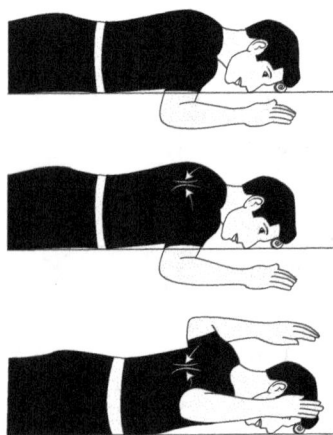

TRUNK EXTENSION—A

Targets: Rhomboid muscles.

Starting Position: Lie prone, with your arms out to the side and your elbows bent to 90 degrees. (You may want to rest your forehead on a rolled-up washcloth to protect your nose or rest your head in the face cradle of a treatment table.)

Action: Holding a weight in each of your hands, squeeze your shoulder blades together and lift your arms 3 to 6 inches toward the ceiling, then lower your arms back down. Start with a light weight (2 lbs./0.9KG) for this exercise. Repeat 8 to 12 times for strengthening, and do 3 sets for endurance.

Focus on: Feeling your shoulder blades squeeze together.

UPPER TRUNK EXTENSION—B

Targets: Middle trapezius muscles.

Starting Position: Lie prone, with your arms straight out to the side. (You may want to rest your forehead on a rolled-up washcloth to protect your nose or rest your head in the face cradle of a treatment table.)

Action: Holding a weight in each of your hands, squeeze your shoulder blades together and lift your arms 3 to 6 inches up toward the ceiling, then lower your arms back down. Start with a light weight (2 lbs./0.9 KG) for this exercise. Repeat 8 to 12 times for strengthening, and do 3 sets for endurance.

Focus on: Making a smooth motion both up and down.

UPPER AND LOWER TRUNK EXTENSION—"Super Hero"

Targets: Multiple trunk extensor muscles including trapezius, latissimus dorsi and gluteus maximus.

Starting Position: Lie prone, with your arms stretched out in front of your head. (You may want to rest your forehead on a rolled-up washcloth to protect your nose or rest your head in the face cradle of a treatment table.)

Action: Holding a weight in each of your hands, squeeze your shoulder blades together and lift your arms 3 to 6 inches up toward the ceiling. At the same time, lift your legs off the floor a few inches. Hold for 2 to 3 seconds, then lower your arms and legs back down. Start with a light weight (2 lbs./0.9 KG) for this exercise. Repeat 8 to 12 times for strengthening, and do 3 sets for endurance.

Focus on: Breathing evenly throughout.

LOWER TRUNK FLEXION—Diagonal Partial Sit-up

Targets: Multiple abdominal muscles including internal and external obliques.

Starting Position: Lie on your back with your knees bent, feet on the floor and hands resting on either side of your head.

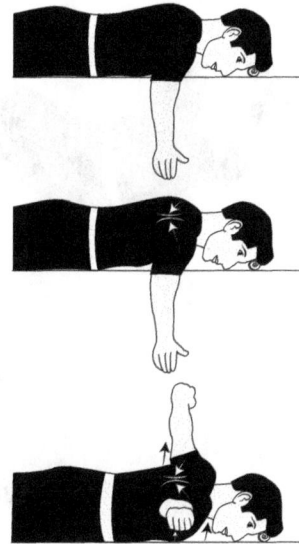

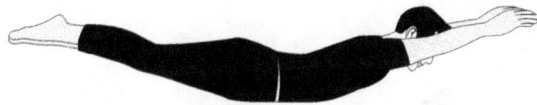

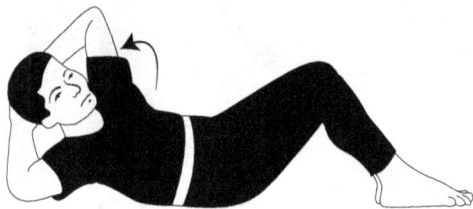

Action: Lift your head and left arm as you gently twist to the right, until your left shoulder blade lifts off the floor. Don't pull with your hands; lead with your shoulder. Hold for 1 to 2 seconds, then return to the start position and repeat to the left side. Remember to breathe during this exercise. Repeat this exercise until you feel fatigued and can no longer lift your shoulder blade. As you get stronger, you will be able to perform more repetitions.

Focus on: Smooth movement. Don't jerk.

LOWER TRUNK FLEXION—Leg Lowering

Targets: Multiple abdominal muscles including rectus abdominus and external obliques.

Starting Position: Lie on your back with your knees bent, feet on the floor, and hands resting on your abdomen.

Action: Press your back into the floor as you straighten your left knee so it is suspended in the air; keep your back pressed into the floor as you slowly lower your straightened left leg to the floor. Bend that leg and return to the start position, then repeat with your right leg. Repeat with each leg 10–12 times. Remember to breathe during this exercise. If you feel your back start to arch away from the floor as you lower your leg, bend your knee and return to the start position. As you get stronger, you may want to add an ankle weight.

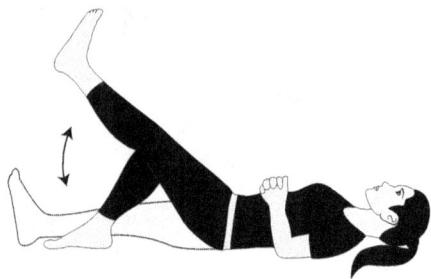

Focus on: Keeping your back pressed into the floor.

Note: Can be done with a 1 lb. or 2 lb. ankle weight on the lifted leg for progressive strengthening.

HIP ABDUCTION

Targets: Hip abductor muscles including gluteus medius and gluteus minimus.

Starting Position: Lie on your right side with your top (left) leg straight and your bottom (right) leg slightly bent.

Action: Slowly lift your top leg toward the ceiling, being careful not to roll toward your back (it helps to keep your toes pointed slightly toward the floor as you lift your leg). Make sure that the lifted leg remains in line with the rest of your body to best engage the target muscles. Repeat 10–12 times, then roll onto your left side and repeat with the other leg. Add an ankle weight as your strength improves, starting conservatively with a one or two-pound weight.

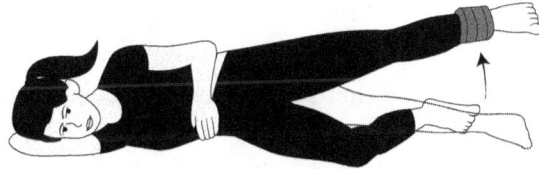

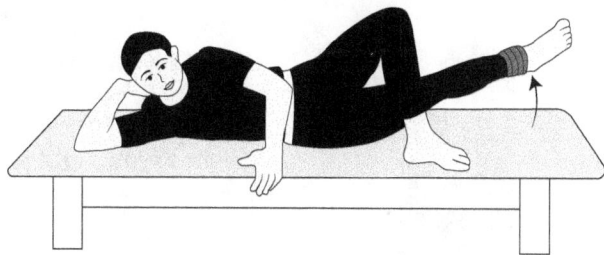

Focus on: Keeping your pelvis perpendicular to the floor.

HIP ADDUCTION

Targets: Hip adductor muscles including adductor magnus, brevis and longus.

Starting Position: Lie on your right side with your bottom leg straight and your top (left) leg bent at the knee, with your left foot on the floor or table in front of your right leg.

Action: Slowly lift your bottom (right) leg toward the ceiling. Repeat 10–12 times, then roll onto your left side and repeat with the other leg. Add an ankle weight as your strength improves, starting conservatively with a one or two-pound weight.

Focus on: Keeping your bottom knee straight.

Feel free to add in other standard core exercises from time to time. Exercises like planks, bridges, squats, or wall squats will help with not only core strength but also balance and stability of your stance as you work.

Upper Extremity Strengthening

The next two exercises will strengthen multiple muscles in your shoulders and arms in a modified proprioceptive neuromuscular facilitation (PNF) pattern. Manual therapists who are just starting to practice will find them particularly helpful in building strength to perform job tasks.

If you have been practicing for a while, your hands and arms are already heavily used and tight as a result of your work. While you do need strong hands and arms to do your work, it is important to find a balance between strengthening your hands and arms and allowing them some much-needed rest. Be aware that strengthening has the potential to overwork your hand and arm muscles and increase your risk of injury. At the same time, by not performing any hand/arm strength training, you could lose the benefit of the joint protection that strong muscles can provide. Use any symptoms you may develop as a guide, and remember to also perform stretching exercises for these muscles.

You will already get some benefit to your arms by doing the upper trunk exercises in the previous section. Those exercises will strengthen your distal arm muscles, since you will be holding weights in your hands. If you want additional upper extremity strengthening exercises, please see the Frequently Asked Questions section at the end of this chapter.

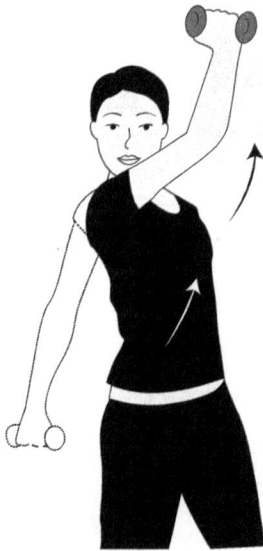

UPPER EXTREMITY STRENGTHENING—Diagonal Pattern A

Starting Position: Sit or stand, holding a 3-pound (1.4 KG) weight in your right hand. Start with your right hand above your left shoulder, elbow bent, palm facing behind you.

Action: Moving slowly and evenly, pull your arm across your body in a diagonal motion, ending with your right hand against your right hip, elbow straight and your palm facing the floor. Then lift your arm back to the starting position with the same smooth motion. Repeat with the left arm. Repeat 10–12 times.

Focus on: Maintaining a slow, even pace in both directions.

UPPER EXTREMITY STRENGTHENING—Diagonal Pattern B

Starting Position: Sit or stand, holding a 3-pound (1.4 KG) weight in your right hand. Start with your right hand against your left hip, elbow bent, and your palm facing the floor.

Action: Moving slowly and evenly, lift your arm in a diagonal, twisting motion, ending with your right hand above your head, palm facing left. Keep your elbow fairly straight as you move your arm. Then pull your arm back to the starting position, tracing the same smooth arc of motion. Repeat with the left arm. Repeat 10–12 times.

Focus on: Maintaining a slow, even pace in both directions.

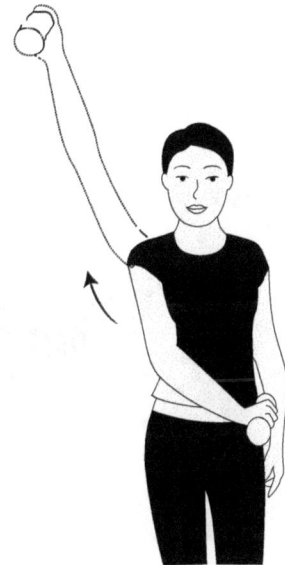

Balance Exercises

Balance exercises help increase body awareness and strengthen core muscles. They also help you maintain a healthy stance as you work. To improve your balance, consider adding some of these balance exercises into your weekly routine.

CONTROLLED LUNGES

Starting Position: Stand with your feet shoulder width apart and hands on your hips.

Action: Take one large step forward with your right foot. Slowly dip down, keeping most of your weight on your back leg and your knees in line with your feet (not out to the side). Stop before your back knee touches the floor. It's important to keep your front knee behind the toes of the front foot, then slowly return to the starting position. Repeat with your left foot forward. Perform 8–12 repetitions with each leg forward. Each repetition

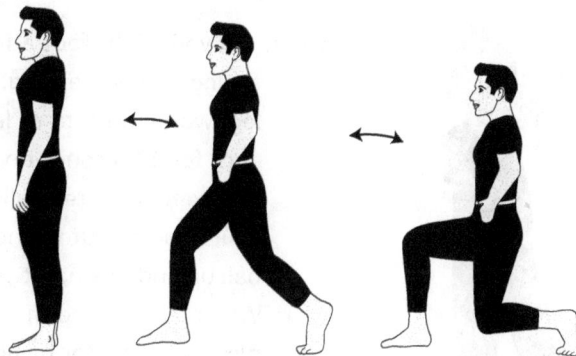

should be smooth and controlled and your upper body should always remain erect. If your knees hurt when you perform this exercise, don't dip down as far and keep your weight on your back leg.

Focus on: Dipping down instead of forward.

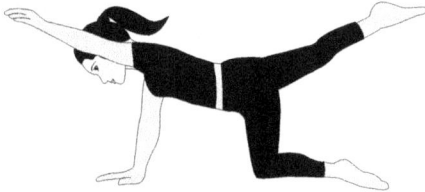

QUADRUPED LIFT

Starting Position: Get onto your hands and knees. If possible, perform this exercise on a stability ball to reduce the pressure on your hands and wrists.

Action: Lift one arm up, elbow straight, keeping your spine in a neutral position (don't let it fall into a swayback position). Be sure to breathe normally. Hold for 3–5 seconds, then return to the starting position. Repeat with the other arm, then with each leg, maintaining a neutral spine each time. When you can consistently maintain a neutral spine while lifting one arm or leg at a time, you are ready to then lift your left arm and right leg up at the same time, still maintaining a neutral spine posture. Relax, then repeat with the right arm and left leg.

Focus on: Maintaining a neutral spine position.

SINGLE LEG STANDING

Starting Position: Stand on a level surface.

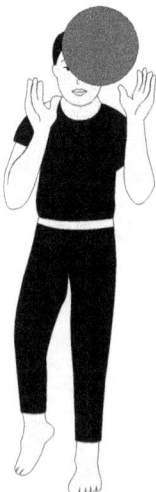

Action: Lift your right foot a few inches off the floor so that you are balancing on your left leg. See how long you can balance on your left leg, working up to at least 30 seconds. When you are able to balance for 30 seconds on each leg, try any of the following to make the exercise more challenging: close your eyes; lift your arms over your head or out to the side; do backwards shoulder circles; toss a ball up and down; lift your heel up and down; or stand on a pillow. When adding one of these challenges, try it first in a doorway or next to a chair for balance support.

Focus on: Keeping your body more or less vertical.

Note: To make this exercise more challenging, you can stand on an exercise balance pad or a bosu (both available for purchase online).

Stretching Exercises

These stretches are designed to increase the supply of oxygen and nerve impulses in your tissues by stretching the muscles of the back, neck, legs, shoulder and chest, as well as those of the arm. They will also increase circulation to the proximal muscles, so they will be ready to support the use of your arms. By increasing circulation and lengthening muscle fibers, stretching makes the tissues more pliable and less likely to tear. Since the front of a manual therapist's body tends to be overworked and tight, stretches are included to address that problem in particular.

Unlike strengthening exercises, stretching exercises can be done every day and even multiple times a day. Since one of the side benefits of stretching is increased blood flow to the muscles, you can refresh yourself by stretching at least one muscle group between each treatment session you give. When choosing which stretches to do on a given day, listen to your body and stretch the parts of your body that feel the most restricted or tight. Performing different stretches and mixing up the order can help keep your workout routine fresh and interesting.

As we age, we lose flexibility in our connective tissue, so stretching becomes even more important. Older practitioners will need to

Warming Up vs. Stretching

There is often confusion about the difference between warming up prior to work or sports participation and stretching exercises like those shown here. The purpose of warming up is to put your muscles and joints through their range of motion before you stress them in your work activities. This reduces your risk for injury.

Stretching, on the other hand, is designed to maintain and/or increase the length of your muscles, and is most effective when you have recently used your muscles to do an activity. Both warming up and stretching increase the blood flow to your muscles.

Because your muscle tissue is not as pliable first thing in the morning due to lack of adequate circulation, it is better to do specific stretching exercises later in the day or after some aerobic activity to rev up your circulation and make your tissues more pliable to get a more effective stretch.

hold a stretch for a longer period of time to get the same benefit. Start with a 30-second hold; if you are in your 40s, hold for 40 seconds. If you are in your 50s, hold for 50 seconds, and so on for a maximum hold of 60 seconds.

All of these stretches should be done within an active, pain-free range of motion. Go into each stretch slowly so you have time to pay attention to the sensations you feel. Practice slow, even breathing while you perform the stretches. Move into each position to the point where you begin to feel a good stretch. Do not try to force the stretch past this point. Do not bounce. Hold the stretch for 30 to 60 seconds. If you feel discomfort, you have stretched too much; back off a bit. If you feel sharp pain, you may be injured. Discontinue stretching until you have been evaluated by a healthcare professional for a possible injury.

WRIST FLEXOR STRETCH

Targets: The muscles on the palm (volar) side of your forearm that flex your wrist and fingers.

Starting Position: Sit or stand. Start with your right elbow bent to 90 degrees and your palm facing down.

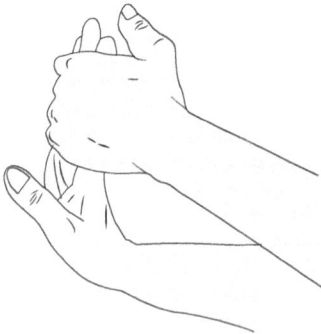

Stretch: Place your left hand on your right palm so that it covers the upper palm and at least the MCP and first IP joints of the fingers of the right hand. Bend your right wrist back so your fingers are pointing to the ceiling. If you feel a stretch in your forearm at this point, hold it there. If you need more of a stretch, slowly straighten your right elbow until you feel a stretch through your forearm. Do not stretch to the point of putting the wrist into hyperextension. Repeat with the left side.

Focus on: Keeping a steady pressure on your palm and fingers as you stretch, and keeping the wrist you are stretching in line with its forearm.

WRIST EXTENSOR STRETCH

Targets: The muscles on the dorsal side of your forearm that extend your wrist and fingers.

Starting Position: Sit or stand. Start with your right elbow bent to 90 degrees and your palm facing down.

Stretch: Use your right hand to bend your left wrist so your fingers are pointing to the floor. If you feel a stretch in your forearm at this point, hold it there. If you need more of a stretch, slowly straighten your right elbow until you feel a stretch through your forearm. Do not stretch to the point of putting the wrist into hyperflexion. Repeat with the left side.

Focus on: Keeping a steady pressure on your hand as you stretch, and keeping the wrist you are stretching in line with its forearm.

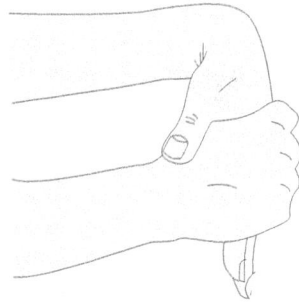

FINGER STRETCH

Targets: The intrinsic muscles in your hand.

Starting Position: Sit or stand. Start with your fingers straight and touching each other. You may rest your forearms on a table if that is more comfortable.

Stretch: Spread your fingers and thumb apart as wide as they will go, hold for a few seconds, then return to the start position. You can stretch the fingers of both hands at the same time.

Focus on: Keeping your wrist in a straight (neutral) position.

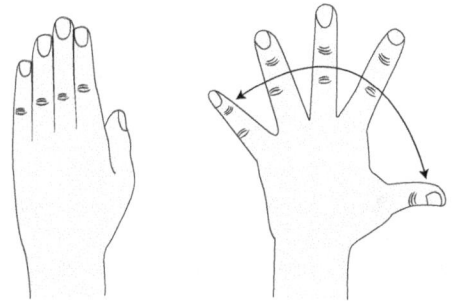

THUMB FLEXOR/ADDUCTOR STRETCH

Targets: The adductor pollicis and flexor pollicis muscles in your thumb.

Starting Position: Sit or stand. Place your right thumb on the dorsal side of your left thumb, for support, and your right fingers on the palm side of your thumb, near the tip.

Stretch: Stretch your left thumb away from the palm of your hand by press-

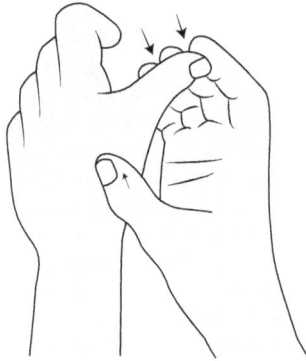

ing on your thumb with your fingers as you counterbalance with your right thumb. Keeping the thumb on the same plane as your palm will emphasize the adductors, as illustrated here; stretching more perpendicularly and dorsally will emphasize the flexors. Relax. Repeat with the other hand.

Focus on: Doing this stretch gently. It is very important to protect your CMC joint as you perform this stretch and keep your wrists straight.

THUMB OPPOSITION STRETCH

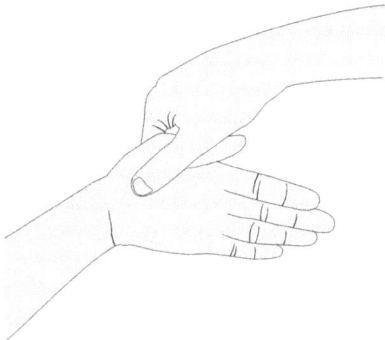

Targets: The opponens pollicis muscle in your thumb.

Starting Position: Sit with your left elbow flexed and your left forearm resting against your body. Grasp your left thumb with your right fingers and place your right thumb on the palmar side of your left thumb at your MP joint.

Stretch: Stretch your thumb by "rolling" the thenar eminence dorsally, away from the palm of your hand. Relax. Repeat with the other hand.

Focus on: Keeping your wrist straight as you stretch.

Neck Stretches

Manual therapists are susceptible to neck injury, often as a result of looking down at their clients for extended periods of time. By stretching and exercising the neck and shoulders, you can counteract the tension and strain put on your neck. You can also work on counteracting the internal rotation of the shoulders that often results from working with your arms in front of your body for long periods.

Starting Position: Sit in a chair, with your feet flat on the floor, your lower back supported, and your hands in your lap. Raise your chest so that your head and shoulders fall naturally into a neutral position. After each stretch you will return to a neutral head position, looking straight forward with your chin level. The neck is delicate and can be easily injured, so do each of these stretches in a slow, controlled manner. Do each stretch once to the left, then once to the right.

EAR TO SHOULDER

Targets: Lateral neck muscles including upper trapezius, scalenes and sternocleidomastoid.

Stretch: Keeping the shoulders level and facing squarely forward, bend your head to the right so the right ear moves toward the right shoulder. Hold where you begin to feel the stretch. Return your head slowly to neutral, then do the same motion to the left.

Focus on: Keeping your nose pointed straight ahead, not twisting the head.

NOTE: To increase this stretch, lay the hand of the arm on the same side on your bent head and let the weight of your hand pull the head a bit farther into the stretch.

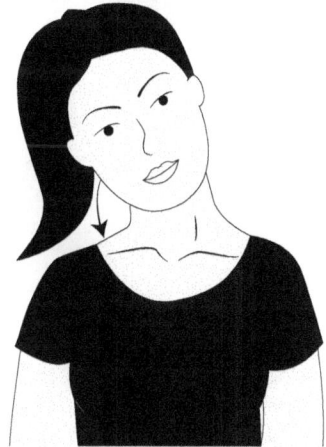

LOOK OVER YOUR SHOULDER

Targets: Neck rotator muscles including upper trapezius, longus colli and scalenes.

Stretch: Keeping the shoulders level and facing squarely forward, turn your head to the left as if you were trying to look over your left shoulder. Hold where you begin to feel the stretch. Return your head slowly to neutral, then do the same motion to the right.

Focus on: Keeping your chin tucked in, rather than jutting out, as you stretch.

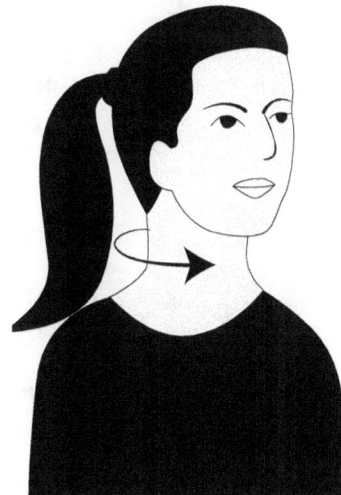

NECK NOD

Targets: Neck flexor and extensor muscles including sternocleidomastoid and splenius capitis.

Stretch: Start with your hands clasped behind your neck for gentle support. Slowly bend (nod) your head down toward the upper part of your chest until you feel the stretch. Return your head to neutral, then slowly extend your neck by moving your head backward to look at the ceiling until you feel a stretch or until your forehead is parallel with the ceiling. Hold, then return to neutral.

Focus on: Keeping your hands "soft."

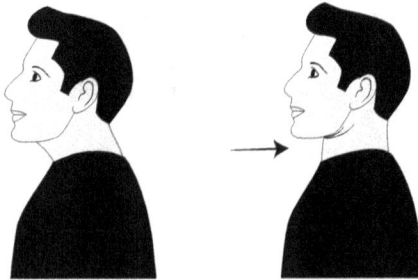

CHIN TUCK

Targets: Neck extensor muscles including splenius capitis and semispinalis capitis.

Stretch: Glide your head straight back on your neck as if you were creating a "double chin." Return to neutral. This stretch is especially good if you have a forward head posture.

Focus on: Keeping your chin level as you glide. It can be helpful to place two fingers on your chin to gently nudge it into retraction.

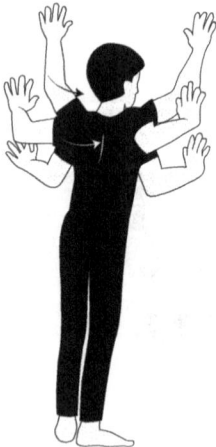

PECTORALIS MAJOR STRETCH—Corner Stretch

Targets: Pectoralis major muscle (upper fibers for higher positions, lower fibers for lower positions).

Starting Position: Stand in a corner of a room, facing the walls. Place your hands on either side of the walls, above your head.

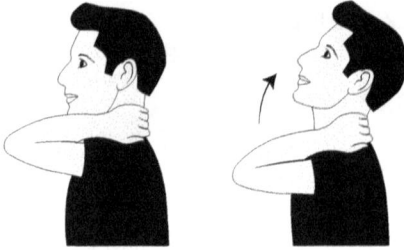

Stretch: Lean into the corner until you feel a stretch in the muscles in your upper front chest. Return to standing position. Repeat this stretch, lowering your hand position each time so you stretch different sections of your muscle.

Focus on: Standing no more than one step from the wall, because the farther you stand from the corner, the more your body weight has to be supported by your hands and wrists.

BACKWARDS SHOULDER CIRCLES

Targets: Upper and middle trapezius, rhomboids and levator scapulae.

Starting Position: Stand or sit on the edge of a chair with your arms relaxed at your sides.

Stretch: Shrug your shoulders up, then back, then down, then up again to where you started, making several large "circles" with both shoulders in a backwards direction.

Focus on: Although this is not technically a stretch, it is an excellent exercise if you tend to have a forward shoulder posture (common among manual therapists).

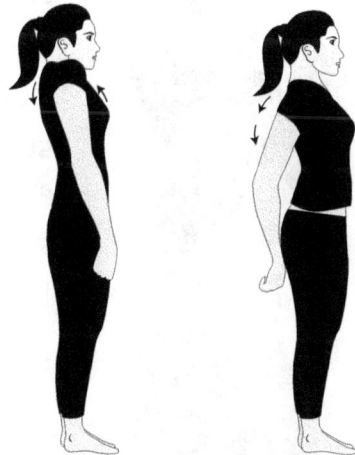

LATISSIMUS DORSI STRETCH

Targets: Shoulder adductor muscles including latissimus dorsi and teres major.

Starting Position: Lie supine with your body centered on your treatment table and your arms straight by your sides. Bend your knees to flatten your lower back against the table.

Stretch: With your thumb pointing up, raise your right arm straight up and over your head. The thumb will now be pointing at the floor. Keep your arm straight (do not bend your elbow). Hold your position when you feel the stretch in the latissimus muscle. Lower your arm and repeat with the other arm.

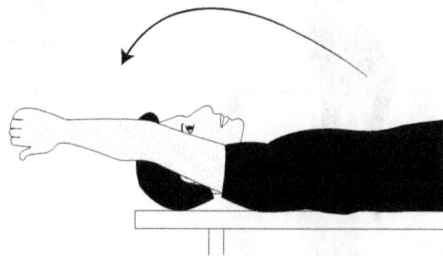

Focus on: Keeping your low- and mid-back flat against the table as you lift the arm. If your back starts to flex, return your arm to the point where your back is flat on the table again and hold the stretch at that point. You may also bend the opposite knee from the arm you're lifting to help keep your back flat against the table.

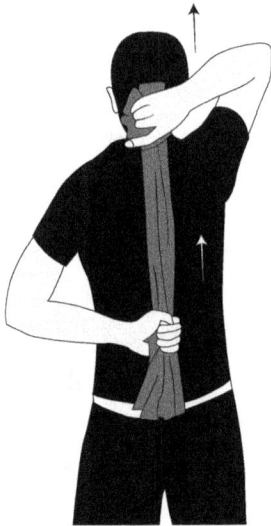

SHOULDER ROTATION STRETCH

Targets: Shoulder internal and external rotator muscles including infraspinatus and deltoids.

Starting Position: Stand with your right arm up and your left arm down, holding onto a towel behind your back.

Stretch: To stretch your right external rotators, pull down on the towel with your left hand. To stretch your left internal rotators, pull up on the towel with your right hand. Switch arms to stretch the shoulder muscles of the opposite side.

Focus on: Keeping the towel in a vertical orientation.

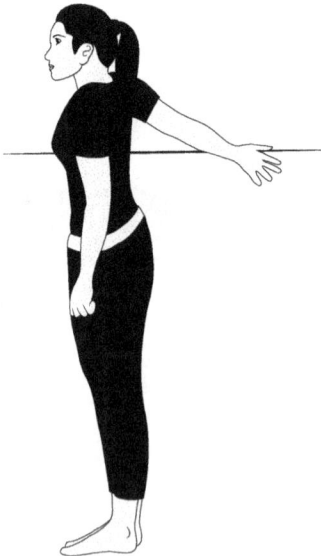

ARM AND SHOULDER STRETCH

Targets: Shoulder adductor, neck rotator and elbow flexor muscles, pectoralis major and minor.

Starting Position: Stand next to a wall with your right arm out to the side and your body slightly turned away from your arm.

Stretch: Gently twist your upper body away from the wall until you feel a stretch throughout your right arm. Hold. Switch sides to stretch your left arm and shoulder.

Focus on: Keeping your shoulder against the wall as you stretch and keeping your scapulae relaxed.

NOTE: Try moving your arm higher or lower on the wall to stretch different fibers of your upper extremity muscles.

PRONE PRESS-UP

Targets: Intervertebral discs and abdominal muscles.

Starting Position: Lie prone with your hands at shoulder height.

Stretch: Press up your upper body until your arms are straight, leaving your hips on the floor. Repeat this press-up 3 or 4 times, holding each one for 3 seconds at the top of the stretch. (Note: if your hands bother you when you perform this stretch, do the Standing Trunk Extension stretch below instead and omit this one.)

Focus on: Feeling the stretch in each part of your spine as you press up.

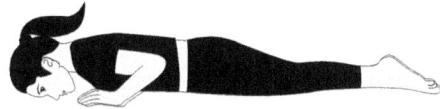

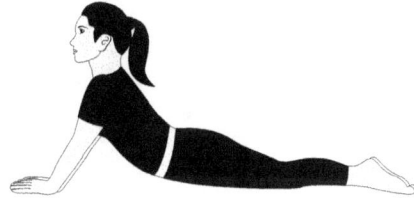

STANDING TRUNK EXTENSION

Targets: Intervertebral discs and abdominal muscles.

Starting Position: Stand with your feet shoulder-width apart and your hands on your hips.

Stretch: Bend backwards as far as is comfortable for you without fear of losing your balance. Repeat this stretch 2 or 3 times, holding each one for 3 seconds.

Focus on: Keeping your head level and looking straight ahead, not up toward the ceiling.

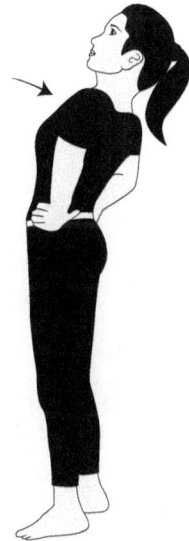

FOAM ROLLER UPPER BODY STRETCH

A foam roller is an excellent tool to assist you in stretching parts of your body in a different, but effective way. To stretch your upper back and shoulders, place the foam roller on the floor in a vertical orientation; lie down on it in a supine position with your head resting at one end and the base of your spine on the other end of the roller. Let your arms fall to the sides and feel the stretch in your pectoralis and arm muscles. Your feet should be on the floor so your knees should be bent, which will help you keep your back flat on the roller. Hold for as long as you are comfortable doing so.

HAMSTRING STRETCH

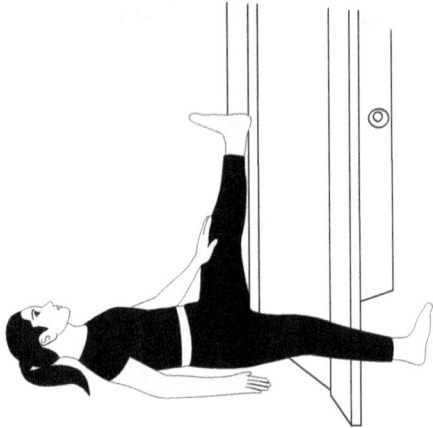

Targets: Medial and lateral hamstring muscles.

Starting Position: Lie on your back in a doorway with the door open. Lie close to the base of the doorframe, at a distance that allows you to comfortably lift up the leg closest to the doorframe and rest your heel against the frame. Let the other leg stick out through the open door.

Stretch: Scoot or slide your buttocks closer to the doorframe until you feel a stretch in the back of your leg. Repeat with the other leg.

Focus on: Keeping your knee straight and your foot relaxed.

NOTE: If you prefer, you can use a yoga stretching strap to do this hamstring stretch. Lying on the floor or a yoga mat, loop the end of the yoga strap around your foot, grab the loop above that one with your hand and, keeping it straight, lift your leg until you feel a stretch. Repeat on the opposite side. A yoga strap is a great tool for stretching. They come with an instruction manual including many different stretches—doing a quadriceps stretch would also be helpful for manual therapists.

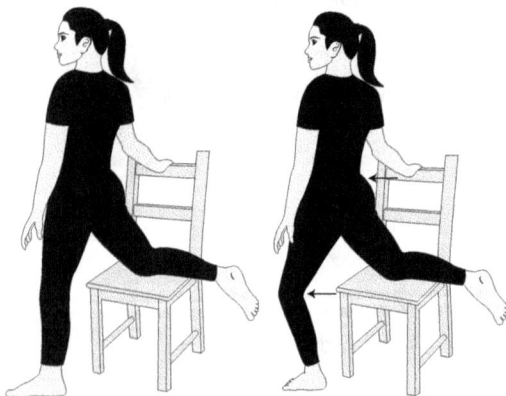

HIP FLEXOR STRETCH

Targets: Hip flexor muscles including quadriceps femoris, iliopsoas and tensor fasciae latae.

Starting Position: Stand next to a chair, placing your right lower leg and knee up on the chair with your foot hanging off the side. Hold the back of the chair with your hand for balance support.

Stretch: Lean forward with your right hip as you bend your standing leg until you feel a stretch in your upper thigh on your "chair" leg. Repeat with the other leg.

Focus on: Keeping your upper body upright as you stretch. Make sure your front knee does not extend farther than your front foot.

CALF STRETCH

Targets: Posterior calf muscles including gastrocnemium and soleus.

Starting Position: Stand facing a wall, with one leg in front of the other and the front knee bent. Place your hands on the wall in front of you for support.

Stretch: Keeping the back knee straight, lean into the wall until you feel a stretch in the back of your calf (gastrocnemius muscle). Hold. If you then slightly bend your back knee and "sink" a bit toward the floor, you will also stretch the soleus muscle in your calf. Repeat with the other leg.

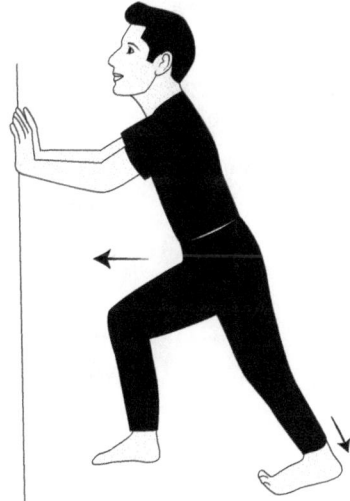

Focus on: Keeping your back toes pointed either straight ahead or slightly inwards.

NOTE: Another way to accomplish this stretch is by using a slant board pushed against a wall.

Body Awareness and Alignment

Movement training can be very helpful for manual therapists, particularly those who have not had experience with dance, sports or other disciplines that teach coordination, grace and ease of movement. Disciplines like The Feldenkrais Method®, Alexander Technique® and T'ai Chi can teach you how to move your body in ways that minimize musculoskeletal stress and encourage overall health. These practices emphasize moving the body as one unit, and using physical properties like weight and joint alignment to help create movement.

As you become stronger and more at ease with your body, you should notice a difference in the way you perform manual techniques. Your strokes should become more even and controlled. Your posture should improve, enabling you to use better body mechanics as you work. You should have greater energy and endurance, and feel less tired at the end of your workday. A feeling of physical strength and grace can be very empowering, and can add a new dimension to your work, both emotionally and physically.

Taking the time to exercise and stretch also gives you a wonderful opportunity to develop your body awareness. Your workout sessions are a time to get in touch with your body, to see how it responds to limited amounts of stress in a controlled situation. As you exercise, focus on your physical reactions to the stretches and exercises you do. Notice which parts of your body move easily, and which feel restricted. Note which muscle groups are tight and which are looser, which are weak and which are stronger.

After you have been working out for a while, you will become intimately familiar with your own body. This increased body awareness will enable you to notice your reactions to the physical work you do as a therapist and empathize with your clients' response to your work.

Organizing Your Workouts

Count on working out at least 3 times a week, using a combination of strengthening exercises, stretches and aerobic conditioning. You will need a day of rest between specific strengthening exercises, but you should be doing some stretching exercises every day and some cardiovascular exercise on most days. The recommended amount of cardio is 150 minutes per week: however, you can break that up into 15 minutes at a time if needed. The benefit will be the same. Add in balance and breathing exercises for a well-rounded, comprehensive conditioning program.

Follow these guidelines as you put together your workout schedule:

- Fit your workouts into your lifestyle. It will be easier for you to stay active if you exercise at convenient times of the day and choose activities you enjoy.
- Do at least 5 minutes of low-intensity aerobic exercise just prior to strength training to warm up your muscles, whether you will be doing only strengthening exercises or combining strengthening and aerobic work in your workout session.
- Don't do strength-training exercises for the same muscle group(s) on consecutive days. (Note: aerobic, balance, breathing and flexibility exercises are fine to do every day.)

- Stretching will be most effective if done after strength training or after aerobic conditioning. Try to schedule stretching later in the day when circulation is better and muscle tissues are more pliable.
- If you stop working out for a period of time and then start again, back off from the level you were at when you stopped and gradually increase back to that level to reduce your risk of injury.
- Your heart rate tends to stay elevated longer if you do aerobic work right before strength training, thus maximizing your cardiovascular benefit.
- Balance exercises are a nice way to finish an exercise session; do a few before starting your stretches.

Suggested Workout Schedules and Sample Routines

The sample weekly routines on the following pages are meant to be a guide; modify them as needed to fit your lifestyle and schedule. During the "stretch" sections, concentrate on the parts of your body that feel particularly tight. If you are pressed for time, think about ways you can add exercises into your daily routine: take the stairs rather than the elevator; park farther away from your home or work; talk with friends or listen to music on a hands-free phone while you walk or ride a stationary bike; or stretch your forearm muscles while you wait in line.

FOR THE BEGINNER: If you are considering a career as a manual therapist and are not physically active right now, you will need to improve your strength and conditioning before you start a training program such as massage or physical therapy school. Do at least 30 minutes of aerobics, 6 days a week, starting slowly and working up to a moderate level of intensity (breathing hard, but still able to carry on a conversation).

Concentrate on the core and arm exercises in this chapter, being careful to leave a day between strengthening a given muscle group. Start with the minimum amount of weight. As a beginner, it is even more important to stretch the same muscles you are strengthening at the end of the session, so you don't lose flexibility as you gain strength. Ideally, you should allow 3 months to improve your overall condition before you begin your professional training.

Workday Warm-Up Routine

Here is a 10–15 minute routine you can do before you start your workday or during a break in the day. If you have limited time between treatment sessions, you can do the breathing exercises at the same time as one of the stretches.

- Brisk walk for 5 minutes
- Pectoralis Major Corner Stretch
- Calf Stretch
- Thumb Opposition Stretch
- Lateral Rib Expansion Breathing Exercise
- Wrist Flexor Stretch
- Wrist Extensor Stretch

If you have only 5–10 minutes, do the following:

- Pectoralis Major Corner Stretch
- Thumb Opposition Stretch
- Wrist Flexor Stretch
- Wrist Extensor Stretch

Fitting Quick Breaks Into Your Workday or During a Treatment Session

Taking small breaks to consciously relax and stretch during your workday is important for preventing injury, even if it's only for a minute or two at a time.

- Three deep, slow breaths while you apply oil to your hands (encourage the client to breath with you, to help them relax and reduce muscle guarding)
- Calf stretch as you lean in to apply pressure to the client's back or thigh muscles
- Shoulder rolls as you move from standing to sitting
- Neck stretches and a corner stretch as you wait for your next client or patient.

End-of-Day Routine

Before you leave work, relax with a few stretches:

- Backwards Shoulder Circles
- Thumb Adductor/Flexor Stretch

Workout Schedule Option 1

MONDAY	TUESDAY	WEDNESDAY	THURSDAY	FRIDAY	SATURDAY	SUNDAY
Walk 30 min.	Swim 40 min.	Walk 50 min.		Walk 30 min.	Bike ride 1 hr.	Run 30 min.
Stretch	Stretch	Stretch	Stretch	Stretch	Stretch	Stretch
Leg and trunk strengthening		Leg and trunk strengthening		Leg and trunk strengthening		
	Balance exercises		Balance exercises		Balance exercises	
Breathing exercises	Breathing exercises	Breathing exercises	Breathing exercises	Breathing exercises	Breathing exercises	Breathing exercises
	Arm diagonals		Arm diagonals			

Workout Schedule Option 2

MONDAY	TUESDAY	WEDNESDAY	THURSDAY	FRIDAY	SATURDAY	SUNDAY
Breathing exercises	Balance exercises			Swim 30 min.		Walk 10 min.
Run 20 min.					X-country skiing	
Stretch	Stationary bike 40 min.		Pilates class	Leg and trunk strengthening	Balance exercises	Stretch
		Stretch		Stretch		
Walk 10 min.	Leg and trunk strengthening	Breathing exercises	Arm diagonals			Stationary bike 20 min.
Arm diagonals	Stretch	Walk 30 min.			Stretch	

Workout Schedule Option 3

MONDAY	TUESDAY	WEDNESDAY	THURSDAY	FRIDAY	SATURDAY	SUNDAY
T'ai Chi class	Breathing exercises	Balance exercises	Walk 10 min.		Arm diagonals	
Stretch			Leg and trunk strengthening		Stretch	Breathing exercises
	Run 40 min.		Stretch	Stationary bike 30 min.		Stretch
	Arm diagonals	Stretch		Stretch		
Balance exercises			Walk 20 min.		Ballroom dancing	
Walk 30 min.	Stretch	Water aerobics 30 min.	Balance exercises			

211

- Arm Stretch
- Standing Trunk Extension

Try starting the day with a home routine which will also help with your self-care and injury prevention. See Appendix C for a detailed Morning Self-Care Routine.

Frequently Asked Questions About Conditioning

Q: **Aren't push-ups a good exercise for core strengthening? Why aren't they listed?**

A: Push-ups are excellent for core strengthening. They are not listed here because the hand position for push-ups can place quite a bit of stress on your shoulders, wrists and forearms. Since these are over-worked and over-stressed areas for manual therapists, other exercises were chosen.

Q: **I'm just starting out in my profession and I'm worried that I don't have sufficient strength in my hands and arms. What exercises do you recommend for me?**

A: In addition to the two arm-strengthening exercises listed in this chapter (which are important in preparing for hands-on work), you can try some of the following:

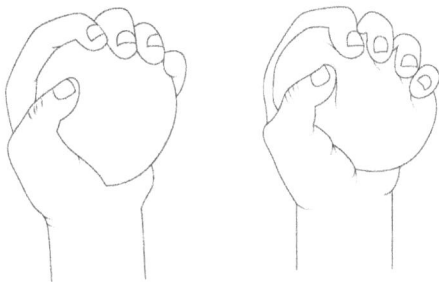

SQUEEZING A BALL

Starting Position: Hold a medium firm ball or some medium level exercise putty in the palm of your hand. Keep your wrist in a neutral position (neither flexed nor extended).

Action: Squeeze the ball or putty with all of your fingers and thumb, hold for 3 to 5 seconds, then relax. Work up to 3 sets of 8 to 12 repetitions, every other day. Using a variety of objects to squeeze will help you develop strength throughout the range of motion of the finger flexors.

WRIST CURLS—Flexion

Starting Position: Sit at a table or desk so the dorsal surface of your forearm is supported and your hand is off the edge, palm facing up.

Action: Hold a weight and slowly curl your wrist up, making sure your forearm stays on the table. Hold for 3 to 5 seconds, then relax. Work up to 3 sets of 8 to 12 repetitions, every other day. Start with a 1-pound (0.5 KG) weight; when you can do 3 sets of 12 repetitions with 1 pound, increase the weight but decrease the number of repetitions until you can again do 3 sets of 12 repetitions.

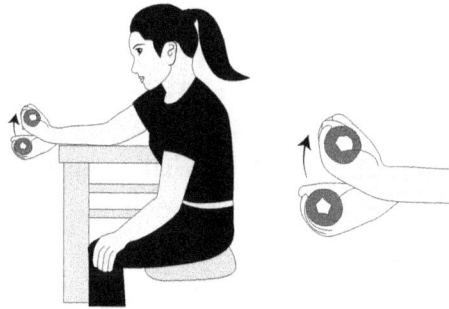

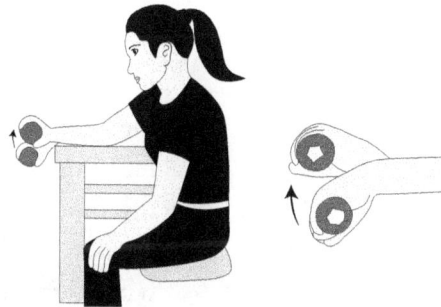

WRIST CURLS—Extension

Starting Position: Sit at a table or desk so that the volar surface of your forearm is supported and your hand is off the edge, palm facing down.

Action: Hold a weight and slowly curl your wrist up, making sure your forearm stays on the table. Hold for 3 to 5 seconds, then relax. Work up to 3 sets of 8 to 12 repetitions, every other day. Start with a 1-pound (0.5 KG) weight; when you can do 3 sets of 12 repetitions with 1 pound, increase the weight but decrease the number of repetitions until you can again do 3 sets of 12 repetitions.

Q: Why don't you have more leg strengthening exercises listed?

A: The cardiovascular (aerobic) exercise you do as part of your conditioning program will give you much of the leg strength you'll need for your work as a manual therapist. The muscles on the sides of your hips, which help to stabilize your core muscles when you work, don't get as much strengthening with aerobic exercise, so exercises for those muscles are specifically mentioned in this chapter. If you want to add more strengthening exercises for your core or hips in your personal routine, you certainly can.

Q: **What about Pilates classes? Or yoga? Wouldn't those be good for me?**

A: Yes, those are both good activities that emphasize breath control and body awareness, although in different ways. Use common sense in classes; some yoga positions can be stressful to hands or knees, and most Pilates classes assume a moderate to high level of overall fitness.

Q: **Should I join a gym? If I do, what equipment should I use?**

A: You don't have to join a gym to get and keep your body in shape for your work. All the exercises listed here can be done on your own. That said, many people find motivation in a gym environment. If joining a gym helps you to exercise on a regular basis, then do it. Some gyms offer group classes in body awareness techniques like yoga and T'ai Chi. If you want to use the weight machines at a gym, schedule an individual session with a gym employee to show you how to use the equipment. Bring this book with you and try to do the same or similar strengthening exercises on the gym equipment. Be careful to minimize hand and wrist effort, including the gripping often required for shoulder or trunk equipment.

Q: **What if I'm over 40 and just starting out?**

A: The musculoskeletal aging process varies greatly from any given individual to another. In general, as we age, our muscles lose strength, our joints become less lubricated and our connective tissue loses elasticity. If you are beginning a career as a manual therapist after age 40, it will be particularly important to condition your body (including strength, balance, aerobic conditioning, flexibility, etc.) prior to starting your professional education program.

Q: **I tried the Leg Lowering exercise and it made my back hurt. Should I continue doing the exercise?**

A: No. Stop doing any of the specific strengthening exercises if they cause pain. For this particular exercise, be sure to keep the stable leg bent with the foot on the floor or table. If doing the exercise still makes your back hurt, you may want to consult with a physical therapist or exercise physiologist to see how you can modify the exercise so it is comfortable for you, or substitute another exercise that strengthens the same group of muscles without discomfort.

1. Matthew Solan, Executive Editor, *Harvard Health Publications*, "Do More for Your Core," https://www.health.harvard.edu/staying-healthy/do-more-for-your-core, November 1, 2023.

12

Planning for Career Longevity

You have seen how important it is to take your musculoskeletal health and overall well-being into consideration as you schedule and perform your treatment sessions each day and each week. In addition to thinking about your health in the short-term, you should also consider how you can stay healthy throughout your career. Statistics indicate a high rate of injury among experienced manual therapists due to the ongoing physical demands of their work over time.

Another reality is that we are all getting older. Aging brings with it a gradual decline in strength and flexibility, and a slowing of the body's ability to recover from physical exertion. As our physical capabilities decline, the likelihood that the demands of our work will exceed them increases.

Now is the time to prepare yourself for these eventualities by considering your career choices while they are still options rather than necessities. For example, you could use your continuing education as an opportunity to learn modalities or subspecialties that place less stress on your body. Lymphatic drainage, craniosacral technique, gait analysis, positional release, and other modalities that do not require maintaining pressure or making forceful, repetitive motions can give your hands and arms a break and also add to the range of tools you have available to treat clients. One of the benefits of incorporating new modalities into your practice is learning the assessment techniques that they use. A good client assessment will allow you to focus your treatments, so you can achieve the same or better results with less work.

You can also consider changing your work environment to a specialty area that requires less intensive hands-on treatment of clients; for example, a PT might move out of an intensive rehabilitation or pediatric specialty to work in a sports medicine clinic where a greater percentage of time is spent on exercise instruction and administrative duties. A massage therapist could choose to work in a spa where part of each session would be spent on treatments like hot stone therapy or aromatherapy that do not require hand force or repetitive motion. Massage therapists can also incorporate less hand-intensive modalities, like lymphatic drainage, breathwork or Reiki, into their work, at least for a portion of each session. Training in these other modalities is readily available and can help you earn continuing education credits. With, rehabilitation therapists can incorporate more ergonomic assessment and discussion into their work with clients. Refer to page 71 for a discussion of ergonomic assessment techniques you can use in your practice.

Finally, you can consider expanding your career beyond treatment as a way of reducing your dependence on hands-on work for your income. You could teach at a school training program or in continuing education workshops, or work in management or administration of a group practice, clinic or spa. As an experienced practitioner, you have more to offer than just a pair of hands, and the sooner your career goals reflect that, the longer your career may last. Many healthcare professionals transition from direct client care to teaching, research or administrative functions as they progress in their careers, both to take advantage of possibly higher-paying positions that their years of experience can help them attain, and to spend less time doing physically demanding work.

Massage therapists may consider working part time in another career. Keeping massage as a part-time career can give you something to fall back on if you are physically unable to keep up with the rigors of a full-time massage practice. Keeping another part-time job can be a good approach when you are just starting to practice, since it allows you to build your practice slowly and not take on too much hands-on work all at once. Just be sure that your second job does not involve some of the same risk factors that are present in massage work.

Research and writing in your field of specialization offer additional career opportunities while reducing your dependence on hands-on treatment work for your livelihood. Think about your career not just in terms of what you know now, but as a constantly progressing process of learning new skills and increasing your breadth of knowledge. Doing so will give you more flexibility and options in your career, with the eventual goal of moving away from doing primarily hands-on treatment.

Being Prepared for the Possibility of Injury

Even if you use the best possible ergonomics and body mechanics, and pay strict attention to your general health and personal fitness, the physical demands of your work can still result in injury. We talked earlier about developing an "injury prevention mindset." Being prepared for injury, if it occurs, is a part of that mindset. It makes sense to consider in advance how you might deal with the impact of an injury on your finances, and how you would go about treating injury. Preparing for the possibility of injury can help you avoid anxiety and give you the peace of mind that comes with knowing you are financially covered and know how to treat an injury that may occur, so you can resume a normal work and home life.

Looking Into Workers' Compensation, Health Insurance and Disability Insurance

Consider in practical terms what would happen if you develop an MSD as a result of your work. A serious tendon injury could require radically cutting back on the number of clients you see. A case of carpal tunnel syndrome could require surgery followed by several months or more of recovery time. Think about your current situation: would you be able to go 1 or 2 months without working and still pay the bills?

One of the best things you can do to protect yourself is to carry enough insurance. With a good health insurance plan, you will more likely seek treatment early on if you develop symptoms. If you work for someone else, you may be covered by workers' compensation insurance that will cover the cost of medical treatments and lost wages if your condition is work-related. You may be able to buy workers' compensation insurance for yourself even if you are self-employed, although some private insurers may not offer coverage for sole proprietors. In the U.S., every state has a mechanism for purchasing workers' compensation if you are turned down by private insurers. Contact the state agency responsible for administering insurance in your state for more information. In many other countries, injuries are covered under the healthcare system regardless of where they occur, so workers' compensation insurance may not be necessary. It pays to take the time now, while you are still healthy, to find out how treatment of work-related injuries is covered in your area, and to what extent. You may need a supplemental or umbrella insurance policy to cover costs your other plans do not cover. One important form of insurance that many people neglect to carry is long-term disability insurance, which can help make up for lost income if your injuries are not covered by workers' compensation or other insurance.

> **Recognizing symptoms and getting treatment early is the best way to keep a minor condition from turning into a serious or chronic condition.**

Knowing How to Recognize Symptoms and Treat Injury if it Occurs

Do you know how to differentiate between the aches and pains we all occasionally experience, and symptoms that require medical attention? If you start to develop worrisome symptoms, are you aware of the different treatment methods that are available and effective for MSDs? Even if you have no symptoms at this point, it is critical to know the specific types of injuries that manual therapists are prone to, and understand what causes them. By doing so, you can recognize them and pay attention to them early in their onset when treatment will be more effective and recovery will be easier.

In Part Three, you will learn how the body responds to injury and find specific guidelines to help you recognize symptoms that require treatment. You will also find numerous treatment options that have been proven to be effective in treating MSDS, including allopathic, holistic and complementary approaches. Armed with this knowledge, you will be able to make informed decisions about your care that can help you heal more quickly and minimize disruption to your work and personal life. Most importantly, you will learn the importance of seeking appropriate treatment as early as possible, to keep minor injuries from turning into serious or chronic conditions. This knowledge will also be very valuable in your work with clients or patients.

PART THREE

Injury, Treatment and Recovery

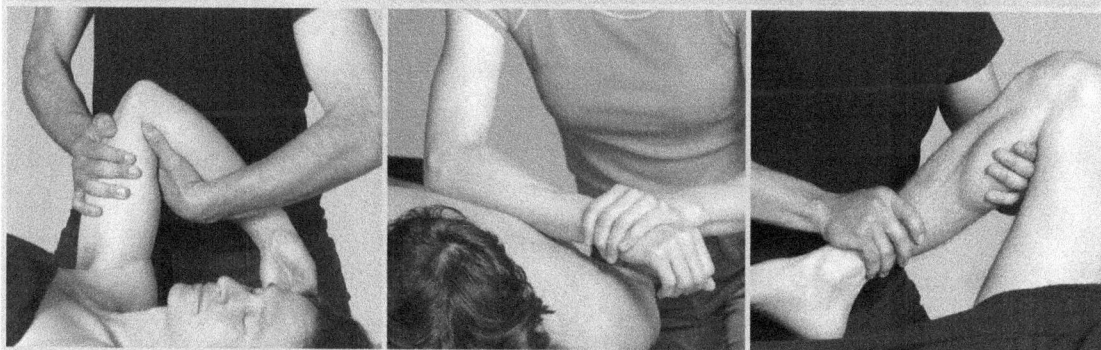

Injury, Treatment and Recovery

Given the number of risk factors that manual therapists face in their work, some practitioners will inevitably become injured. Despite your best efforts to use the principles of ergonomics, good body mechanics and the other self-care tactics mentioned thus far in this book to protect yourself from injury, you may still develop an MSD. The ups and downs of life and the pressures of work can interfere with even the best intentions and most careful surveillance of lifestyle and work habits. In day-to-day life, it is very difficult to avoid every risk factor and perfectly control your work environment, schedule and activities away from work to stay 100 percent symptom-free. Life intervenes, things come up, distractions disturb your awareness, and you can end up with enough exposure to risk factors that symptoms or injury can become an issue.

Symptoms can arise at any stage of your career, including during your initial training. Recognizing, assessing and treating symptoms early and appropriately is your best strategy for staying on your career path with the least amount of disturbance or lost time.

13

Understanding and Responding to Symptoms

If you start to experience symptoms, review the principles of ergonomics in Part Two to make sure you are following them as much as possible to avoid causing any further damage. Renew your focus on good body mechanics and pay particular attention to how you schedule clients and how many demanding treatments you give each day. Getting enough rest will be even more important as you focus on healing. You may find that being more vigilant with these prevention methods will resolve your symptoms. Hopefully you will be able to identify a specific cause for your symptoms, and addressing that cause will alleviate those symptoms. For example, you may find that using certain techniques aggravates your symptoms, and finding alternatives for those techniques makes the symptoms go away.

It is also possible that you have been following all of the injury prevention principles correctly, but some non-modifiable risk factor, such as a prior injury or a genetic predisposition, has caught up with you and is causing new symptoms. Whatever the cause, it is important to keep using the injury prevention techniques you have already learned, to help keep your symptoms from progressing.

It is equally important to seek treatment from a qualified healthcare provider if your symptoms continue or progress, since putting off treatment can lead to a chronic and potentially debilitating injury. It can be difficult to determine when medical treatment is necessary, and many people hesitate too long before seeking evaluation by a healthcare provider. In this chapter, you will learn how to differentiate between the minor symptoms practitioners can experience in a physically demanding job, and more significant symptoms that indicate that you may be injured. You will also see how these symptoms arise when body tissues are stressed to the point of injury.

Recognizing the Typical Symptoms of MSDs

Musculoskeletal symptoms can range from the mild aches and pains that can accompany any physical effort to more serious symptoms that indicate a disorder requiring medical evaluation. The key to protecting your health is to remain attentive to your body, so you can recognize the very first signals it sends you, even if they are mild. These signals can indicate that something is wrong and needs to be addressed, whether that means changing your techniques, getting more rest, scheduling fewer clients or seeking treatment. By learning to notice symptoms early on, you can take the necessary steps to address the causes and treat symptoms quickly and effectively. Responding early and appropriately when symptoms arise is the best way to avoid chronic or serious injuries later on.

There are a number and variety of symptoms that can accompany MSDs. You may feel a sense of heaviness or fullness in the injured area. Tingling sensations are typically a sign of nerve impingement, and can sometimes progress to a sensation of burning pain and even numbness. Muscular symptoms resulting from injury range from weakness and fatigue to guarding, hypertonicity and spasm.

The most common symptom by far of MSDs is pain. It is often the first symptom that arises when injury occurs. Much of this chapter is devoted to a discussion of pain and its underlying mechanisms, to help you better understand this fundamental and sometimes complex symptom.

Table 6. Typical Symptoms of MSDs

- Muscular weakness or fatigue
- Muscle spasm, hypertonicity or guarding
- Hypersensitivity (e.g., being touched on the affected area is unpleasant or intolerable)
- Pain during activity, for example, when working or performing everyday activities (e.g., opening a jar, door knob, car window or faucet, brushing your hair or teeth, writing)
- Pain following activity
- Tenderness
- Aches
- Burning
- Twinges
- Crepitation (popping or clicking when joints move)

- Numbness and tingling (paresthesias), especially when it awakens you at night
- Feeling of fullness, heaviness or congestion of the affected area
- Involuntary or uncoordinated movements (e.g., tremors, twitches, tics, sudden flexion/extension of fingers, inability to hold objects steady in the hand)
- Clumsiness
- Loss of function
- Hesitation to use a limb to hold objects or support your weight
- Protecting the affected area, holding it stiffly
- The realization that the affected part of the body has not felt "normal" for a while, like it did previously

You may have some of these symptoms and not others; some symptoms may go away or may be replaced by new symptoms. The presence of even a single symptom is reason enough for concern. Certain symptoms can indicate a serious injury, illness or condition, and should be evaluated and treated without delay.

Table 7. Symptoms That Require Prompt Medical Attention

- Intense pain*
- Any pain that lasts more than 7 days in a row
- Inflammation that is moderate to severe, or lasts more than five days in a row
- Unexplained clumsiness, weakness or loss of function*
- Any numbness, tingling or burning sensations

- Pain that radiates down an arm or leg
- Symptoms that wake you up at night or prevent you from falling asleep
- Changes in skin color
- Symptoms that change or worsen rather than improving.
- New bowel/bladder dysfunction*

*Requires immediate medical attention

Everyone has musculoskeletal symptoms from time to time. The most common are the aches and pains that can develop after a hard workout, too much yard work, a bad night's sleep, or a taxing day at work. As you get older, you may find that the aches and pains begin a little sooner, and take a little longer to go away. Many people lump aches and pains together without making a distinction between them. Understanding what causes these symptoms will help you distinguish whether they are the aches that come about as a side effect of hard work, or the pain that can be an early indicator of injury.

Muscle Aches

Muscle aches during activity are caused by a build-up of metabolites, or byproducts of the process the body uses to liberate stored energy from glycogen (the substance that gives us energy to do work). All muscle contractions produce metabolites, but higher levels are produced when glycogen is metabolized anaerobically (without oxygen) during static loading or very high-effort activities. In these situations, metabolites are produced at a higher rate than they can be flushed out.

The most talked-about metabolite, especially among athletes, is lactic acid, but lactic acid is not the culprit in burning sensations or muscle fatigue as once thought. It is the build-up of other metabolites, which are acidic in nature, that causes the burning sensation, and it is likely that excess calcium leaking into the muscle causes fatigue. Fatigue is a protective mechanism that prevents the muscle from damaging itself. Gently moving the affected area, massaging the area, or doing whole-body aerobic activities such as walking will typically help flush out metabolites and allow the muscles to replenish energy stores.

Lactic acid has also been found blameless for muscle aches that occur a day or two after a hard effort, sometimes referred to as delayed onset muscle soreness (DOMS). These aches may be caused by a combination of localized chemical changes caused by other metabolites and, most significantly, minor damage to muscle tissue (microtrauma). Microtrauma initiates an inflammatory response as part of the body's repair process. It is thought that the greatest amount of microtrauma occurs during eccentric contractions, when a muscle is lengthening while under tension. It is still unclear if warming up before a hard effort or stretching afterwards can prevent DOMS. Muscle aches are only a concern if they become chronic. Repeated microtrauma through overuse of the same muscle-tendon units can produce trigger points, and eventually can cause physiological changes that result in injury.

As a general rule, you should not be experiencing DOMS as a result of your manual treatment work. While you may occasionally push yourself too hard at work and end up feeling muscle soreness a day or two later, you should not be working to this extent on a regular basis. If you find that you experience DOMS frequently or regularly, you will need to figure out what aspect of your work—scheduling, techniques, postures, etc.—is causing your soreness. Ongoing muscle soreness should be a warning sign that you are doing something that could eventually lead to injury.

Pain

Any discussion of injury and symptoms will necessarily include some discussion about pain, since it is the most common indicator of injury. Pain is a remarkably complex issue. The word "pain" can be a very subjective term that is used differently by different people. Pain is defined by the International Association for the Study of Pain (IASP) as, "An unpleasant sensory and emotional experience associated with, or resembling that associated with, actual or potential tissue damage."[1] The fact that their definition includes both a sensory and emotional component reflects recent scientific findings related to how our bodies process pain signals.

Causes of pain can be mechanical (compression, inflammation, cuts, punctures), thermal (heat or cold), electrical, chemical (external, such as a caustic chemical, or internal, such as acidic metabolites), and visceral (heart attack, kidney disease). Pain signals are transmitted by small-diameter nerve fibers known as nociceptors, which are different from the larger-diameter fibers used to carry motor signals to the muscles. The pain signals that these small nerve fibers carry help to protect you from injury, such as when you pull your finger back from a hot stove. Nociceptors in an injured area often develop an increased sensitivity due to local chemical changes. For example, a person who has been badly sunburned will experience very high levels of pain from even a light touch. This hypersensitivity to pain protects us from further injury while the body heals.

Repeated stimulation of any nerve enhances the pathway for nerve signals. If an area suffers trauma repeatedly, such as a muscle that is overused or a tendon that is stressed to the point of damage, the nociceptors in that area may become hypersensitive. This hypersensitivity may be accompanied by additional chemical changes that tend to maintain this level of hypersensitivity, even though the initial symptoms are gone and any injury has healed. This phenomenon may be part of the formation of trigger points in muscle and fascia and could be a precursor to chronic pain syndromes.

Be sure to pay attention to any pain you may feel. Some types of pain signal that you need to seek medical treatment; other types of pain indicate that something you are doing needs to be changed so it doesn't lead to injury. Generally speaking, pain that is short-lived, steadily diminishing and does not greatly limit function or prevent a good night's sleep does not necessarily indicate you are injured. Pain associated with injury requiring ongoing medical treatment is often stronger, may go on for weeks, months or even years, and can come and go, stay constant or increase over time. It is also more likely to restrict movement, cause weakness and atrophy of muscles and disrupt sleep. Pain that does not resolve quickly, even if it is not constant but lasts over a period of weeks or longer, is always a sign that treatment is necessary.

During your recovery from injury you may feel some pain during treatment. A certain amount of pain is normal under these circumstances and generally does not indicate further injury. Tissues and nerve endings can be irritated as part of the therapeutic process, and putting up with some pain may be necessary in order to make progress.

Bear in mind that the experience of pain is subjective, and each person will have a different idea of when their pain becomes an indication of injury. With increased understanding and awareness of your body, you will start to get a sense of the point at which your aches and pains become the early signals of injury. This awareness will help you evaluate the symptoms you are experiencing and decide whether you need to rest, adjust your activity or seek treatment. If you have any doubt about whether the pain you feel is a cause for concern, it is always best to err on the side of caution and start addressing the causes of your pain as quickly as possible. You run the risk of developing a chronic pain condition if you allow your pain to continue untreated.

Chronic Pain, Non-Specific Pain and Pain Memory

Trauma and pain do not always go hand in hand. Trauma can occur without pain: when intervertebral discs are damaged, for example, you may not feel pain because the discs are poorly innervated. It is fairly common for diagnostic tests to show bulging discs in patients who have come in for unrelated conditions, and who report no pain in the area. While pain is usually a good initial indicator of trauma and the threat of injury, disorders in nerve cell function can result in pain that is not related to injury. In fact, chronic pain is often non-specific, meaning that upon examination, the initial injury is no longer present, but the nociceptors remain overly sensitive to stimulation.

A phenomenon known as "pain memory" may be the reason. Pain memory occurs when repeated peripheral pain signals result in physiological changes at the level of the spinal cord. These physiological changes can actually perpetuate the sensation of pain long after the original trauma has healed. Intense pain from surgery or severe acute trauma, for example, may cause these physiological changes to the spinal cord in as little as 24 hours.[2] However, there is some evidence that lower levels of pain, if sustained over a period of weeks or months, may also cause pain memory to develop. Pain memory probably originated as an important survival mechanism, so that even the simplest of organisms could remember to avoid potentially harmful exposures. In humans, it has the unfortunate effect of causing chronic pain.

Chronic pain can cause muscle guarding, changes in movement patterns, muscle imbalances, postural issues and psychological distress. The nervous system is closely tied to the immune system, and long-term pain and stress may result in suppressed immune function. The body's ability to heal itself can be diminished, making re-injury more likely. This truly vicious cycle can continue until the hypersensitivity to pain is addressed and the emotional and psychological aspects of chronic pain are dealt with.

The Emotional Side of Pain

We saw previously that pain signals travel from nociceptors to the spinal cord to the part of the brain that can trigger a reflex, such as when you pull your hand away from a hot stove. Those same signals also reach the emotional and decision-making centers of the brain. The fact that pain signals travel to multiple centers in the brain is probably related to the importance of responding to pain as a survival mechanism.

Pain causes a number of different emotional reactions. People who experience acute pain can become fearful and anxious about the pain they feel and its causes. Think of a small child who learns to fear the doctor after her first inoculation. People with acute injuries can develop a fear-avoidance response to pain, which leads them to cease all activity that causes discomfort. While this reaction may help the healing process in the short-term, over the long run the lack of activity will actually slow healing, causing atrophy and loss of range of motion. The fear-avoidance response is especially common in people suffering from low back pain. In response, the medical community has stopped recommending bed rest for this type of injury and instead recommends a return to normal activities as soon as possible.

Chronic pain is associated with anxiety and depression, as well as stress and PTSD.[3] Depressed people tend to take a more passive approach to dealing with pain, either by not seeking treatment or not taking an active role in treatment. They may look instead for a healthcare practitioner to "fix them," which in turn can cause disappointment and feelings of hopelessness when a cure is not simple and immediate. These experiences can further intensify the emotional reaction to pain, causing cycles of chronic pain and depression that are often referred to as a "downward spiral."

The Cognitive Side of Pain

In addition to traveling to the pain and emotional centers in the brain, pain signals also travel to the decision-making center. There is some evidence that chronic pain affects our ability to make decisions, and may even result in diminished cognitive abilities, such as memory problems, later in life. When decision-making abilities are impaired, it may be the emotional side that takes over when dealing with chronic pain.

Never Ignore Pain

As you can see, pain is not always easy to define or understand. Pain can be a serious symptom, and in most cases, the presence of pain should compel you to avoid activities that may be causing it. Symptoms of pain may also require attention from a healthcare provider. At the same time, some pain may not be related to an injury and avoiding activity may actually be detrimental to the healing process.

With any pain you feel, regardless of the cause, one thing is certain: you must pay attention to the pain and address it in some way. Without evaluation from a qualified healthcare provider, you cannot determine whether the pain you feel is non-specific or due to an identifiable underlying cause that could be an MSD, but could also be a disease. Some diseases mimic musculoskeletal pain, and only a qualified healthcare practitioner can distinguish between the two and make an accurate diagnosis. Even non-specific pain requires treatment to avoid the difficult, long-term emotional and cognitive effects of chronic pain.

When Symptoms Signal Injury

If your symptoms are mild, and you can identify the causes of the symptoms and change those factors in your practice, your body mechanics or your activities outside of work, you may find that your symptoms diminish and eventually go away. If your symptoms are more intense, or if they do not go away even after you make these adjustments, it is time to start considering the possibility that you may be injured.

The word "injury" is another term that can be hard to define. Perhaps the most practical way to define injury is *any physical damage to the body that impedes or prevents you from performing normal or desired activities.* You could consider that you are injured and in need of medical attention when your symptoms have reached the point that any of the following statements applies to you:

- You are no longer able to perform the number of treatments or the types of treatments that you usually do as part of your studies or practice without experiencing symptoms.
- You are limited in any of the normal tasks of daily living (e.g., cooking, cleaning, dressing and personal hygiene)
- You are no longer able to participate in a sport or hobby you enjoy
- You are unable to get a good night's sleep.

Symptoms associated with MSDs are the result of a series of specific physiological changes that occur in the musculoskeletal system in reaction to the risk factors you saw in Part One. Learning more about the physiology of injury will help you better understand your symptoms and the treatment you will receive, and also inform your work as a healthcare professional with your own clients or patients.

How Your Body Responds to Injury

In Part One, you learned about the weak links, those parts of the body that are most vulnerable to injury. You saw how these weak links could be stressed by exposure to risk factors at work and off work, resulting in trauma to tissues. Every type of tissue in the body has a limit of how much stress it can tolerate and still remain structurally sound and function normally. Beyond that limit, the tissue will break down or fail. When the exposure to risk factors exceeds that threshold, the trauma—either sudden or repeated—overwhelms the body's ability to heal. The result is injury.

The importance of early treatment becomes very clear when you look at the complex physiological processes that are set in motion if you wait too long to seek treatment. Damage to the musculoskeletal tissues happens more quickly and insidiously than most people imagine. While most of this damage is reversible, some cumulative injuries can become severe and long-lasting, and even cause permanent disability.

> Damage to the musculoskeletal tissues happens more quickly and insidiously than most people imagine.

Exposure to Risk Factors and Microtrauma

In Chapter 3 you saw that your risk of injury is modified by four important variables—the frequency, intensity and duration of exposure, and exposure to several risk factors at the same time (see page 42). The frequency with which you perform a repetitive motion, the intensity of force you use or how awkward your postures are, and the number of hours per day and per week that you perform manual techniques will all determine your risk of injury. Enough exposure to risk factors singly and in combination can create small tears (microtrauma) in the muscle, tendon and ligament fibers.

Injury and Re-Injury

Microtrauma in itself does not necessarily lead to injury. In fact, it is a normal part of the wear and tear the musculoskeletal system undergoes every day. A key factor that keeps microtrauma from progressing to injury is healing time. Body builders, for example, are instructed to take a day off between weight-lifting sessions to give their muscles time to rest and heal the microtrauma that is part of building muscle. The amount of healing time needed will vary from individual to individual.

> **How Minor Injuries Turn into Major Ones**
>
> - Ignoring your symptoms
> - Delaying treatment
> - Trying to "work through the pain"
> - Not attempting to figure out what is causing your symptoms
> - Continuing to do the same technique or carry the same workload that is causing your symptoms
> - Not taking time off to recover
> - Making no changes to hobbies, sports and activities around the house that aggravate your symptoms.

Repetition of trauma without adequate healing time, often referred to as "overuse," has a cumulative effect on the muscles and connective tissues. This phenomenon is often referred to as the "injury/re-injury cycle": you injure yourself, and before your body has had the time to heal, you re-injure yourself. As the trauma continues unabated, the injury becomes more and more severe.

When microtrauma has progressed to a sufficient level to trigger pain receptors or cause other reactions in the tissues, your body

> **By the time you feel pain or other symptoms, your tissues may already be damaged.**

starts sending you signals in the form of symptoms. By the time you are able to perceive these symptoms, tissue damage may have already started taking place. Catching the injury early, stopping the trauma and getting appropriate treatment can prevent the vicious cycles of inflammation, injury and re-injury.

Inflammation

Recent research has shown that inflammation is more likely to be present in sudden onset and/or acute injury rather than the types of slow-onset MSDs that manual therapists experience. For example, examination of painful tendon tissues has not shown inflammation to be present. For this reason, we now refer to tendon injury as "tendinosis" instead of "tendinitis" (-"itis" refers to inflammation).[4]

With sudden or acute trauma, the body responds to injury on several levels. On the most basic level, trauma damages or kills the cells that make up the muscle, fascia, tendon, ligament and other connective tissues. As the cell membrane loses its integrity, the contents of the cell spill out into the surrounding tissue. The contents include chemical mediators that trigger the body's inflammatory response, producing acute inflammation in reaction to this local injury. The inflammatory process sets in motion a series of changes in the tissues as the body begins to repair itself and replace damaged tissue with healthy tissue.

There are five principal signs of an inflammatory process:

1. Swelling (edema)
2. Heat
3. Redness
4. Pain
5. Loss of function

One, several or all of these signs may be present at any one time. In addition to these signs of inflammation, you may experience other symptoms associated with acute musculoskeletal injury (see Table 7 on page 225). Any of these symptoms, alone or in combination, can be an indication that tissue damage has occurred.

If there is adequate blood flow in the affected area, the chemical mediators and dead cell tissue are washed away and flushed into the general circulation. Anything that impedes circulation to the area (static loading, tension, lack of physical conditioning, smoking, etc.) will impede healing in the area.

Scar Tissue

Tissue repair begins early in this process. Muscle and connective tissue cells are permanent cells that, once destroyed, cannot regenerate. Instead, the body replaces the original tissue with connective tissue patches, in the process we know as scarring. Scar tissue serves to reattach the portions of tissue that have been torn. New scar tissue is weak; with time and relief from the trauma that caused the injury, the scar tissue becomes a structural part of the soft tissues around it.

Given enough time and rest, the inflammation will dissipate, an appropriate amount of scar tissue will form, and the area will heal properly. Although scar tissue is permanent, it does not have to greatly affect function. However, if you re-injure the affected area, you will cause the formation of additional scar tissue. If the injury is to a tendon, degeneration of the collagen fibers, another type of fiber in the tendon, may occur. This process can result in chronic tendinosis. Repeated trauma without adequate healing time can cause this process to progress to the point of chronic tendinopathy, referred to as tendinosis.

Considering the nature of muscle and tendon tissue, this overabundance of scar tissue can cause as many problems as it was originally intended to fix. Muscles and tendons are made up of fibers that run parallel to each other. This formation allows them to slide smoothly over each other as the muscle or tendon contracts. Scar tissue, on the other hand, tends to form unevenly, with collagen fibers crisscrossing each other in every direction, forming a messy patch of fibers lying on top of each other. Massage or gentle mobilization techniques can help straighten out these fibers in young scar tissue, helping to restore movement and relieve pain.

Scar tissue also lacks the functionality of the tissue it replaces. A section of muscle that has been replaced with scar tissue will not be able to contract and will not be as flexible as it was before, making it weaker and more easily re-injured. If the injured area is immobilized or left untreated, the scar tissue can cause the muscle fibers to adhere to each other, binding them together so they are no longer lying parallel to each other. Once the fibers no longer move independently of each other, even a small effort that normally would recruit a smaller number of fibers will involve the entire group of fibers that are stuck together. What would ordinarily be a simple and efficient muscle contraction will now require a larger effort, leading to fatigue. Where the adhesions form, the fibers no longer glide smoothly over each other, but instead rub against each other, creating friction that can cause inflammation and degeneration of collagen fibers, another essential component of tendon tissue.

Scar tissue can also tack the muscle to other structures in the area, such as bone. As the scar tissue matures, it hardens, stiffens and contracts, forming hard masses or adhesions at the points where the fibers have stuck together. If hard, stiff scar tissue forms near or at a joint, it can interfere with the movement of the bones at that joint. Many manual therapists address adhesions and scar tissue masses as part of their daily work. These are sites of past injury from overuse or other trauma.

Repeated microtrauma from overuse and the resulting development of scar tissue and degeneration of collagen fibers are common to many musculoskeletal disorders throughout the body. While the location and type of tissue being affected varies, the underlying causes are very often similar. You will find more detailed information about specific MSDs in Chapter 14.

Seeking Evaluation of Your Symptoms

No one wants to be an alarmist or run to the doctor for every small ache and pain. On the other hand, you have seen that manual therapists have a high incidence of injury. Once the injury process begins, changes occur in the tissues that can cause long-term symptoms and even disability. It is clear that seeking appropriate healthcare evaluation and treatment for symptoms at the first suspicion of injury is the best way to keep them from turning into chronic injuries with long-term consequences.

Evaluation and treatment need to be both early and appropriate:

Table 8. Symptoms That Can Signal a More Serious Condition

Certain symptoms that sometimes accompany musculoskeletal pain can be an indication of a more serious condition. These symptoms include:

- Unexplained weight loss
- Frequent feelings of fatigue
- Abdominal pain
- Loss of bowel or bladder control
- Nausea
- Headaches
- Dizziness
- Fever
- Depression

Three Good Reasons to Seek Early Treatment for Symptoms

1. A better medical outcome

Early treatment for musculoskeletal disorders is more likely to result in a successful outcome with few or no chronic symptoms. Treatment early in the progression of a disorder tends to be conservative: moist heat, ice, rest and over-the-counter pain medications are commonly recommended early treatments. Later treatments can be more invasive, possibly involving injections, surgery and extensive rehabilitation. Pain is more likely to become chronic if left untreated for longer periods of time, and may be accompanied by loss of range of motion and weakness. Conditions involving impingement or entrapment of nerves, such as thoracic outlet syndrome or carpal tunnel syndrome, can be particularly difficult to resolve. If left untreated for too long, these conditions can cause permanent nerve damage and muscle tissue atrophy.

2. A better emotional outcome

Chronic pain is very frequently associated with anxiety, depression and fear/avoidance of any activity that causes or aggravates symptoms. These emotions can prevent an injured person from seeking appropriate treatment, and may lead to continuing cycles of pain, depression and feelings of helplessness. Seeking early treatment, on the other hand, is the first step in taking an active role in the prevention of chronic physical and emotional symptoms.

3. A better financial outcome

Early treatment leads to less time off work, both in the short and long term, and smaller medical bills. Instead of months off to recover from a serious injury, early treatment may only require a few weeks off, or none at all. You may only be required to reduce the amount of hands-on work you do for a short time, while making changes to work techniques to avoid aggravating symptoms. Early, conservative treatment is not only more likely to be effective, it is also much less expensive than the more intensive treatments that chronic conditions can require.

early because there will be a much better chance of a positive outcome, and appropriate because there are many possible causes for pain and other symptoms, and musculoskeletal injury is only one of them. For example, the most common causes of back pain are muscle strains and ligament sprains. Less common but more serious conditions can also cause low back pain, such as degenerative disc disease, arthritis of the spine, kidney disorders, abdominal aortic aneurysm and tumors. Seeing a healthcare professional who is qualified to recognize a wide range of disorders and diseases and do differential diagnosis is an essential part of your treatment. He or she will be able to rule out these conditions, or give you an appropriate referral for treatment if such a condition is present. You will learn more about making appropriate healthcare choices to evaluate and treat symptoms and injury in Chapter 15.

For all of these reasons, it is always better to be cautious and seek advice from a healthcare professional sooner rather than later. Even low-level, bothersome symptoms are a good reason to get an evaluation. If you have any doubt or question about any symptoms you are experiencing, there is no reason to wait and worry. Seeking early treatment will reduce your anxiety about your symptoms, helping you to heal more quickly. It is better to be told that nothing is wrong and relieve your anxiety than to wait too long and develop an acute condition that could become chronic.

1. International Association for the Study of Pain Website, https://www.iasp-pain.org/publications/iasp-news/iasp-announces-revised-definition-of-pain/
2. Sun-Ok Song and Daniel B. Carr, "Pain and Memory," *International Association for the Study of Pain: Pain Clinical Updates*, 1999; 7(1): 1–7.
3. Arne Wynds, Jolien Hendrix, Astrid Lahousse, et al, "The Biology of Stress Intolerance in Patients with Chronic Pain—State of the Art and Future Directions," *Journal of Clinical Medicine*, 2023 Mar 14;12(6):2245. doi: 10.3390/jcm12062245
4. Evelyn Bass, LMT, "Tendinopathy: Why the Difference Between Tendinitis and Tendinosis Matters," Massage Department, Southeast Medical Clinic, Juneau, Alaska, USA

14

Injuries Common to
Manual Therapists

M usculoskeletal disorders are very common in the general population, and are second only to colds and flu as a cause of missed work days. A description of all of the musculoskeletal disorders that exist would fill an entire book by itself. This chapter concentrates on those specific conditions that are most common among manual therapists.

Any of the soft tissues in the body—muscles, fascia, tendons, ligaments, cartilage, bursae, nerves and blood vessels—can be subject to injury due to overloading of the tissue. In the general population, upper extremity MSDs tend to be relatively uncommon, while back injury is very common. As you saw in Chapter 2, eight out of 10 American adults will experience back pain at some point in their lives.

The hand-intensive nature of manual practice produces a higher than average occurrence of upper extremity MSDs among manual therapists. Risk factors like bending and lifting also cause back and neck injury among these practitioners. Manual therapists most frequently report injury to their thumbs, shoulders, lower back, neck and upper back and wrists: the weak links you saw in Chapter 2. In this section, you will learn about specific injuries to those weak links and how they occur, categorized by the type of body tissue involved in each injury.

The injury descriptions here are intended to provide an overview of each disorder and make you aware of their typical symptoms. If you are experiencing any of these symptoms, try to avoid the temptation to assume that you are suffering from that disorder. Instead, read on to Chapter 15 where you will learn how to find an appropriate healthcare provider who can give you more detailed information and evaluate your symptoms.

Muscle and Fascia Injury

Injury to muscle and the surrounding fascia can occur suddenly, such as a muscle strain or tear from a fall, or due to repeated contraction, especially when the muscle is fatigued. Muscles rarely become injured as a result of a single contraction. A muscle is more likely to fail, or lose the ability to contract, before it can generate enough force to tear itself. As you saw earlier, small tears in muscle and fascia tend to repair themselves with scar tissue, which can lead to adhesions, affecting range of motion and the overall condition of the muscle. Small tears can also lead to pain and eventually tissue degeneration, which further limit muscle function. Pain in muscle and fascia can sometimes become chronic, persisting well after the initial injury has healed.

Fascial scar tissue and adhesions can have effects well beyond the site of injury. Fascia is continuous throughout the body, connecting muscles, tendons, bones, skin and even internal organs. The tendon that connects a muscle to a bone does not stop at the musculotendinous junction, but instead continues as the fascia that separates the muscle into compartments, bundles or individual fibers, re-assembling at the other end to form another tendon. The connective tissue of the tendons is also continuous with the periosteum that surrounds the bone, which then connects to other tendons and myofascia. Anything that limits the movement of fascia in one part of the body is going to restrict movement across that entire segment, if not that entire side of the body.

Fascial changes can go beyond the connective tissue itself. Contained within the fascia is a viscous substance called "ground substance." This material actually has the ability to change its state in response to stress, both physical and emotional, going from fluid to gel-like to solid. This ability to change state may be part of a protective mechanism, as it helps fascia to stiffen, taking some of the load off of muscle tissues. This same mechanism that is protective with short-term, infrequent exposure to stress can have negative consequences with repeated exposures. Overexposure to physical and emotional stressors can result in constriction, stiffening and drying of fascia. This process can create adhesions in the fascia, and these adhesions can stick to muscle fibers and other structures.

Myofascial Pain Syndrome

The main feature of myofascial pain syndrome is the presence of trigger points. Trigger points are small, highly localized points of hypersensitive tissue located within a taut band of muscle. Trigger points are characterized by the fact that they elicit referred pain. For example, trigger points in the upper trapezius may cause headaches.

There are a number of theories about the physiological basis of trigger points. One theory asserts that they are caused by localized biochemical changes and ischemia when a muscle is overloaded. Supporting this theory is the fact that trigger points are common among sedentary workers, due to the static loading of sitting for long periods and the resulting ischemia in their muscles. They are also common among workers whose jobs require repetitive motions, since the level of activity in a particular muscle group may overwhelm the local circulatory system's ability to replenish electrolytes and flush out metabolites. Another theory is that small muscle spindles are over-activated by adrenaline during physically and emotionally stressful events and these overactive muscle spindle fibers are what comprise the taut bands of muscle. Bands in which trigger points occur are not tight due to typical causes, such as spasms or voluntary muscle contraction. In this way, trigger points may also develop as a secondary effect of an acute injury.

There are two types of trigger points: those that are "active" and painful at rest, and those that are "latent" and only painful if pressure is applied on the point. Both active and latent trigger points can cause muscle hypertonicity, loss of range of motion and muscle weakness. All of these could also be predisposing factors for MSDs, especially if the repetitive motions or static loading that caused them continue. Secondary or satellite trigger points can also exist, producing referred pain in muscle fibers that have been asked to compensate for the loss of function in the muscle fibers where the primary trigger points are located. As trigger points spread in this way, they can cause pain and limit function in an entire quadrant, or even half of the body, significantly altering posture and movement. Widespread trigger points throughout the body are the primary symptom of myofascial pain syndrome. Diagnosis of myofascial pain syndrome can be difficult, since symptoms of this syndrome can mimic other disorders, such as bursitis or tendinosis.

Trigger points can be effectively treated with direct pressure, which first causes ischemia, and then, when pressure is reduced, an increase in localized blood flow. Other treatments include injection of a mild, local analgesic, "dry needling" (similar to acupuncture), or spraying with a coolant and stretching the affected muscle fibers. Each of these techniques is more effective if followed by passive and then active stretching of the muscle fibers.

Fibromyalgia

Unlike myofascial pain syndrome, the painful points of fibromyalgia do not typically cause referred pain. They are termed "tender points" to distinguish them from trigger points. While fibromyalgia can involve widespread pain, the tender points can also be localized to a particular area. Fibromyalgia has a number of other associated symptoms, which do not occur in all patients. The more common symptoms are fatigue, sleep disturbances, depression and gastrointestinal disorders. There are several more specific disease processes that have similar symptoms, so it is critical to rule out other conditions before beginning any type of treatment.

There are a number of theories about what causes fibromyalgia, but none are conclusive at this time. Because fibromyalgia is still somewhat controversial and poorly understood, it has proven difficult to treat. Massage may relieve the tender points, and gentle exercise has been shown to reduce symptoms. Memory foam mattresses are sometimes recommended to relieve pressure points and help reduce sleep disturbances. Biofeedback, counseling to deal with the emotional issues related to chronic pain, and stress reduction techniques may also be effective in lessening the perception of pain. Several medications now exist that are purported to relieve symptoms.

Tension Neck Syndrome

The neck is a common site of MSDs. These disorders are often caused by working with your neck in flexion for long periods, like looking down at your clients or patients throughout the day. Doing this fatigues the posterior neck muscles. Try to trust your palpation skills so you only need to look down occasionally at your hands or your client/patient. Working with the shoulders hunched or rounded with your head jutted forward fatigues those same muscles. These working positions cause tension in the upper trapezius as well as in other smaller muscles in the upper back and neck. Symptoms resulting from these postures are associated with a common condition known as tension neck syndrome. The symptoms of this injury include chronically tight and sore muscles in the neck and upper

---

Perpetuating Factors for Myofascial Pain

There are a number of factors that may cause myofascial trigger points, or the tender points associated with fibromyalgia, to linger in the tissues. These factors include:

- Poor posture
- Repetitive motion
- Static loading
- Muscle overuse or disuse
- Structural abnormalities (e.g., asymmetry)
- Hypermobility

- Thyroid disorders
- Chronic infections or allergies
- Poor nutrition
- Non-restorative sleep
- Depression/anxiety
- Obesity
- Smoking

Many of these factors are the same as the risk factors for musculoskeletal disorders you saw in Part One. The steps that are used to prevent MSDs from happening in the first place can also help ensure that these disorders do not recur later on.

shoulders, often combined with pain, burning sensations and reduced range of motion. Other symptoms of tension neck syndrome can include fatigue of the neck muscles and headaches or migraines due to referred pain. Neck pain and loss of range of motion can lead to awkward postures, for example, if the sufferer twists at the torso to make up for the lack of ability to turn the head. Fortunately, symptoms of tension neck syndrome have been shown to respond well to ergonomic adjustments in the workplace, manual therapy and improved body mechanics and posture.

Non-Specific Back Pain

While lower back conditions such as disc bulges, disc herniations, sciatica and micro-fractures do cause pain, most low back pain is considered non-specific and unrelated to these pathologies. X-rays and MRIs reveal no obvious physical disorder, yet the sensation of pain is real and sometimes debilitating. Non-specific low back pain can start as a simple muscle strain, but it frequently becomes chronic, possibly due to hypersensitivity of nociceptors (see page 227). Non-specific back pain is poorly understood, and therefore difficult to treat.

Low Back Pain and Injury

The most prevalent MSD in the general population is low back pain. Approximately 80 percent of adults experience at least one episode of low back pain in their lifetimes, and about half of them will go on to have at least one more episode. Low back pain is one of the main reasons that clients seek treatment by manual therapists; it is also a significant risk among healthcare professionals themselves.

Most low back pain is minor, caused by simple muscle strains. These strains are caused either by sudden trauma, such as slipping and falling, or more gradually, by repeatedly working in awkward postures such as bending and twisting, or from heavy, frequent or awkward lifting. In fact, many people in the general population above the age of 30 have degenerative disc bulges without any functional impairment or pain. More serious injuries can result from long-term exposures to these risk factors, or sudden, intensive exposure to a major risk factor like heavy lifting.

Tendon and Tendon Sheath Injury

Tendons are very strong strands of tissue that connect muscle to bone. They are particularly vulnerable to injury by the nature of their structure and the way they function. Tendons attach muscle to bone near the fulcrum of movement (the joint), so they are under great mechanical stress. If this stress is amplified by repetitive or improper use, the tendons are likely to tear. Tendons are also poorly vascularized and poorly innervated. Damage to a tendon is not felt as quickly as to a muscle, so tears may happen before the nervous system can respond and ease tension on the tendon. With their limited blood supply, tendons heal slowly from microtrauma. There is potential for uneven scarring and the subsequent formation of adhesions, as well as degeneration of collagen fibers. Since the scar tissue is weaker than the original tissue, the chances of re-injury are increased.

Overuse Syndrome

The term "overuse syndrome" is alternately used to refer to a group of disorders, such as tendonosis and carpal tunnel syndrome, and to a particular condition, first described in musicians, that arises when the upper limbs are overused during hand-intensive activities. In overuse syndrome, signs and symptoms are present that do not match any specific disorders. While achiness, diffuse pain or feelings of fullness may be present in the area, typically in muscle tissue, there is no inflammation, tendon damage, or other easily detectable sign that would lead to a specific diagnosis.

While overuse syndrome was the most commonly listed diagnosed condition in the survey of American massage therapists cited in Chapter 1, it was not clear from the survey whether these therapists were given this diagnosis by their healthcare providers in place of a more specific diagnosis, or if an actual diagnosis of overuse syndrome was made because no objective signs of a more specific condition were present.

If you are diagnosed as having overuse syndrome, it is best to clarify the diagnosis with the healthcare provider to see if a more specific condition could be causing the symptoms. At this point, you may need to consult a more specialized practitioner who can make a more specific diagnosis and help create an effective treatment plan.

Treatment for overuse syndromes typically includes resting the affected area, using hydrotherapy, receiving manual therapy and taking pain relieving medication. Once the symptoms are under control, the injured area can be stretched and strengthened by a rehabilitation professional as part of an exercise program that is carefully monitored to avoid recreating the original symptoms. Finding effective treatments may be a process of trial and error, particularly if you are not able to get a more specific diagnosis. Be sure also to reduce or eliminate any activities that aggravate or perpetuate the symptoms.

In areas where the tendons pass through other structures, such as at the carpal tunnel in the wrist, the tendons are surrounded by sheaths of connective tissue that are lubricated with synovial fluid. When tendons are overused, particularly in awkward postures or when pulled repeatedly across bony structures, they can become injured. Injury in tendons or tendon sheaths is referred to as tendinosis or tendinopathy. With the exception of sudden, traumatic injury, tendon injuries are usually not felt until they have become chronic. They involve degenerative changes to the tendon without the presence of inflammation.[1] These are the tendon MSDs usually experienced by manual therapists.

The characteristic symptom of tendon and tendon sheath injury is localized pain ranging from mild to severe. Pain generally is worse with movement and better with rest. The more tendon fibers are torn, and the more degeneration of collagen fibers has progressed, the worse the pain and the longer the healing time will be. Pain may radiate distally or proximally. Some loss of function may occur as a result of edema, pain or build-up of scar tissue in a tendon. For example, if tendinopathy occurs at a joint, it may restrict movement. Tendinopathy can become chronic tendonosis without adequate healing time, or if the injury/re-injury cycle is set in motion.

Wrist Tendinopathies

Irritation and cumulative microtrauma and degeneration of the tendons and tendon sheaths of the fingers and wrists are common among people whose work involves repetitive hand and wrist motions combined with force, a group that includes most manual therapists. Injury can occur to the flexor tendons that pass through the carpal tunnel, to the extensor tendons that pass over the carpal bones at the back of the wrist, or to the flexor and extensor tendons that attach at the wrist itself. Common symptoms of wrist injuries include stiffness and pain when the tendons are under tension, such as when gripping or applying pressure with your palm, or when they are moving through the sheaths, such as when bending your wrists or moving your fingers.

Rotator Cuff Injuries

The muscle-tendon group that makes up the rotator cuff of the shoulder is a frequent site of tendonosis. Particularly at risk are the supraspinatus muscle and its tendon, which can be damaged through repeated contact with the acromion during shoulder flexion and abduction. The most common symptom of a rotator cuff injury is pain in the shoulder that is often worse at night. Injury to a rotator cuff tendon combined with bursitis is referred to as impingement syndrome. Referred pain from trigger points and injuries in the neck is commonly felt in the shoulder, which can make diagnosis of conditions in this area difficult.

Epicondylosis

Repeatedly gripping or making wrist motions while pronating or supinating the forearm with the addition of force, or repeatedly carrying heavy objects in one hand can damage the flexor or extensor tendons near their respective epicondyles of the elbows. Pain, accompanied by damage to the tendons at the epicondyles is often mislabeled "epicondylitis," even though this condition very often presents without inflammation, and is therefore technically a tendonosis condition. Epicondylosis is also associated with the practice of certain sports, so lateral epicondylosis is commonly termed "tennis elbow," while medial epicondylosis is known as "golfer's elbow."

De Quervain's Tendinopathy

Damage to the tendon sheaths at the base of the thumb commonly occurs from repetitive gripping, causing a condition known as "de Quervain's tenosynovitis," although it is really a tendinosis of that tendon sheath. This degeneration keeps the tendons from moving smoothly through the sheaths, causing pain and discomfort while gripping, supinating or pronating the hand, or when making a fist. Bending the wrists while gripping increases the risk of developing this disorder.

De Quervain's is a good example of a disorder for which strength is not necessarily a protective factor. In fact, men with greater grip strength may be more likely to suffer from this disorder than other men, because they tend to overuse this strength in their work. Splinting the thumb may help to rest the muscle-tendon units involved. This type of tendinosis is becoming common among people who use their thumbs repetitively to type text messages on their cell phones as they are holding the weight of the cell phone, gripping it with bent wrists. This injury has become known colloquially as "texter's thumb."

Intersection Syndrome

Tendons lying a few inches proximal to the dorsal wrist can become irritated as they cross under muscles that abduct and extend the thumb. Repeated wrist extension causes the radial wrist extensor tendons to rub against the thumb abductor and extensor muscles, causing inflammation and pain. This condition is called intersection syndrome, because it occurs where the two sets of structures meet. It is also sometimes referred to as "squeakers" due to a squeaking noise during combined movements of the wrist and thumb.

Trigger Finger

Repeated and sustained tendon movements through a synovial sheath while in an awkward posture, such as using a single finger to squeeze the trigger on a powered massage tool, can result in formation of a nodule on the tendon. As the tendon attempts to slide through the sheath, the nodule can get stuck, limiting movement of that finger and creating a condition commonly known as trigger finger. Thickening of the tendon or its sheath (hypertrophy) from inflammation or repetitive use creates even more rubbing and friction, and additional injury.

Bursa Injury

In areas near joints where tendons cross over bones and ligaments, the tendons are protected by fluid-filled sacs known as bursae. While there are many bursae throughout the body, the ones most commonly injured are in the shoulder, elbow, hip and knee—areas of the body that move the most. Injury to a bursa is correctly called bursitis, because inflammation has been shown to play a role in it. The pain and inflammation from bursitis can be difficult to differentiate from other conditions, such as tendonitis. In fact, these disorders often co-exist.

Shoulder Bursitis

In the shoulder, tendons are pulled across the bursa during arm movements, particularly when the shoulder is flexed and abducted (a very common working position for manual therapists). Repeated irritation of the bursa from tendon friction, particularly in an awkward posture, can cause inflammation and pain. When this inflammation reaches the stage of injury, it is called bursitis. Bursitis is more likely to occur if inflammation is already present in the area, or if there are long-term postural problems that increase pressure on a bursa.

Bursitis in Other Locations

In the knees, inflammation of the prepatellar bursae can be caused by the prolonged or repeated pressure of kneeling. Bursae in the elbows can become inflamed in a similar manner by leaning on them.

Ligament, Cartilage and Joint Injury

Ligaments are fibrous tissues that connect bone to bone. Tears to ligament fibers that are large enough to cause inflammation and pain are called sprains. While sprains most often occur from a sudden traumatic event, such as a fall, they can also occur from repetitive loading. Working while bending forward at the waist, for example, can eventually sprain the paraspinal ligaments. Injuries to ligaments along the spine are considered to be one of the most common causes of low back pain.

Since ligaments have a poor blood supply, they are slow to heal and prone to re-injury. A mild overstretch resulting in a minor tear of a ligament will cause some pain and inflammation; this will often heal slowly but with no lasting damage. Repeated damage can cause adhesions or tight ligaments, which can greatly reduce range of motion and cause conditions like "frozen shoulder."

The incomplete healing that can occur with larger tears can lead to joint instability and eventually to joint injury. Most of your joints are held in place by a combination of muscles, tendons and ligaments. If you subject a part of your body to more force than the muscles in the area can counteract, or if you sustain that force to the point where muscles fatigue, your muscles will no longer be able to help stabilize the joint. The forces will then transfer to the ligaments, which may not be strong enough to take the load without damage.

Repeated trauma can also weaken ligaments over time, making them lax and creating instability in the joints they cross. Joint instability in turn can cause the bones in the joints to move out of their normal positions, creating spots of increased pressure on the cartilage that separates and cushions the articulations between bones. Cartilage tends to thin as we age anyway, and this increased pressure can cause additional wear to the joint. Scar tissue in the joint cavity can also change the synovial fluid there. The amount of fluid decreases and the remaining fluid become less viscous, so it provides less cushioning to the bones of the joint. All of these processes can eventually result in painful bone-on-bone contact, osteoarthritis and degenerative joint disease (DJD).

IP, MCP and CMC Joint Osteoarthritis

The weight-bearing joints of the body, such as the hips and knees, are a common osteoarthritis location in the general population. Manual therapists often turn their fingers into weight-bearing joints, repeatedly using straight or extended fingers to apply direct downward pressure. In fact, lining up the joints and leaning in with body weight is often recommended as part of good body mechanics. While lining up the finger and thumb joints can reduce the amount of muscular effort required to hold a position, this technique should still be used with caution. By lining up these joints, you will be concentrating the pressure on small surfaces, where cartilage damage is more likely to occur than in the larger joints of the body, such as the elbows. Excessive exposure to this type of joint loading can damage cartilage in the interphalangeal (IP) joints, and eventually cause osteoarthritis, particularly among older people.

The thumb is a very common location of injury because it tends to be overused. Osteoarthritis of the thumb can occur because of this overuse, but other factors can also contribute to it. As you remember from Chapter 2, the CMC joint is a fairly loose saddle joint that allows for considerable movement. It is stabilized by a number of muscles and ligaments that hold it in the proper position during movement or static loading. When you use your thumb to apply more pressure than the strength of your muscles can sustain, there is a tendency for the thumb to go into hyperextension at either the MCP or CMC joint.

Over time, these poor joint positions can result in microtrauma to the ligaments at the base of the thumb, causing laxity of the joint. Laxity in turn can result in subluxation, or partial dislocation, at the CMC joint. At this point, forces on the thumb are not evenly distributed, and damage to the cartilage in the joint can occur, increasing the likelihood of osteoarthritis over time.

Even using the thumb in a good position can result in damage to the cartilage at the MCP or CMC joints if enough pressure is applied with the tip of the thumb. Remember that for every pound of force you apply with the tip of your thumb, 10 to 12 pounds of force can be generated at the base of your thumb. This pressure at the CMC joint can be even higher among women, who tend to have a smaller contact surface with the trapezium, the carpal bone at the base of the thumb, concentrating forces on a smaller area. With repeated damage, over time and with advancing age, the cartilage of the CMC joint can wear away, resulting in osteoarthritis. Symptoms include joint stiffness, inflammation and pain at the base of the thumb during pinching activities.

Disc Injuries

The intervertebral discs are a highly vulnerable part of the spine. The discs consist of an outer ring, or annulus, of tough, fibrous connective tissue, and a center, or nucleus, of a gel-like substance. They are quite strong, capable of absorbing hundreds of pounds of compressive force. The discs provide some shock absorption between the vertebrae, and allow the spine to be quite flexible. As long as you maintain the natural curves in your spine, and are standing upright in a neutral or near neutral posture, the force of compression on the discs is concentrated straight down and is evenly distributed around the fibers in the disc. When you bend forward, backward or to the side, you compress the discs unevenly and reduce their ability to withstand this compressive force.

Manual practitioners commonly bend forward at the low back or neck as they work. These positions compress the discs in the anterior spine and force them to expand posteriorly. The discs can also be compromised during twisting motions, which stress some of the discs' fibers while other fibers go slack. Heavy lifting, even when done with good body mechanics and correct posture, can also exceed the compressive force limits of the discs. The most frequent locations of disc injury are in the low back, specifically at L4/L5 and L5/S1. This portion of the spine acts as a fulcrum for movements of the torso, and absorbs most of the stress of bending and lifting.

With repeated exposure to any of the risk factors mentioned above, tears can occur in the disc's outer fibers, leading to a loss of overall disc height and a condition known as degenerative disc disease. Since the discs do not have their own blood supply, these small tears are slow to heal. While many people have tears in their disc fibers, most actually do not suffer pain or any other symptoms of injury. If the tears are concentrated in one part of the disc, the weakness in that area can allow the nucleus of the disc to bulge outward. Disc bulges can gradually worsen, sometimes to the point where they press on nerve roots and cause pain. If enough pressure is placed on nerve roots along the spine, symptoms of nerve compression, such as numbness and tingling running down the arm (with cervical disc involvement) or leg (with lumbar disc involvement), can develop. Complete tears through the fibers can cause the disc to herniate or rupture, resulting in a serious condition that may require surgery.

The neck can be injured in much the same way as the lower back. The cervical spine is the most flexible part of the spine, and even though the forces operating on it are not as substantial as on the lower back, the stress placed on the intervertebral discs can nevertheless exceed their strength. Working with a forward-head posture or constantly flexing the head while looking down at the client can, over time, put enough pressure on the cervical discs to cause disc bulging. Disc bulges in the cervical spine can impinge nerve roots, causing referred pain, numbness and tingling in the shoulder, arm, hand or head (see page 254 for more on nerve impingement injury).

Injury to Vertebral Bodies

Strenuous work like lifting clients can damage the vertebrae themselves. Micro-fractures found in the endplates (the cartilage on the top and bottom of each intervertebral disc) are thought to result from heavy lifting and other concentrated forces on the spine. Like the rest of the disc, the endplates are slow to heal, and repetitively placing stress on already weakened endplates can result in cumulative damage. Since the discs get their nutrition from the endplates, damaging them can eventually lead to degenerative disc disease.

Nerve Injury

While the nervous system is often described as being separate and distinct from the musculoskeletal system, gradual-onset nerve injuries very often have a musculoskeletal component. As the nerves leave the spinal cord and branch out to all of the areas of the body, they intertwine with muscles, run alongside tendons, and slide across ligaments and bones. Along the way, these musculoskeletal structures can irritate and inflame the nerves. For this reason, nerve injuries are included in most discussions of MSDs. While nerve injuries have unique symptoms, the methods that are used to prevent them are much the same as those used to prevent any MSD.

Nerves can be damaged by direct compression (either repeated or a single, traumatic event), by loss of blood supply, and by vibration. Nerves are typically compressed in places where nerves lie between hard structures like bone, or pass through or between softer, but still unyielding structures like muscle, tendon, ligament or fascia.

Compression is more likely to occur in tight spaces in the body such as the carpal, cubital, radial or tarsal tunnels, or the thoracic outlet. Nerves that run just below the skin, for example those in the hypothenar eminence or the tips of the fingers, are prone to compression injury because their location is so superficial. Contact stress, caused by actions such as using the hand as a hammer, can damage both the superficial nerves and the blood vessels of the hand. Bulging vertebral discs (typically found in the cervical or lumbar spine) can compress nerve roots coming off the spinal cord.

When muscles and tendons are overused, the resulting hypertrophy or chronic hypertonicity can compress nerves that run through or near them. Nerve sheaths can also become irritated and inflamed by overuse, or by direct trauma to the sheath or the joint it passes by. Inflammation can cause edema, which can place pressure on nerves and impair their functioning. Trauma or injury to the nerve can cause enough inflammation to create scar tissue around the nerve. The scar tissue can cause the nerve to adhere to surrounding structures, compressing the nerve at that location. Scar tissue from a previous injury can also compress or irritate a nerve. Vibration to the hands and arms, for example, when working with power tools, can directly damage nerves and the blood vessels that feed them.

When nerve damage first occurs, it often causes inflammation, which can hinder circulation to the nerve and slow healing. The reduced local circulation can further damage nerves by depriving them of nutrition. Inflammation and irritation of a nerve can be quite painful, and can produce a significant amount of muscle guarding and loss of function of

---

Double Crush Syndrome (DCS)[2]

DCS is a clinical condition that usually involves multiple compression sites along a single peripheral nerve. Impingement of a nerve at one site is thought to increase the likelihood of developing a subsequent nerve impingement or other MSD at another site along the nerve pathway, usually distal to the original impingement site. For example, if you have a bulging disc in your neck that is pressing on a nerve root that feeds the arm, you may develop another nerve impingement at the elbow or wrist. Researchers believe that this phenomenon, often referred to as "double crush syndrome," happens because the original impingement reduces the conduction of nerve impulses and increases tension on the nerve. The reduced nerve impulses may result in atrophy and weakness in distal tissues fed by the affected nerve, while the reduced elasticity in the nerve causes irritation and inflammation each time you move the affected body part.

After years of doubt, the consensus among researchers is that double crush syndrome is a proven phenomenon and we are certain that proximal nerve compression can cause distal referred pain. Since proximal nerve compression can cause distal symptoms, either directly or indirectly, it is very important to look at the entire nerve pathway when diagnosing distal pain syndromes, particularly in the upper extremity. Performing a carpal tunnel release surgery, for example, may not relieve symptoms if the true source of the pain is impingement at the elbow, thoracic outlet or cervical spine. Common tests for DCS include nerve conduction studies (NCS), ultrasound studies and electromyography (EMG).

the distal upper or lower extremities. For this reason, it is often difficult to diagnose distal pain syndromes when nerve compression is involved.

Repeated damage to a nerve can cause paresthesias, with sensations of numbness, tingling or burning. If left untreated, damage to the nerve fibers can become extensive enough to affect nerve function, reducing the speed of the nerve impulses as they pass through. This can lead to further symptoms of numbness, heaviness and even a total loss of sensation in the areas the nerve supplies. It can also lead to atrophy of any muscles that are innervated by the damaged nerves. Nerve damage to this extent can be permanent.

Sciatica

Sciatica is caused by compression of the sciatic nerve at the point where it leaves the spine (L4/L5). Common symptoms of sciatica are pain, numbness and tingling that radiate down the leg, following the path of the sciatic nerve as it travels down the back of the leg to the foot.

Sciatica is often caused by a disc bulge that presses on the sciatic nerve. It can also happen when a vertebra slips forward (often at L4/L5), in a condition known as spondylolisthesis. Certain activities can cause or aggravate sciatica, including holding or frequently moving in and out of awkward postures such as bending or twisting at the waist, prolonged sitting without good lumbar support, and heavy or awkward lifting. Degenerative disc disease can also cause sciatica by narrowing the opening from which the sciatic nerve leaves the spine and compressing the nerve at that point.

As with any nerve disorder, when symptoms of sciatica appear, it is critical to seek treatment as soon as possible. Your healthcare practitioner will need to rule out more serious conditions, definitively diagnose the sciatica, and begin

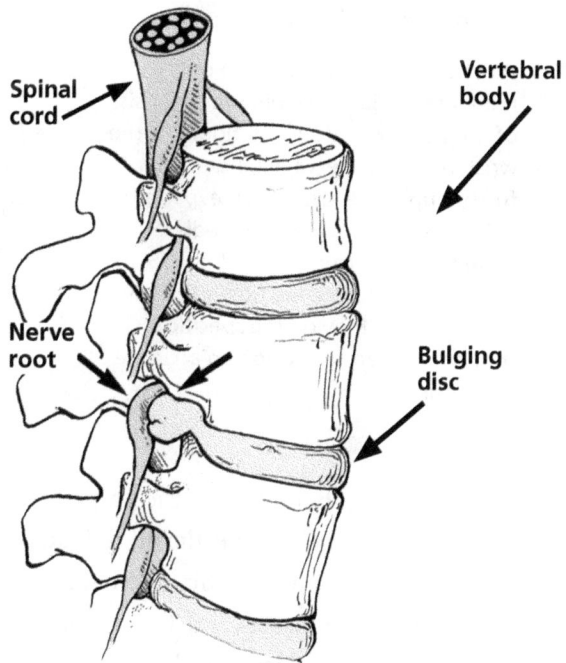

Spinal cord

Vertebral body

Nerve root

Bulging disc

Bulging Vertebral Disc

treatment quickly to prevent permanent nerve damage.

Another condition can mimic the symptoms of sciatica. Piriformis syndrome, in which the sciatic nerve is compressed as it passes under or through a tight or hypertonic piriformis muscle in the buttocks, can cause the same symptoms as sciatica without any spinal nerve root involvement. Piriformis syndrome is common among workers who do heavy lifting (such as manual therapists who lift clients), and those who sit for long periods of time as they work (such as therapists who specialize in reflexology).

Carpal Tunnel Syndrome (CTS)

Carpal tunnel syndrome (CTS) has been widely discussed in the media, and it is likely that it has been over-diagnosed as a result. Despite its notoriety, CTS does not appear to be a very common condition among manual therapists. Only a small percentage of practitioners reported a CTS diagnosis in the survey of American massage therapists (Chapter 1).

Not All Wrist Pain is CTS

Wrist pain can be a symptom of a number of MSDs, including tendonosis of the flexor or extensor tendons at the wrist, as well as nerve impingement further up in the arm. If you experience pain in your wrist, don't immediately jump to the conclusion that it is CTS, nor let any healthcare practitioner tell you it's CTS unless they do the specific tests that are needed to provide an accurate diagnosis.

CTS most often occurs among workers who use a combination of high hand forces like applying pressure with the palm or gripping, repetitive motions and awkward wrist postures. While these risk factors are certainly present in hands-on treatment work, they are more likely to result in much more common injuries that cause symptoms at the wrist, such as flexor or extensor tendonosis, than CTS.

The exact cause(s) of CTS are still not completely understood. The carpal tunnel is a very small, oval passageway in the wrist, bounded by the carpal bones and the transverse carpal ligament, also called the flexor retinaculum (see illustration on page 257). Passing through this fixed space are the nine tendons of the forearm flexor muscles and the median nerve. If the amount of space in the tunnel is decreased by factors such as mechanical pressure, edema or hypertrophy of the tendon or tendon sheaths, the increase in pressure in

AREAS OF NERVE COMPRESSION: THE UPPER EXTREMITY

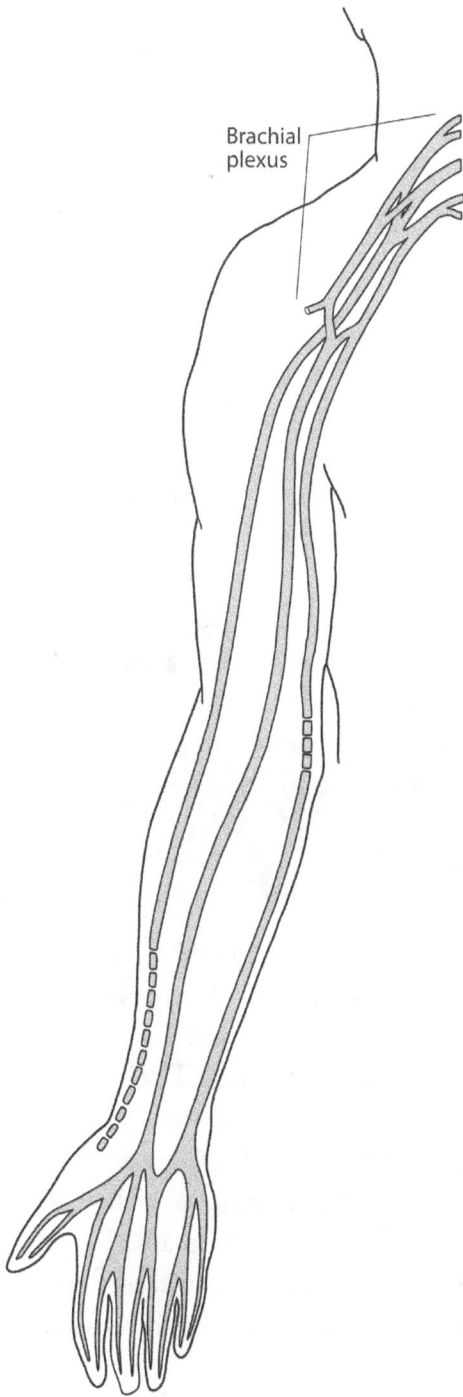

Brachial plexus

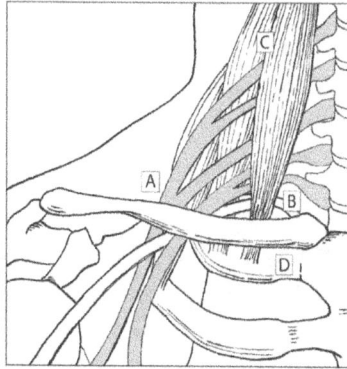

THORACIC OUTLET

The brachial plexus nerve bundle (A) and blood vessels (B) supplying the arm and hand are compressed in the area between the scalene muscles of the neck (C) and the first rib (D). The brachial plexus branches near the front of the upper arm to form the median, radial and ulnar nerves.

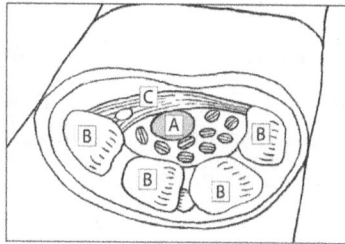

CARPAL TUNNEL

Compression of the median nerve (A) can occur at the wrist, where it passes through a canal formed by the carpal bones (B) and transverse carpal ligament (C).

© ENBeade 2007

the space can compress the median nerve. Even minor inflammation of a few of the flexor tendons can create enough edema to impinge the nerve. During pregnancy, increased fluid volume and retention can increase pressure on the median nerve in the carpal tunnel, causing CTS symptoms that typically resolve following the pregnancy.

Certain hand and wrist positions can also create pressure on the median nerve. Holding the wrist in flexion for a sustained period of time, for example, particularly with gripping, can compress the median nerve against the transverse ligament.

The classic symptoms of CTS are paresthesias (tingling, burning, numbness), pain and weakness of the hand. Paresthesias and pain are felt in the palmar aspect of the wrist radiating into the hand, the thumb, index finger, third finger, and the adjoining half of the ring finger (corresponding to the innervation pattern of the median nerve). Depending on the severity of the compression of the nerve, these fingers may lose some or all feeling and function. Shaking the hands can temporarily relieve these symptoms. It is common for CTS sufferers to be awakened by pain in the night, and to experience more pain in the morning than in the evening. A feeling of fullness or tightness in the wrists may precede other symptoms, and should be monitored carefully. If left untreated, the pressure on the nerve can permanently damage it and cause atrophy of the muscles it innervates, such as the thenar eminence.

Thoracic Outlet Syndrome (TOS)

The thoracic outlet is an opening at the base of the neck bordered by the anterior and middle heads of the scalene muscles, the first rib and the clavicle. Through this opening run arteries, veins and the brachial plexus nerve bundle, all of which continue down the arm. The brachial plexus divides to form the median, radial and ulnar nerves. Anything that narrows the space in the thoracic outlet, such as inflammation or hypertonicity of the scalenes or pectoralis minor, elevation of the first rib, depression of the clavicle, or presence of an extra rib at C7 (also known as a cervical rib, a rare, congenital abnormality) can cause compression of the brachial plexus, as well as impingement of the arteries and veins.

Gradual onset is most common in TOS that results from overuse. Repetitive motion in sustained poor postures, such as a forward head position or rounded shoulders, has a cumulative effect over time, causing pressure on the brachial plexus.

The primary symptom of TOS is pain in the cervical and supra-scapular regions, which may radiate down into the triceps, then the inner arm, the medial forearm and the ulnar side of the hand. The pain may be shooting, dull or generalized. Diminished nerve impulses due to compression can cause paresthesias and, eventually, weakening and atrophy of distal muscles along the nerve route. Diminished blood flow to the arm caused by compression of arteries can deprive the arm of the circulation needed to efficiently heal injuries. The hand may become cold or very pale as a result. Reduction in nerve impulses leads to a progressive decrease in dexterity and fine motor control.

TOS is not a common disorder, and it often presents with symptoms that are similar to other disorders, such as CTS or a bulging cervical disc. For this reason, there is a potential for patients to be misdiagnosed. The presence of nerve impingement at the thoracic outlet makes double crush syndrome more likely to occur. Pinpointing the exact site of entrapment with the help of a specialist is very important if you are experiencing symptoms.

Less Common Nerve Injuries

While they are not frequently reported by manual therapists, there are other types of nerve injuries to be aware of. Any nerve injury can be serious, since damage to nerves can cause permanent loss of feeling and function. Some of these nerve injuries have symptoms that mimic other conditions, so they may be difficult to diagnose. Disorders such as reflex sympathetic dystrophy (RSD), while rare, can be particularly serious. Any nerve disorder that is diagnosed and treated early in its onset will respond better to conservative treatment and be less likely to become chronic.

Radial Tunnel Syndrome

The radial nerve can become impinged near the elbow, where it passes through a small opening, the radial tunnel, underneath the supinator

TABLE 9. Common Injuries Reported by Manual Therapists, by Location

Back injuries	Most often caused by	Typical symptoms
Muscle strains and ligament sprains	Static loading while bending at the waist Heavy, frequent and awkward lifting	Pain Inflammation Loss of range of motion (ROM)
Sciatica	Disc bulge pressing on nerve roots	Pain in lower back, hip Numbness or tingling radiating down leg
Non-specific pain	Unknown	Localized and referred pain
Neck injuries	**Most often caused by**	**Typical symptoms**
Tension neck syndrome	Static loading while bending at the neck or elevating the shoulders	Burning sensations, hypertonicity, pain
Disc bulges	Sudden injury (e.g., whiplash), long-term awkward postures such as forward neck flexion	Localized and referred pain Numbness and/or tingling radiating down arm
Thoracic Outlet Syndrome	Tight muscles (pectoralis minor, scalenes) Repetitive arm movements in awkward positions, especially with shoulder flexion or overhead movements Presence of a congenital cervical rib Elevated first rib	Pain, sometimes referred to shoulder Numbness and/or tingling radiating down arm Reduced circulation and edema in arm
Shoulder injuries	**Most often caused by**	**Typical symptoms**
Rotator cuff tears, tendinopathy	Sudden injury Repetitive arm movements in awkward positions, especially with shoulder flexion or overhead movements	Shoulder pain Loss of function Loss of ROM Inflammation
Shoulder bursitis	Repetitive arm movements in awkward positions Tight muscles pulling tendon across bursa	Shoulder pain Inflammation Loss of function Loss of ROM
Impingement syndrome	Same as rotator cuff tendonosis, bursitis	Shoulder pain Inflammation Loss of function Loss of ROM
Frozen shoulder	Adhesions Tight ligaments	Loss of ROM

TABLE 9. *(Continued)* **Common Injuries Reported by Manual Therapists, by Location**

Elbow injuries	Most often caused by	Typical symptoms
Epicondylosis	Repetitive wrist bending and forearm rotation while gripping with force	Pain at lateral or medial elbow
Radial tunnel syndrome	Repetitive hand motions with bent wrist or rotated forearm Tight muscles over the radial nerve	Pain at the lateral elbow and dorsal forearm—often mimics tennis elbow Fatigue and weakness of muscles in back of hand
Hand/wrist injuries	**Most often caused by**	**Typical symptoms**
Tendinopathy	Repetitive gripping or hand motions with bent wrist or in combination with hand force	Pain in the wrist and hand Degeneration of collagen fibers in tendon Loss of grip strength and ROM
Carpal tunnel syndrome	Repetitive gripping or other hand motions with bent wrist in combination with hand force Edema in the carpal tunnel due to pregnancy	Numbness and tingling of the thumb and first three fingers Pain in the wrist, hand and fingers, sometimes referred back up the arm Loss of grip strength and ROM Left untreated, can lead to permanent muscle atrophy
Intersection syndrome (Also known as "squeakers")	Repetitive wrist and thumb extension Tight thumb muscles irritating wrist tendons	Pain just proximal to the dorsal, radial wrist
Pronator Teres Syndrome	Compression of the median nerve at the elbow or just distal to it.	Pain and numbness at the wrist, and weakness of the Flexor Pollicis Longus (FPL) and Flexor Digitorum Profundus (FDP), leading to a loss of dexterity
Finger/thumb injuries	**Most often caused by**	**Typical symptoms**
DeQuervain's tendinopathy	Repetitive, forceful gripping or wringing motions	Pain at the base of the thumb on the radial aspect of the wrist
CMC joint osteoarthritis	Forceful, repetitive thumb motions and pinching, particularly with the thumb in extension Joint laxity due to ligament damage Advancing age	Pain at the base of the thumb Inflammation Loss of function and ROM
IP joint osteoarthritis	Repeated use of the fingers to apply downward pressure with force Advancing age	Pain in the finger joints Inflammation Loss of function and ROM

muscle. Tight muscles in this area can press the nerve against bone or connective tissue. Repetitive hand motions, especially when done with a bent wrist or rotated forearm, may increase the likelihood of radial nerve irritation. Chronic irritation of the nerve leads to radial tunnel syndrome, causing pain around the outside of the elbow that may be mistaken for lateral epicondylosis.

Ulnar Neuritis and Cubital Tunnel Syndrome

The ulnar nerve runs underneath the medial epicondyle of the elbow. It is often referred to as the "funny bone" when it is struck accidentally. Repeated pressure on this nerve, for example by resting your elbows on a hard surface, can irritate the nerve and cause tingling sensations down into the ulnar side of the hand. This condition is alternately referred to as ulnar neuritis or cubital tunnel syndrome.

Complex Regional Pain Syndrome

Complex Regional Pain Syndrome (CRPS) is characterized by hyper-sensitivity to pain (allodynia) following an injury, particularly one that involves a period of immobilization, such as a broken bone or carpal tunnel syndrome. Typical symptoms include constant, moderate to severe pain accompanied by burning sensations, inflammation, changes in skin color and temperature, limited range of motion and sweating. CRPS is essentially a disorder of the sympathetic nervous system, which continues to transmit constant pain messages well after the initial trauma has healed. Increased sensitivity to pain is thought to be due to changes in the local biochemistry of the tissues, especially the chemicals associated with pain signals, as well as vasoconstriction.

Treatments for CRPS typically involve attempts to reduce or shut down the nerve signals from the area with neuropathic medications or nerve blocks. There is only a brief window of opportunity, perhaps as short as a few weeks, to diagnose and treat CRPS, after which it can become chronic and resistant to treatment. The condition may even spread to other parts of the body if not controlled early, complicating treatment.

Pain conditions such as CRPS which have the potential to become chronic are best treated by a pain specialist. Once the pain has been controlled, the patient can undergo a therapy program to help further reduce pain and restore normal function. As with many other pain disorders, research is focusing on the underlying causes of the condition, so that more effective treatments can be discovered.

Facing the Possibility of Injury and Seeking Treatment

It can be difficult for manual therapists to admit they may have an injury. As healthcare providers, manual therapists promote health and well-being. It seems incongruous for a healthcare practitioner to be in anything less than perfect health.

Manual therapists tend to concentrate on their clients' health and put their own health aside. They do not talk much about injury among themselves, and when they do, the discussion is often tinged with fear or shame. Students can fear admitting they are injured, since they are trying to keep up with classmates who seem able to concentrate only on learning techniques and helping their clients. Professionals may fear losing their job or appearing less capable than their colleagues in the boss' eyes. Some therapists try to ignore their symptoms, hoping that they will just go away. Others subscribe to the idea that they can "work through the pain." They put off treatment, saying they just need to get through the next quarter at school or the next week with a full workload and then they will take a rest. Practitioners and students who are able to continue working despite their symptoms often get positive feedback, while those who cannot may fear they will get little support.

Unrealistic expectations, rationalization and fear only serve to increase the likelihood that injury will occur. Don't take chances with your career and your health. There is nothing shameful about getting injured; as you have already seen, injury is quite a common occurrence among manual therapists. You would not let a client ignore their injury symptoms. You deserve the same consideration.

1. Karim Kahn, et al., "Time to abandon the "tendinitis" myth: Painful, overuse tendon conditions have a non-inflammatory pathology," *BMJ*, 2002; 324: 626–627.
2. William J. Molinari III, John C. Elfar, "The Double Crush Syndrome," *Journal of Hand Surg Am.* 2013 Mar 5;38(4):799–801. doi: 10.1016/j.jhsa.2012.12.038 https://pmc.ncbi.nlm.nih.gov/articles/PMC5823245/

15

Diagnosis and Treatment of Injuries

To properly treat your symptoms, you will need to work with a diagnostician to determine all of the following:

1. What type of injury has occurred? (diagnosis)
2. At what point did symptoms first occur? (onset)
3. What is the extent of the injury? (severity)
4. Why did you get injured? (cause)

Your first tendency may be to try to make these determinations yourself. Some manual therapists possess the level of training necessary to assess symptoms and diagnose MSDs; for others, such determinations are outside their scope of practice. Whatever your scope of practice, objectivity is essential in making an accurate assessment and diagnosis. For this reason, healthcare practitioners are routinely discouraged from assessing and diagnosing their own conditions. For any treatment to be successful, it is important to first be assessed by a skilled, objective healthcare practitioner who can rule out any non-musculoskeletal condition or disease process that may be causing your symptoms.

If you should become injured as a result of your work, you have a number of options available to you to resolve your injury. Effective treatments are out there; it is just a matter of knowing how and where to find them. If you catch your condition in the early stages, treatments should remain conservative and short term. In this chapter, you will find practical information to guide you through the sometimes confusing process of diagnosing and treating a work-related MSD.

Getting a Diagnosis

To obtain successful treatment, you must first be assessed by a knowledgeable, objective healthcare practitioner. Medical doctors (MDs) have the most extensive training, scope of practice and licensure to accurately and expertly assess and diagnose your condition. In some countries or states, other medical professionals including naturopathic doctors, osteopaths or physical therapists also have these qualifications.

Although your diagnosis may come from a healthcare professional other than an MD, it is important to involve an MD in your treatment. MDs have the widest-ranging scope of practice, which allows them to

---

The Pitfalls of Self-Treating Symptoms

As a healthcare practitioner, you may be tempted to try to treat yourself, perhaps to avoid incurring medical costs, especially if you are not insured. You may feel that you have the knowledge to adequately treat your symptoms by yourself. Treating yourself may seem like the easiest and fastest way to make an annoying and upsetting problem go away quickly.

If you have been experiencing symptoms for longer than a week, it is unlikely that home treatments like ice packs and over-the-counter pain relievers will have much effect. Relying on these self-treatments can also waste valuable time while your injury worsens. Just as objectivity is essential to accurately evaluate and diagnose MSDs, it is equally as important in prescribing proper treatment. If you do try to self-treat and your symptoms worsen during that time, or if new symptoms appear or recur as soon as you resume activities, seek medical attention right away. Early treatment of MSDs is critical to a good outcome.

TABLE 10. Healthcare Practitioners Who are Commonly Licensed to Diagnose MSDs (varies by jurisdiction: check with your local health department for more information).

• Physicians (MDs and medical specialists of all types)	• Osteopaths (DOs)
• Physician Assistants (PAs)	• Doctors of Physical Therapy (DPTs)
• Nurse Practitioners (NPs)	

take all aspects of your health and history into account in treating your injury. They can diagnose and prescribe medications and order x-rays or blood work to help in the diagnostic process.

The first step in making a diagnosis is to rule out non-musculoskeletal conditions or disease processes. It is important to confirm that an MSD is the real cause of your symptoms, since a number of serious illnesses, such as rheumatoid arthritis, kidney disease or cardiac conditions can cause similar symptoms to those associated with MSDs. Once the necessary examinations and tests have been done to make this determination, the healthcare professional you see should be able to provide at least a preliminary diagnosis that can be used to start you on a treatment plan.

Your general family physician or primary care provider (PCP) is your first resource, and should be able to both rule out non-musculoskeletal causes for your symptoms and make a preliminary diagnosis of your condition. If your case is more complicated or difficult to diagnose, or if your usual physician does not have enough experience with MSDs to properly diagnose your condition, they should refer you to a healthcare professional with more in-depth knowledge of MSDs to get a more specific diagnosis: for example, a physical medicine and rehabilitation physician (sometimes called a physiatrist).

An exact diagnosis may take longer to pinpoint, and can remain elusive for a time. Medical science does not yet completely understand all aspects of MSDs. Your symptoms may come and go, or be atypical and difficult to classify. In nerve impingement injuries, it can be difficult to determine the exact site of nerve compression, since symptoms can be felt at any point along the nerve pathway. Trigger points may cause referred pain that is difficult to trace to its origin. There may also be a number of injury processes going on at the same time, and these different processes can present a confusing, overlapping array of symptoms. A more exact diagnosis may become evident as you go through your treatment. During a course of treatment, it is helpful for other types of practitioners or specialists to get involved, to provide additional information that can help uncover the true diagnosis for your injury.

Selecting a Primary Care Provider (PCP)

Particularly when you catch symptoms at an early stage, your family doctor or primary care physician may be able to adequately diagnose and treat you and/or refer you to an appropriate manual therapist for further treatment. Whether it is your family physician or another healthcare practitioner, it is critical to select one knowledgeable and sympathetic professional to be your primary care provider (PCP) for your MSD. Your PCP is the person who will develop a treatment plan for your injury, provide ongoing evaluation and advice, and coordinate your care with other practitioners involved in your treatment. You should meet with your PCP regularly to discuss all aspects of your treatment, evaluate your progress, and make any necessary adjustments to keep you on the road to recovery.

> Your primary care provider (PCP) is the healthcare professional you select to develop your treatment plan, advise you and coordinate your care throughout the treatment of your injury.

It is most effective to select a PCP with a broad scope of practice who can perform a complete differential diagnosis and refer you to specialists if necessary. Your PCP should ideally be a highly trained medical professional who is well versed and completely up-to-date on MSDs and the best treatments for them.

There are a number of healthcare practitioners who are well qualified to treat MSDs, and would be good candidates to be your PCP. Sports medicine physicians, physiatrists, physicians who are hand specialists and rehabilitation medicine physicians all have extensive training in treating the musculoskeletal system. Orthopedists are more frequently consulted for spinal conditions such as bulging discs. Specialists such as these should be able to further refine your diagnosis and suggest the most effective treatments. You can find these specialists through professional associations for their specialties, or you can get a referral

Stay Open to Different Modalities

There is a natural tendency to seek treatment from colleagues you trust in your own profession. Massage practitioners may seek treatment from other massage practitioners, or from another alternative healthcare professional. American massage therapists surveyed tended to seek out non-traditional practitioners and treatment for injury symptoms. Physical therapists may be more likely to get treatment from a physical therapist, or from an allopathic physician. In reality, since MSDs are usually caused by a number of different factors, a single treatment modality will likely not hold all of the answers for successfully resolving the symptoms and injury. Every modality can contribute to the healing process, so keeping an open mind when you seek treatment can lead to a better outcome.

from a hospital or university that has an occupational medicine, physical medicine and/or sports medicine department.

During your first visit with a prospective PCP, they should do a thorough exam and ask you questions about your work and symptoms. Then ask them the following questions to determine if they have the necessary skills and relevant experience you are looking for:

- Do you feel that you can give me a preliminary diagnosis at this time? (To see if they already suspect or know what kind of injury you have.)
- What is your approach to treating this type of injury? (To confirm that the provider has a well-defined approach, including any tests that may need to be done or any referrals to other practitioners.
- Do you customize treatment specifically for each patient? Or ask if they use a standardized treatment plan for all MSD patients.)
- What tests do you usually do as part of your diagnosis? (To see if the provider has the necessary skills to make a differential diagnosis, adequately assess your levels of pain and other symptoms, and evaluate the impact your symptoms are having on your work life and other activities.)
- What other healthcare practitioners do you usually work with in treating this type of injury? (To see if the provider refers out to physical therapists, hand therapists, massage therapists, etc.; in other words, if the provider takes a multidisciplinary, team approach rather than recommending that you work only with them or just prescribing medication or another single-treatment method.)

If you feel at all unsure about their responses, you can ask for a referral or find someone else on your own. If you do choose to begin treatment with this person, remember that you can leave at any time, and transfer your records to another provider you feel is better qualified to treat your condition.

Once you find a healthcare professional with the right qualifications to be your PCP, you will want to make sure that they ask you the right questions and listen attentively to your responses. They should want to know much more about the injury than just where it hurts and how long it has been a problem. A full medical history should be taken, including a history of past injuries and illnesses, the treatments you have tried so far for this condition (what worked/didn't work), and what medications you are taking. Other tests may be added, to obtain more information. Some of these tests are quite simple; others may be invasive, painful or expensive. Ask your provider what benefits they feel the test results will offer in gaining a better understanding of your injury and creating a treatment plan for it, to help you determine if you should go ahead with the test.

In addition to a medical history, the provider should want to know all about your work: what type of work you do (massage therapy, physical therapy, using instruments or equipment, doing adjustments, etc.); how many clients you see in a day and in a week; how long you have been practicing; which techniques make the symptoms worse; and what kind of work environment you practice in (home office, medical office, clinic, hospital, etc.). Questions about your lifestyle—eating, sleeping and exercise habits, tobacco and alcohol use—are also appropriate and can help the provider get a better picture of your overall health.

After obtaining all this information, the provider should perform a complete examination, including the affected areas, and also evaluate your overall posture and stance. They should also look for possible proximal pathology that may be contributing to or causing your distal pain and/or injury. If your wrist hurts and the provider looks only at your wrist, suggest an evaluation of your neck and shoulder as well. If the provider balks at this idea, find another one who has a better understanding of MSDs and respects your desire to take an active role in your own care.

If you become dissatisfied with the way the provider is handling your case, it is always best to let them know you are not satisfied with their approach and explain exactly what you would like them to do instead. Then give the provider a chance to respond. If you have not been given a thorough work-up as mentioned above, if you feel the provider really doesn't listen to you, or if you still feel uncomfortable with your treatment plan after the second or third visit, move on. Remember that it is your prerogative to change healthcare providers. As a consumer of healthcare services, you have a right to competent, compassionate and effective treatment. One word of caution, though—avoid frequent changes in providers, especially if the reason for changing is that you are not getting better as quickly as you would like. Patients who frequently disrupt their own treatment plans in search of a quick cure have been shown to be more likely to develop chronic conditions.

In any case, it is always helpful to obtain a second opinion, to get another perspective on your condition. You should plan on getting a second opinion, particularly if you are diagnosed with a condition that could threaten your ability to function at home or at work, like sciatica or tendinosis.

Although finding a good PCP is very important, you also share in the responsibility for your treatment. No healthcare professional can help you if you don't follow their advice, if you withhold information or don't communicate effectively with them, or if you self-treat along with the prescribed treatments and don't coordinate those treatments with your PCP. The PCP you choose will be your ally in resolving your injury, not a miracle worker who will magically make everything better. Working with your PCP on an equal footing will empower you and facilitate proper treatment of your condition.

Filing a Workers' Compensation Insurance Claim

If you are already covered by workers' compensation insurance, or if you work for an employer who carries it, you can file a workers' compensation claim for your injury. You may not be covered if you work as an independent contractor. If you are not sure whether you are covered, ask your employer.

During your first visit to a healthcare professional about your condition, you should determine together whether your injury was work-related. If you are covered, workers' compensation insurance may pay for all necessary medical treatment if your condition was caused or aggravated by your job. This insurance may also pay you partial wages for the time that you are absent from your work. The ability to take paid leave from your job will give you the time you need to recover from your injury.

Determining the Cause of Your Injury

To properly treat your injury, you must determine what caused it. MSDs are usually caused by a combination of factors. Some of the most common of these are a heavy workload or a sudden increase in your workload, overuse of one part of the body (like the thumbs), or improper technique, particularly awkward positioning. It is in these situations that you have the kind of intensity, duration, frequency or combination of exposures to risk factors that often leads to injury (see Chapter 3). Any pre-existing characteristics you may have and experiencing stress at home or on the job are other common factors that contribute to causing injury. By understanding which of these factors may have caused and/or contributed to your injury, you can start to modify those factors so you can heal your injury and avoid re-injury.

As you begin treatment, it can be helpful to consult with experienced colleagues in your profession who can watch you work and

---

Questions to Ask Yourself to Identify the Possible Cause of Your Injury

- Did I make any change in my work habits, schedule, environment, workload or technique?

- Was I under more stress than usual at the time the symptoms arose?

- Have my body mechanics deteriorated, due to inattention, distraction or other reasons?

- Has the state of my general health deteriorated or changed, putting me at risk for injury?

- Do I have a healthy lifestyle (eating well, sleeping enough, not smoking, etc.)?

It may not be possible to identify just one or two causes of your injury. Most injuries are caused by exposure to multiple risk factors, and it can be very difficult to say which one is the most significant contributor to your symptoms. You may have to temporarily stop exposing yourself to as many factors as possible that could be contributing to your injury (work, sports, hobbies, pro-inflammatory foods) until your symptoms subside. Then you can slowly re-introduce each of these elements, while carefully monitoring yourself for the recurrence of symptoms.

evaluate your technique, posture and body mechanics. They can point out movements and positions that may be putting too much stress on the injured body part, and suggest alternative techniques that are less stressful to your body. Using the information in this book as a guide will be helpful. They can also evaluate your standing and sitting postures as you work, as well as certain movement patterns that may be contributing to injury. You can then bring your findings to your PCP, who can use them to formulate as specific and accurate a diagnosis as possible and develop an appropriate treatment plan for you.

Developing a Treatment Plan

With a preliminary diagnosis in hand, your PCP should work with you to create a treatment plan that includes short-term symptom relief, rehabilitation of the injury, and changes in your work or other aspects of your life to help you avoid re-injury while you are healing. If your injury is mild and you are able to determine what caused the injury and stop doing it, you may be able to keep working while you are in treatment. Otherwise, your PCP will likely recommend that you lighten your workload or take time off from work for a prescribed period of time. How long you will need to curtail your work activities will depend on the extent and nature of your injury. If you have been referred to a physical, occupational or massage therapist, that person may help you identify and change the aspects of your work or other activities that caused your injury, rather than your PCP.

Components of a good treatment plan should include:

- Defining functional treatment goals
- Deciding which modalities to incorporate
- Deciding whether temporary work cessation or work restrictions are necessary
- Creating timelines and checkpoints, with periodic progress evaluations
- Referring out to appropriate specialists as necessary
- Planning for reintroduction to work, if time off from work was part of the treatment plan

A Sample Course of Treatment for MSDs

The exact treatment you receive for your condition will depend on your diagnosis and the recommendations of your PCP. This sample course of treatment illustrates how a multidisciplinary team of healthcare professionals can work together with you to resolve an MSD. You can use this example as a basis for discussion of the relative merits of each of the treatments described.

Your evaluation begins with a visit to a qualified healthcare professional (usually a physician) to rule out underlying diseases, get a diagnosis, begin any medications if necessary (pain relievers, etc.), and start to develop a treatment plan. If necessary, the physician will refer you to a specialist (a sports medicine physician or doctor of physical therapy, for example) to help pinpoint a more specific diagnosis and suggest possible treatments.

At this point, you select either your original doctor or one of the specialists to be your PCP. Your PCP will create a treatment plan for you, based on an evaluation of your condition and the recommendations of the specialists you have seen. You will check in with your PCP periodically throughout your treatment, at intervals decided between the two of you.

Your treatment plan may include practitioners in several modalities, each one addressing a different aspect of your symptoms or rehabilitation. For example, you may see a rehabilitation therapist for further assessment to verify the diagnosis and treatment plan.

A physical therapist can also prescribe strengthening and flexibility exercises and advise you on hydrotherapy and other types of home care. You may see an occupational therapist to fit you for a splint or support if needed. Some rehabilitation therapists may also give you advice on ergonomics for your practice. At the same time, you might see a massage practitioner to reduce overall muscle tension, eliminate trigger points, release myofascial tissues and adhesions, and relieve stress. The goal is to reduce your overall pain level so you can complete your therapy without significant restrictions to your movement, work and lifestyle.

You may consider consulting other complementary healthcare specialists such as a naturopath, who can prescribe natural alternatives for pain and inflammation relief; an acupuncturist, who may be able to help relieve pain; or a biofeedback practitioner, who can help you identify and reduce unhealthy stress and muscle tension patterns. Be sure to inform your PCP of every complementary treatment you are receiving.

For certain conditions like CTS or bulging discs that do not respond to other treatments, you may need to consult a surgeon. Your PCP should make that determination and refer you to an appropriate surgeon.

If your injury becomes chronic, seeing a mental health counselor or psychotherapist can help you deal with the emotional issues that chronic MSDs commonly bring up.

Depending on the nature and severity of your symptoms, your PCP may recommend either work restriction or a temporary work cessation. This is intended to give your body time to heal and avoid any work situations that could aggravate your condition. If you work for an employer, it is best to involve them at this point so you have their buy-in for these changes to your work routine. As your treatment progresses, part of the plan may be a gradual reintroduction to work, hopefully with the goal of resuming full work activities over a period of time.

Coordinating Care/Treatments

Your PCP is likely to refer you to other healthcare practitioners who will assist in your treatment. A holistic, team approach to injury treatment is usually quite effective. However, when a number of practitioners become involved in your care, it can get confusing to remember who performed what treatment or who prescribed what medication. Make sure that your PCP helps you coordinate the different aspects of your treatment plan, and keep them informed of all the treatments you are receiving. Your PCP can then make sure that your treatments do not conflict with each other. Keeping a log of your appointments with each practitioner is another useful habit to get into. For each appointment, note the treatments that were done and any medications that were prescribed. Your PCP may recommend a multidisciplinary approach to your treatment which combines a number of treatments at the same time, such as massage or physical therapy combined with medication and behavioral therapy. This kind of approach is most effective when prescribed by an experienced healthcare provider who has seen proven results by combining treatment methods.

Staying in Charge of Your Treatment and Recovery

Although your PCP will help coordinate your care, you are the person who should ultimately control the process of rehabilitation of your injury. Ask any questions that come up for you during your treatment, even if they seem insignificant. Write them down before your appointments, so you are well prepared to begin a discussion with the practitioners who are providing your care. Ask what results you can expect from each type of treatment, and request an estimate of how long your recovery might take. Usually it is not possible to predict exactly how much time an injury will take to heal, but you should be given some idea of when you might expect to start seeing improvement. Monitor your own progress, and if you feel you are not getting better or that a particular treatment is not working, ask your PCP to reassess your treatment plan and discuss other options with you. Be your own advocate. Taking an active role will make you feel empowered and aid in your recovery.

Conservative Treatment of MSDs

The primary goals of injury treatment can be summarized in the "Five R's":

1. Relieving pain
2. Reducing inflammation (if present)
3. Relaxing muscles
4. Restoring function and range of motion
5. Re-educating posture and movement

A good treatment plan will be multifaceted to address each of these goals.

If you seek medical attention early in the development of symptoms, your treatment plan should remain fairly conservative, non-invasive and short-term. In this section, you will find information about the most common conservative treatment methods for MSDs. These treatment options are widely available and usually quite effective at this stage of injury. They are relatively low risk, and can be tried out singly or in combination on a trial-and-error basis, so you can see which are effective for treating your injury and which are not. You may find that

---

How Those Around You Influence Your Recovery

How we deal with injury depends greatly on our beliefs about injury and pain. Your beliefs may reflect attitudes you learned from your family, friends and teachers, or from healthcare practitioners who have treated you. These attitudes may help or hinder your healing.

An inadequate level of support can produce feelings of helplessness and a loss of control over what is happening to you. Passive, depressive, fearful and avoidant behaviors can set in and continue the cycle of chronic physical and emotional pain. On the other hand, having a good support network and a positive attitude can help you cope better with injury, pain and treatment and recover more quickly. An individual who takes an active approach to their symptoms, gets early treatment, keeps a positive attitude toward recovery, and seeks out supportive friends and caregivers will certainly have a better outcome than someone who takes a passive, avoidant approach.

a treatment that worked well at one stage of your recovery no longer works at a more advanced stage, or vice versa. Staying flexible and trying new or different treatments will help facilitate your recovery. Keep an open mind as you consult with the healthcare professionals involved in your treatment. Each modality has something unique to offer in the treatment of MSDs.

Side Effects and Efficacy of Treatment Methods

Some of the conservative treatments that have few side effects have been shown to be quite effective; for example heat or massage, which work very well to relieve non-specific back pain. The efficacy or safety of other treatments, such as certain herbal treatments, has not been supported by high-quality medical studies.

On the other hand, most of the treatment options with a higher potential for side effects, such as prescription drugs or surgery, have been shown to be effective in most cases. However, their side effects can sometimes be quite serious; for example, permanent scarring, infection or other complications from surgery. Most medical professionals will therefore recommend a conservative course of treatment before moving on to treatments that involve more risk.

Resting the Injured Part of the Body

If your work is causing or aggravating your symptoms, you may need to take some time off to allow your injury to heal. In some cases, you may be able to simply reduce your workload; in others, it may be necessary to stop working completely for a period of time. When you are not working, try to rest your injury as much as possible.

Figure 5. Common Injury Treatments in Order of Increasing Potential for Side Effects

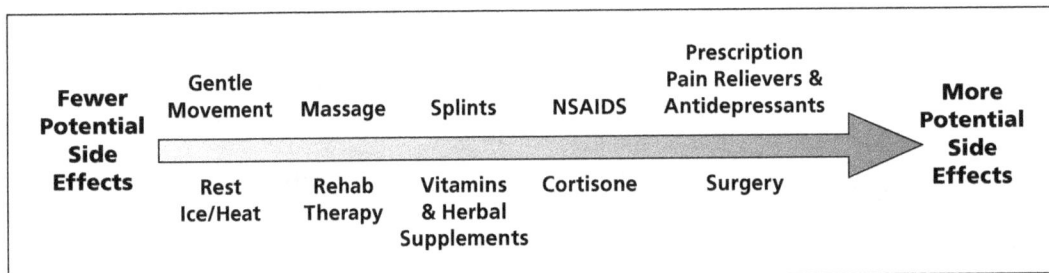

It can be difficult to decide to take time off from your work. In addition to the short-term loss of income, there is also a concern about losing clients or endangering your job. If you are experiencing significant symptoms, chances are you will not be doing your best work at that time. You may end up being more focused on your own pain than on the needs of your clients, and they will likely notice the difference. If taking time off is essential to properly treat your injury, choosing to continue working instead may put your career, as well as your health, in danger. It is important to weigh the long-term risks of not giving yourself the rest you need to heal your injury with the short-term difficulties of taking time off work.

You will need to strike a balance between resting the injured part of your body and finding a healthy level of physical activity. Continuing to gently move the injured body part will increase circulation, flush out waste products from your tissues, and maintain strength, flexibility and range of motion. In the past, bed rest was recommended for conditions such as low back pain, but studies have shown that inactivity actually prolongs healing time. Disuse can cause muscle atrophy and hypertonicity; it also reduces circulation, which impedes healing. Atrophy occurs very quickly, often within a few weeks. As a result of atrophy and reduced blood flow, the tissues become weak and irritable, and even the smallest motion can cause pain. Returning to normal activities, as long as those activities do not include physical demands that can aggravate the injury, will help you recover more quickly. The most effective treatments combine some amount of rest with a specifically designed exercise program that maintains muscle tone and promotes adequate circulation.

Having Realistic Expectations about Recovery

When they begin treatment of an MSD, clients/patients tend to think of recovery as a straight line: they move from treatment to treatment, making consistent improvement in each session. This improvement builds upon itself, and after a number of sessions, they arrive at the end point of the straight line: full recovery.

In reality, treatment looks like a long, squiggly line, sometimes moving upward, sometimes moving downward, and sometimes moving sideways. Clients/patients advance, then have a setback, then advance again only to find themselves at a plateau for a while. This dance of advancement, setbacks and plateaus often continues all the way through treatment. They do finally get to an end point, but may not be fully recovered by then. It may take additional time after formal treatment has ended for the pain or discomfort to go away completely, or for the mobility to return to what it once was. Sometimes, the injured part of the body never returns to full function and mobility without any pain, that feeling as if the injury never happened. That can happen, but it's probably best to set realistic goals for yourself to avoid disappointment or feeling discouraged when setbacks occur. Better to make any necessary adjustments in your schedule, techniques, or any other factor that originally contributed to your injury so it doesn't hinder you in the future.

Complementary or Alternative Healthcare Treatments

Many people find the treatment they receive from complementary healthcare practitioners to be as, if not more, effective than traditional treatment methods. The benefits of massage therapy, for example, have been well documented.

Discuss alternative therapy options with your PCP, and then let them know when you start receiving other types of care so they can coordinate the different treatments you are receiving. An increasing number of physicians and other allopathic practitioners are open to having their patients try alternative treatments as an adjunct to medical treatment. Some allopathic physicians are now practicing what is termed "integrative medicine," which incorporates proven treatments from naturopathy, osteopathy, acupuncture, massage and other alternative modalities into their own practice, or by referral to other practitioners. If prescribed by a physician, some of these treatments, including chiropractic and massage therapy, may be reimbursed by your health insurance policy.

Biofeedback

Biofeedback specialists monitor the physiological signals of the body, such as muscle tension, heart rate, blood pressure and brain waves.

They use those signals to help clients learn to consciously control what are otherwise involuntary functions. By becoming attuned to the physiological reactions of your body, biofeedback can help you recognize and reduce muscle tension and the associated feelings of anxiety and stress. In conditions where muscle tension is the cause of pain symptoms, biofeedback can be effective in reducing pain. In chronic pain conditions resulting from other causes, biofeedback can help you learn to control your perception of, and reaction to, pain signals.

Exercises in biofeedback sessions may include visualization, meditation and deep breathing. The exact mechanisms by which biofeedback works are not well understood, and it may not be effective for all MSDs or chronic pain conditions. Biofeedback is more likely to be effective when symptoms are related to excess muscle tension, such as low back pain with significant muscle guarding and tension neck syndrome. When performed by a trained professional as part of a treatment plan, biofeedback can be an effective treatment and help reduce the need for medication.

Treatments that Can Only be Prescribed by Your PCP or a Specialist

Rehabilitation Therapy: Physical Therapy, Occupational Therapy and Hand Therapy

Patients with MSDs are often referred to physical or occupational therapists for treatment. Physical therapists help clients correct postural problems, relieve symptoms and regain strength, mobility, flexibility and function using myofascial release and other types of soft tissue massage, strengthening and stretching exercises, and passive joint mobilization. Occupational therapists retrain patients to work and function in a manner that will prevent injury and re-injury. Hand therapists are either OTs or PTs who specialize in the treatment of upper extremity disorders, including injuries to the hand, wrist, elbow and shoulder.

These rehabilitation professionals have been trained to administer effective treatments for MSDs, including hydrotherapy, ultrasound, myofascial release and other types of soft tissue work, strengthening and stretching exercises, gait and/or postural analysis, and passive joint mobilization. Hand therapists also create custom-made splints and braces, if necessary. If your posture is implicated in your injury, a rehabilitation therapist can prescribe specific exercises and stretches and posture/movement re-education to correct it as part of your treatment. These professionals can also perform physical assessment and testing to help further determine or refine a diagnosis and decide which treatment methods will be most effective.

You should see a rehabilitation therapist on a regular basis, usually one to three times per week. These therapists can be very helpful not only in delivering treatment, but also in encouraging and reassuring you as you heal and recover from your injury. Since you see them often, you can develop a strong relationship with the therapist, who can become your cheerleader, an ally in your recovery.

Choose a rehabilitation therapist who specializes in treatment of musculoskeletal disorders. You may need to call several practitioners and ask them if they regularly treat MSDs and if they incorporate manual therapy (the best ones do), to find the most experienced professional to treat your injury. If your injury is to your upper extremity, a certified hand therapist may be the most appropriate rehabilitation therapist for you.

Exercise, Stretching and Mobilization

The exercises and stretches you saw in Chapter 11 were designed for manual therapists who are symptom-free. For an injured manual therapist, rehabilitation therapists will usually prescribe a set of exercises and stretches specifically designed to treat that person's injury. Many experts believe that exercise should be started as early as possible in injury treatment. Some physical therapists feel that MSD patients should start exercising as soon as mild exercise can be performed, even if there is still pain when doing them. Exercise counteracts muscle atrophy from disuse, and stretching and mobilization help restore range of motion and avoid abnormal scar tissue formation. Your rehabilitation therapist will design an exercise program tailored to your needs. Stick to this program, and do not supplement it with your own exercises: some exercises or stretches may be counterproductive and contraindicated at certain points in your treatment.

Strengthening exercises are contraindicated in the first, acute stages of injury. The repetitiveness of strengthening exercises may in itself exacerbate your injury. Since it is often difficult to determine the right time to start exercise, rely on your therapist to tell you when the time is right.

Rehabilitation therapists will usually do passive stretching and mobilization with you in the early stages of treatment. Passive exercise will be added to your treatment plan as your injury begins to heal. As your injury and symptoms permit, you will start to perform exercises and stretches yourself, with your therapist and at home. It is important to do these exercises consistently. Most likely, part of the reason you were injured was that your muscles were too weak to withstand the intensity of the work that was demanded of them. It may also be that your postural (core) muscles were weak, so you were unable to maintain a healthy working posture. Unless you strengthen those muscles, you will not be up to the demands of your work. Once you are out of rehabilitation therapy, it will be important to maintain and eventually increase your level of fitness and strength to avoid re-injuring yourself.

People who are injured tend to instinctively avoid using the injured body part, to protect it from further injury. This fear and subsequent immobilization contribute to the vicious cycle of chronic pain. One of the goals of rehabilitation therapy is to restore normal movement patterns and get the client to use the injured part of the body again without pain or other symptoms.

Heat and Cold Therapy

Application of heat or ice is often used as part of rehabilitation or massage therapy treatments. Both heat and ice can be used effectively for treating MSDs, but these treatments are sometimes overlooked in favor of anti-inflammatory medication and muscle relaxants.

Generally, ice is used to treat acute injury where inflammation may be present, and heat is used for chronic injury. Heat, especially moist heat, is effective in reducing chronic muscle tightness or muscle spasm, such as in non-specific low back pain or tension neck syndrome, as well as other symptoms associated with MSDs. The application of heat increases circulation to superficial tissues, which makes rigid, contracted muscle tissue more pliable and speeds healing.

Applying heat is contraindicated for the treatment of acute inflammation, or for nerve injuries where inflammation is present and may place additional pressure on irritated nerves. Since heat causes vasodilation, it can increase inflammation in these conditions. Ice is contraindicated for Raynaud's syndrome or any other circulatory problems, since the vasoconstriction that ice application induces would further reduce circulation. Heat can be applied to structures close to the skin using wet towels or damp pads, electric heating pads or microwaveable hot packs, and to deeper structures using ultrasound equipment.

Ice causes temporary vasoconstriction, provoking an increase in blood flow to the tissues. Injuries in which inflammation plays a major role respond very well to ice treatments. Ice therapy can involve direct ice massage, the use of ice packs, or ice water immersion. Direct ice massage to pinpoint specific areas of pain may be more helpful than applying ice to an entire area of tissue, since ice massage brings about a greater increase in circulation to the area, facilitating healing. After ice is applied, the influx of blood to the area will make it stiff and inflexible; it is best to allow the area to return to a normal temperature before treating it further. Ice also can be also used as a natural pain reliever. When you apply ice to the injured area, it becomes numb, and pain diminishes temporarily. Always exercise caution and lay a cloth on the skin first when applying ice to avoid freezing the skin, and when using heat to avoid burning the skin.

Whether to apply heat or ice can be a tough call in many injuries. The musculature around the injury may be quite hypertonic, but depending on the nature of the injury, inflammation may also be present. Some people respond better to ice than to heat, and vice versa. You may need ice application at first, and heat later on. As a general rule, if the area feels hot, ice is most likely the best treatment; if it feels cold and stiff, heat is probably the way to go.

Before treating at home with heat or cold therapy, it is always best to consult your rehabilitation therapist or PCP so they can help you decide which treatment is safe and advisable at a given time. If you would like to supplement the hydrotherapy treatments you receive from the therapist with home treatments, ask them to help you coordinate your efforts with theirs to avoid over-treatment.

Splints and Supports

Rehabilitation therapists, particularly occupational therapists, sometimes prescribe splints or supports to help treat MSDs. There is a big difference between a "splint" and a "support." Supports are used to provide extra stability to weak joints, not to rest injuries. Splints are a rigid medical device prescribed to immobilize a joint to allow it to rest as part of treating a particular condition. If wearing a splint is indicated to treat your injury, it will be selected or custom-designed and created specifically for you by a healthcare professional licensed to dispense and prescribe them. This same professional will monitor your condition and determine how you should use the splint. Splints should not be self-prescribed, nor used preventively.

Splinting has been traditionally recommended for upper extremity injury, to allow an injured thumb, wrist or elbow to rest and recover. Some conditions, notably carpal tunnel syndrome, respond well to the limited use of wrist splints. Night splints help CTS sufferers avoid flexing their wrists as they sleep, since wrist flexion puts pressure on the median nerve and causes numbness and tingling, often waking the sufferer and disrupting restful sleep. These splints are typically designed to be comfortable enough to wear all night without causing irritation. Some CTS sufferers are able to train themselves to sleep with their hands straight between pillows instead of wearing night splints.

For other soft-tissue injuries, wearing a splint can be a mixed blessing. If you wear it during the day and continue to use your hands and arms for normal activities, you may end up fighting against the splint or working with your upper arm in awkward positions, and do more harm than good. While splints do allow an injury to rest, over-dependency on or overuse of splints can cause atrophy and weakness that can hinder your ability to heal. For this reason, use of splints full-time or for long periods of time is not recommended. Given the risks associated with splint use, it is important to closely follow the instructions provided by the prescribing practitioner.

If you wear a splint for any length of time, be on the lookout for diminished muscle size in the injured area and inform the prescribing practitioner if you notice atrophy. If your injury is not severe, you should be able to take the splint off for some time each day and do exercises to keep the muscles toned. If you are severely injured, you may have to put up with some atrophy to get the benefit of resting the injured area.

Another potential problem with splinting is loss of range of motion at the joint. In a soft tissue injury, muscle or tendon tissue can heal solidly together and greatly reduce range of motion. Combining the use of a splint with gentle mobilization and exercise can minimize the formation of scar tissue and keep it from hardening and shrinking while allowing the injury to rest.

Unless specifically prescribed for that purpose, supports and splints should not be used as you work. Splints can weaken muscles and transfer stress to other joints. Supports may also weaken muscles and increase heat in the area, which could increase inflammation if it is present.

If a support is recommended, wrist and elbow supports and neoprene wraps usually can be bought without a prescription at your pharmacy. These supports come in standard sizes, so they may not be exactly the right size for you. A poorly fitting support can be ineffective or even aggravate your symptoms. A doctor or rehabilitation therapist can supply you with adjustable, better-quality supports than those available at the pharmacy. Some insurance policies will cover them.

Massage Therapy

Muscle hypertonicity and spasm often accompany MSDs. The muscles surrounding an injury site contract and go into spasm in an attempt to "splint" and guard the injured area from further trauma. Chronic muscle hypertonicity causes local vasoconstriction, leading to ischemia, further muscle contraction, spasm and pain. Massage can be a very effective treatment in relieving pain and increasing circulation to the injured area.

Massage treatment can include relaxing hypertonic muscles, releasing trigger points, and providing overall relaxation to reduce stress and feelings of anxiety. In fact, reducing pain and emotional stress may be necessary to get the most benefit from strengthening and flexibility exercises that are frequently prescribed as part of rehabilitation therapy. Tight bands of muscles that are associated with trigger points will become tighter and elicit painful symptoms if they are stretched, further reducing range of motion and function and possibly creating a pain fear-avoidance response. It is helpful to be massaged by a practitioner who is skilled at finding and relieving trigger points before beginning therapy that requires a more active patient role, such as stretching and strengthening exercises.

It is best not to massage an acute injury site directly, as any mechanical friction or pressure could cause additional irritation and tissue damage. At this stage, massage can help reduce muscle tightness, spasm or guarding in the areas surrounding the injury.

If the acute injury is to a limb, your therapist can work on muscles one joint proximal to the injury location. For example, if an acute injury to the forearm causes muscle spasm in that area, the therapist can work on the muscles above the elbow to help prevent the upper arm and shoulder muscles from also going into spasm.

Gentle, passive movement of the injured area can keep the tissues flexible and help prevent abnormal formation of scar tissue. Manual lymphatic drainage (MLD) techniques can facilitate removal of metabolic byproducts and edema from the damaged tissues. As this technique involves light pressure, it can be done close to acute injury sites. Once these gentle techniques have had their desired effect, massage in the injured area can be effective in breaking up and realigning scar tissue to restore full range of motion.

Studies have shown that massage can be an effective treatment for many types of MSDs, including low back pain, especially if it is non-specific in origin. In fact, the combination of treating hypertonicity and trigger points, and reducing emotional stress while promoting a relaxation response is ideal for treating many causes of chronic pain. Massage therapists can also use hot and cold treatments (or both, for contrast therapy) to treat the areas around the injury. Massage may also help reduce the symptoms of CTS by relaxing arm muscles to take pressure off the flexor tendons, releasing fascia to allow the tendons and median nerve to move freely, increasing circulation to flush out waste products, and reducing edema. It can also help reorganize scar tissue formation around the carpal tunnel to help open up the space, reducing pressure on the median nerve.

Conditions such as myofascial pain syndrome, which are characterized by widespread trigger points, can be effectively treated with massage therapy. Disorders that are primarily due to static loading and the lack of circulation that accompanies it, such as tension neck

Effective Soft Tissue Treatments for MSDs

There are many types of soft tissue techniques that can be used to treat MSDs, but not all of these techniques are effective for every injury or every person. Here are some of the soft tissue techniques that show promise for treating MSDs.

Trigger Point Therapy: It is likely that trigger points play a role in many musculoskeletal disorders. They share the same perpetuating factors as MSDs, and many of the same symptoms. Treating trigger points can reduce or eliminate the symptoms they cause, such as muscle tension and referred pain, making it easier to get at any underlying conditions. Many massage and rehabilitation therapists treat trigger points. If you suspect that you have widespread trigger points, consider seeing a therapist with advanced training or certification in trigger point treatment, such as myofascial trigger point therapy or neuromuscular therapy. Massage therapists typically treat trigger points through ischemic compression or repetitive strokes in the direction of the muscle fibers. Practitioners with a broader scope of practice can use techniques such as "spray and stretch," where a coolant is sprayed on the skin above the trigger point while a stretch is applied to the muscle, or injection of a pain reliever directly into the trigger point. These techniques may be more effective for patients whose trigger points are too sensitive to be treated with massage techniques.

Myofascial Release: Many manual therapists are trained in myofascial release, which can be helpful in treating the trigger points and adhesions that are associated with MSDs and myofascial pain syndrome.

Myofascial release increases circulation to trigger points in order to deactivate them, and mobilizes the fascia surrounding muscles, both directly through manual techniques and indirectly through active and passive stretching. These techniques restore freedom of movement and balance to an area while relieving pain. A practitioner with training in myofascial release will be able to perform a thorough assessment of your body's fascial tissues, finding restrictions and then stretching the tissues to restore normal function. Since fascia runs throughout the body, many practitioners believe that a systematic, holistic approach to myofascial treatment is most effective. Structural integration methods are an example of this systematic approach.

Structural Integration: There are several variations of deep bodywork that are based on Ida Rolf's theories of structural integration. This type of bodywork typically involves a series of ten treatment sessions designed to release long-held patterns of improper posture and movement. Structural integration includes modalities such as Rolfing®, Zentherapy®, Hellerwork® and Soma Neuromuscular Integration®, each of which brings a slightly different focus to the treatment sessions. Physical release of tight muscles and fascia is often accompanied by emotional release, which can add to the effectiveness of these treatments in dealing with chronic pain.

Active Release Techniques: Another method used to break up adhesions is Active Release Techniques® (ART). In ART, the practitioner locates an adhesion by palpation, and then holds it while the client makes active movements to break the adhesion away from underlying tissue. ART consists of hundreds of protocols designed to address specific conditions, most of which are MSDs caused by overuse. ART may be useful for treating myofascial adhesions, or for freeing nerves that have become trapped by adhesions along their pathways.

syndrome, often respond well to effleurage and myofascial release techniques. Symptoms of thoracic outlet syndrome can be addressed by carefully reducing hypertonicity in the scalenes and pectoralis minor in order to increase the space in the thoracic outlet, taking pressure off the nerve plexus and blood vessels in the area. Tendonitis and bursitis symptoms may be relieved by relaxing the muscles that keep tendons under tension or pull them across bursae.

The value of full-body, relaxation massage in healing injury should not be overlooked or underestimated. People who are injured experience their injury throughout their bodies, not just in the affected body part. Pain, anxiety and discomfort tend to cause a good deal of general muscular tension and guarding, which can slow healing and exacerbate symptoms. Even those conditions that are not directly related to the musculoskeletal system, or are of uncertain origin such as chronic, non-specific pain, may benefit from the reduction in overall physical and emotional tension that massage provides.

Some health plans and workers' compensation systems will pay for massage treatments, although in many cases the massage treatments must be prescribed as part of a treatment plan developed by another health care professional.

Chiropractic Treatment

Chiropractors work to increase mobility and correct misalignments in the spine and other joints. These misalignments are referred to as subluxations. To accomplish these goals, chiropractors commonly perform manipulations called adjustments. Much of the work chiropractors do involves manual techniques, including some soft tissue mobilization, to help vertebrae and other joints move back into their proper position and move freely. The combination of adjustments and soft-tissue work can help reduce pain and spasm along the spine, as well as any of the symptoms that nerve root compression may cause in other parts of the body.

Despite criticism from the traditional medical field, chiropractic has become the most commonly used form of complementary medicine. Chiropractic treatment may be effective in cases of chronic neck or low back pain, particularly if it is related to a subluxation of the vertebrae in that area. A combination of soft-tissue treatment and chiropractic adjustment may be effective for MSDs, as it addresses both the sub-luxations in the spine that may irritate nerves and put muscles into spasm, as well as the tight or imbalanced muscles that may be causing or aggravating vertebral subluxation. Be sure to find an experienced chiropractor who is well versed in treating MSDs.

Osteopathic Manipulative Treatment

Osteopaths (DOs) are fully licensed physicians in many jurisdictions. The focus of their training and practice is typically the musculoskeletal system. DOs practice a form of therapy that treats musculoskeletal impairments through joint manipulation and soft tissue work. While they may treat the spine, their approach is somewhat different from a chiropractor. DOs use a broad range of techniques including strain-counterstrain, muscle energy technique, myofascial release and trigger point therapy. Given their ability to diagnose, use manipulative thera-pies, and in many jurisdictions prescribe medication, an osteopath may be a good choice for a PCP for a musculoskeletal disorder.

Medications

Medication is often used as part of a treatment plan to reduce inflam-mation if present and relieve pain from MSDs. The most commonly used medications that can achieve these effects fall into three categories: non-steroidal anti-inflammatory drugs (NSAIDs); acetaminophen for pain relief if you can't tolerate NSAIDs; muscle relaxers such as robaxin or flexeril; and anti-inflammatory steroids. The type of pain medica-tion you use will depend on your injury and the recommendations of your PCP.

All medications, including those prescribed for MSDs, have side effects that should be considered and evaluated before you begin to take them. When prescribing medication for your injury, your PCP should discuss the possible side effects with you and confirm that any other medications you are taking or conditions you have (including allergies) do not contraindicate use of the prescribed medication.

Non-Steroidal Anti-Inflammatory Drugs (NSAIDs)

Aspirin, ibuprofen and naproxen sodium are examples of NSAIDs that are usually available without a prescription. Acetaminophen (known as paracetamol in some countries) can relieve pain, but has no anti-inflammatory effect. Your PCP can prescribe prescription-strength NSAIDs that may be more effective than the non-prescription versions. Each of these medications works in a slightly different way; you may need to try several (but not at the same time!) before you find the one that is most effective for you. NSAIDs like ibuprofen or naproxen sodium may not be effective in treating conditions such as tendonosis, where inflammation is not the cause of ongoing symptoms, but may be effective for pain relief.

NSAIDs can carry cardiovascular risks and can be irritating or even damaging to the stomach, and should be used with great care. Certain NSAIDs do not interact well with other NSAIDs and should not be taken at the same time.

Taking NSAIDs for the purpose of reducing inflammation is only appropriate if your PCP feels you have a new, acute case of tendinitis. As we said earlier in this book, most experts feel that all tendinopathy is tendinosis with no inflammatory component, NOT tendinitis or another inflammatory condition. If your PCP feels that your particular injury may respond well to NSAIDs, you can certainly give that treatment a try for a few weeks to see if it helps reduce inflammation (if present), in addition to relieving pain.

NSAIDS must be taken consistently for 10–14 days, around the clock, to be effective in reducing inflammation. For example, taking ibuprofen sporadically for a few days will have little effect, because there is no sustained level of anti-inflammatory drug in your bloodstream. Usually it takes a week or two for this type of medication to start reducing inflammation to an appreciable degree if inflammation is present, although it may work within a day or two to relieve pain.

Muscle Relaxers

Pain tends to cause muscle guarding and spasms that can hinder your recovery. Drugs like robaxin or flexeril, to name just a few, can help your muscles relax so your prescribed treatments can have more of an effect.

Anti-Inflammatory Steroids

Cortisone is a synthetic steroid used to reduce inflammation. Cortisone injections are a common treatment for tendinitis if your PCP is certain that is the correct diagnosis, and can be very effective. Often one injection in the right spot can clear up a mild or moderate case of tendinitis immediately. Cortisone injections can be effective enough at reducing inflammation and scar tissue and allowing healing to eliminate the need for surgery for some conditions.

Cortisone injections can have little to no effect on other types of MSDs. If your pain is not related to the presence of inflammation (which is the case with many common MSDs), such as in tendonosis or nerve entrapment due to adhesions, the use of cortisone is not indicated. Cortisone injections, if necessary, should be administered by a specialist, since the medication must be injected into exactly the right place to be effective. If injected directly into the tendon or joint cartilage, cortisone can cause weakness of the tendon or softening of cartilage. For this reason, it is usually injected in the area around a tendon or joint, and not directly into the connective tissue itself.

Typically, a single cortisone injection is given to see if it reduces symptoms before considering further injections. If the first cortisone injection is effective, it is sometimes followed by a booster shot. Your PCP and the specialist who administers the cortisone should help you weigh the benefits and risks of repeated cortisone injections for your condition.

Opioids

Within our nervous systems are receptors for opiates, specifically the endogenous opiates known as endorphins. Endorphins are neurotransmitters that are released in response to pain, binding with the opiate receptors to reduce the intensity of pain sensations and produce a mild euphoria.

Opioids are a class of pain-relieving medications that also bind with opiate receptors. Codeine, oxycodone, hydrocodone or percocet are commonly used opioids. In certain very specific, chronic, intractable conditions, and under the strict supervision of a qualified pain doctor, these medications may be an effective part of a pain-management plan. Bear in mind, and discuss with your PCP, that these medications are HIGHLY

ADDICTIVE and should only be used under extraordinary circumstances. In general, due to the highly addictive qualities of this class of medication, they should be approached with great caution or not prescribed at all.

Other Prescription Medications

In addition to the medications mentioned above, your doctor may prescribe muscle relaxants or antispasmotics for acute muscle spasms. These drugs, such as diazepam or cyclobenzaprine, help reduce the muscle tension, spasms and anxiety that often accompany a musculoskeletal disorder. Antidepressants are another class of medications that can be beneficial in treating musculoskeletal disorders, because they have pain-relieving qualities in addition to their mood-improving effects. These include (among others) gabapentin, tricyclics like amitriptyline, and SNRI's like duloxetine.

Safe Use of Nutritional and Herbal Supplements

Naturally occurring substances are not necessarily safe just because they are "natural." They can interact with each other or with over-the-counter and prescription medications and have significant side effects. High doses of vitamin C, for example, may destroy the body's supply of vitamin B12. A number of herbal supplements can interact with medications for diabetes, blood pressure or the heart, among others. Devil's claw, for example, can affect heart rate, blood pressure, stomach acidity, blood clotting ability and blood sugar. It may also cause allergic reactions, headaches, tinnitus (ringing in the ears), and loss of the sense of taste. It should be avoided by anyone who is pregnant or nursing, and all others should check with a doctor, naturopath or pharmacist for information about possible interactions with other medications, and health conditions for which this supplement may be contraindicated. Be sure to tell your PCP, naturopath and pharmacist about all medications and supplements you are taking, to avoid any potential negative reactions or interactions.

Vitamins and Herbal Supplements

A naturopath can prescribe herbal anti-inflammatory preparations that may be effective for musculoskeletal injuries if inflammation is present. Several naturally occurring substances are thought to have anti-inflammatory properties, including vitamin C in high doses, ginger, turmeric and bromelain (if taken without food). Topical ointments containing menthol (an oil extracted from peppermint) or capsaicin (an extract from chili peppers) may be effective at reducing symptoms of pain. Standardized extracts of herbs such as devil's claw and white willow bark may have both anti-inflammatory and analgesic properties to help reduce symptoms of disorders such as non-specific low back pain. Glucosamine, chondroitin and silicon (which can be extracted from horsetail and nettles) may help repair connective tissue and cartilage.

At this time, there have not been enough well-designed scientific studies performed to determine whether these natural treatments are effective, and a full picture of all side effects they may produce. One issue has become clear from the studies that have been performed on these substances—they do not work for everyone, and they are not highly regulated enough to know if you are getting the real product, and in the dosage indicated on the label. Some patients report very good results anecdotally, while others see no improvement in symptoms. These treatments may also take considerably longer to be effective when compared to over-the-counter anti-inflammatories and pain relievers such as acetaminophen (paracetamol) or ibuprofen.

Surgical Treatment of MSDs

Surgery may be proposed for certain conditions when conservative treatments have not been effective in adequately reducing symptoms or restoring normal function. Surgery is a more invasive treatment, so there is a greater amount of risk associated with it than with more conservative treatments. Some of the potential complications of surgical treatment are swelling, temporary or permanent loss of function, nerve damage, and infection. Even successful surgery can have side effects such as scarring, pain and reduced function that can take time to resolve. Despite these risks, there are conditions for which surgery is the most effective form of treatment.

With some conditions, such as vertebral disc herniation or complete rotator cuff tear, surgery may be the only option that can restore normal function and relieve pain. In the case of true, accurately diagnosed carpal tunnel syndrome that has not responded to more conservative treatments, surgery can completely relieve the nerve impingement. Recovery of feeling and strength in the hand is better if surgery to relieve pressure on the nerve is done as quickly as possible after the onset of symptoms. Recent advances in carpal tunnel surgery, such as endoscopic release, may permit a faster and less painful return to work, leave smaller scars, and conserve grip strength. The quality of endoscopic surgeries can vary, however, and there is an increased risk of complications, such as incomplete release of the transverse ligament or inadvertent damage to the nerve or tendons. Any surgery for CTS can result in complications, so it is imperative to have a conclusive diagnosis from a neurologist before proceeding with CTS surgery. To make their diagnosis, the neurologist should test for median nerve conduction latency at the carpal tunnel and rule out any possible impingement in the upper extremity, thoracic outlet and cervical spine that could be causing your symptoms.

For other conditions, surgery is often ineffective. Surgery is seldom indicated or effective as a treatment for non-specific muscle/tendon injury classified simply as overuse syndrome, since it may cause more problems than it solves. The intrusion of surgical instruments into the

Questions to Ask a Surgeon

- Are there any effective alternatives to surgery?
- What are the potential consequences if I don't have surgery?
- What is the general success rate with this type of operation?
- How many times have you performed this specific procedure?
- What is your success rate with this procedure?
- Will you refer me to rehabilitation following the procedure?
- How long should recovery take?
- When will I be able to return to work?
- Will I lose any strength, range of motion or other functionality?
- Are there any other potential complications or side-effects of this surgery that I should be aware of?

small spaces and delicate structures of the hand, for example, can cause damage and consequences beyond the original injury. As with all treatments, the potential side effects and complications of surgery must be weighed against the possible benefits.

If you consult with a surgeon, be prepared to hear them recommend surgery. Like you, they chose their specialty because they believe it is an effective way to treat people who are ill or injured. Even if you are totally averse to the idea of surgery, a surgeon may be able to give you information that can help you determine the best course of treatment for your MSD.

Before considering any surgery, you must be sure to have an exact diagnosis of your injury. It is important to also get a second opinion from another physician or surgeon with the same specialty as the one you have already seen. Be prepared to do a good deal of research on the surgery that is suggested for your injury. Find out both the general success rate for the type of surgery that you are considering and the individual success rate of your surgeon and other surgeons in your area for that surgery.

As with any healthcare profession, the quality of surgeons will vary. Look for a surgeon who is board certified, as they must meet higher standards. Experience counts a great deal with surgery, and someone who has performed a particular procedure a few hundred times is bound to be more proficient than someone who has done the same procedure only a few dozen times. You may want to work with a surgeon who specializes in the part of the body that you have injured: a hand surgeon, for example, may be the best choice for an injury to the hand or wrist. Ask your PCP or other physicians you already know and trust which surgeons in your area are experienced and have a good reputation. A local hospital may also be able to help with a referral. If there is a particularly good surgeon in your area for your type of injury, his or her name will likely come up more than once as you are making your inquiries.

As a potential consumer of surgical services, you have the right to shop around for the best possible treatment. Just be sure not to put off surgery too long in cases where a delay could result in permanent disability, such as with nerve impingement. Remember, the goal with surgery is to get through it as well and as quickly as possible, so you can begin the rehabilitation and recovery process.

Rehabilitation After Surgery

Surgery is just the first step in the overall surgical treatment process. Following the surgery, your surgeon should give you a referral and prescription for rehabilitation to restore function to the affected area. Rehabilitation is usually performed by a physical therapist, occupational therapist, or physical medicine and rehabilitation (PM&R) physician. The first goals of rehabilitation are typically to maintain or increase range of motion while reducing pain and inflammation to promote healing. Later phases of rehabilitation can involve reorganizing scar tissue and increasing range of motion while building strength and coordination. As you go through rehab, the rehab specialist you see should help you understand what caused your injury in the first place, to ensure that you don't get back into the same bad habits and re-injure yourself.

Returning to Work

If you have taken time off from work to treat your injury, returning to work can be challenging. Injured therapists understandably want to heal as quickly as possible so they can return to a normal life and practice. You may also be feeling financial pressure to return to a full workload right away. Despite these feelings, it is critical to be patient and allow yourself adequate time to recover before returning to work. MSDs typically take months or years to develop, so they usually take a good amount of time to heal. Even if you are not experiencing symptoms at the moment, your symptoms may recur at a future time, particularly if you push yourself to go back to work too soon. Some MSDs have symptoms like irritation and pain that can come and go over time. Certain treatments, like cortisone injections, may relieve symptoms quickly, leading you to believe you are healed and can resume using your hands or arms the way you did prior to your injury. If you do resume your activities before the injury has had a chance to heal, you may re-injure yourself. Going back to square one when you were on the road to recovery is more frustrating and injurious than being conservative and waiting for true healing to occur. For these reasons, it is best to be cautious and gradually work your way back into resuming your work.

Consult with your principle healthcare provider (PCP), as well as the rehabilitation professional that has been treating you, to determine if you are ready to start working again, and how many hours you can work per week. Together you can create a schedule that includes a gradual increase in work time based on how you feel.

As you return to work, be aware that you may encounter some of the same risk factors that caused or aggravated your symptoms. Resuming work activities may bring back those symptoms. You will need to be particularly attentive so you can respond to any symptoms that arise and change your work techniques or ergonomics accordingly. Certainly, no one who has been injured by their work should start working again as though nothing had ever happened, even if their symptoms seem to have resolved. You will need to make changes to avoid those work methods that caused or aggravated your symptoms, as they are the most likely to cause a recurrence. It will also be helpful to reduce your exposure to risk factors in general, perhaps by choosing to do less hands-on work, taking longer breaks between clients or patients, or deciding to use different, less stressful techniques than before—especially as you are first returning to work.

Depending on how much time you had to take off, and how you rehabilitated your injury, you may not have the same level of conditioning for hands-on work as you did before. Even though your rehabilitation may have given you a base of strength and endurance, conditioning is largely activity-specific. You will need to do some actual hands-on treatments to rebuild strength and endurance in the specific muscle groups you use in your work.

Work with your PCP and your rehabilitation therapist to develop a return-to-work plan, which should be coordinated with your employer. The plan may include some initial restrictions on the number of hours you work or the types of treatments you perform, with the understanding that you will be able to increase your work intensity gradually if you remain largely symptom-free. Part of the return to work plan can include an ergonomics evaluation of your work environment and habits, particularly if your rehabilitation therapist or your workers' compensation provider offers this service. If your work caused or aggravated your injury, and you do not make changes to the way you work or the amount of work you take on, you run the risk of re-aggravating your injury and developing a chronic condition. Remember, there are many risk factors that lead to MSDs and cause them to become chronic, and it can be difficult to determine exactly which exposures to avoid. This is a good time to review the risk factors in Chapter 3 and evaluate your exposure to them in your work and other activities, using the risk factor worksheet in Appendix A.

Prior injury is a significant risk factor and one of the primary predictors of a future injury. Once you have had an injury, you are more prone to injury at the same site, due to weakness in the previously damaged tissues. You may also be prone to injury at other sites, due to changes in your movement patterns as you compensate for the loss of function of the previously injured area. Consider a person who has had a knee injury and now finds it difficult or painful to kneel or squat. They will bend at the waist more often than before, increasing the likelihood of injury to their lower back.

It is also important to continue treatment as you start working again. You may be tempted to stop your treatment program once you begin to feel better. If you feel fine except for a twinge here and there, you may not see any reason to continue doing stretches and exercises, using heat or ice, or receiving massage. Since many MSDs can have lingering symptoms, continuing your rehabilitation as a precaution makes sense. This is particularly true if one of the causes of the original injury was muscle weakness or imbalance, poor movement patterns, adhesions, or other vulnerabilities that rehabilitation can address. The goal of rehabilitation at this point is to maintain strength and flexibility, and help keep scar tissue properly oriented to prevent adhesions.

Continuing in Your Profession Following Injury

When you have had a work-related injury, you may doubt your ability to continue in your profession. If you have been injured and are concerned that the symptoms you are experiencing will be a permanent part of your life, you can take some comfort from the results of the surveys discussed in Chapter 1. Of those massage therapists who reported symptoms related to work, almost all reported that their symptoms had either completely resolved, or were only present at a low level. A very small percentage of those with symptoms reported that they still were occurring at a high level or that they had considered leaving their profession because of their symptoms. Many of the respondents reported making other changes, such as reducing the number of massages they did or changing techniques, but for the most part they continued in their profession.

The survey of physical therapists also reported a considerable number of practitioners who had experienced symptoms, and about 1 in 6 changed to a different specialty within the profession or left the profession altogether due to an MSD. Out of this group, however, the vast majority changed specialties and remained physical therapists. Most of the different hands-on practitioners who had symptoms were able to make changes to their practice in order to continue working. Massage practitioners reported changing techniques, changing table height, improving their body mechanics, reducing use of a body part (like their thumbs) while performing massage, and leaving more time between massages to avoid the recurrence of symptoms. In addition to changing specialties, physical therapists more often asked physical therapist assistants to help with physically demanding tasks, adjusted treatment table height and client position, and used more electrotherapy or other less hand-intensive techniques in place of manual treatment. If the injury were to a different part of the body than the upper extremity, for example, the back, they spent more time in positions (e.g., seated on a stool) and avoided lifting as much as possible. Chiropractors were also able to use technology in place of manual methods.

While PTs and chiropractors have a broad range of treatment modalities available to them, and therefore have many options available to them after injury, massage practitioners may feel more limited. After all, massage is primarily a hands-on treatment method, with a scope of practice that limits the use of technology or other alternatives. Despite these limitations, the field of massage is very broad, and massage therapists have a wide range of modalities to choose from that are easier on the practitioner than deep tissue, clinical and Swedish massage. Some modalities, such as lymphatic drainage or craniosacral techniques, require very little pressure to perform and offer more opportunities to work while seated. Others, such as Trager®, muscle energy technique, positional release and strain-counterstrain involve moving and positioning the client rather than repetitive strokes or deep pressure. Reiki and breathwork can also be quite beneficial and attractive modalities for the client, depending on their needs. With some additional training, you can learn one or several of these techniques and incorporate them into your work. You could also become certified in spa techniques, many of which offer therapeutic benefits to clients while being less demanding on the practitioner.

16

When Injuries Become Chronic

With appropriate and timely treatment, and modifications to work, home activities and pastimes to reduce exposure to the risk factors that caused the injury, most MSDs slowly heal. Symptoms subside and eventually disappear. But a small percentage of manual therapists will continue to have ongoing symptoms, even after receiving appropriate treatment and modifying their habits. Some of these practitioners have injuries that are particularly stubborn, and have to cope with symptoms for a while until they eventually go away. Others have injuries that are complex, advanced and/or resistant to treatment. Their symptoms linger on, possibly because they are not able to identify and correct the cause of their injury and end up re-injuring themselves. If they eventually do discover the cause, their symptoms may start to resolve. It is also possible that they have caused irreversible damage to their tissues, and that damage causes ongoing symptoms. Now that their injury has become chronic, these therapists need to think of recovery as a long-term process and make changes in their work and home life to accommodate their symptoms.

A basic tenet of medicine is that most disease is self-limiting. In other words, the body will be able to heal itself from any condition as long as it is not constantly re-exposed to the causes of the condition. In fact, one of the reasons it is difficult to study the relative effectiveness of treatments for various conditions, including MSDs, is that most patients get better over the course of any study regardless of the type of treatment they are undergoing, even if it is a placebo. All that is needed to heal many conditions is the body's own healing ability and the reduction of anxiety that results from dealing with an injury and seeing a medical professional.

Injuries or illnesses that are not self-limiting can become chronic. Once a musculoskeletal disorder begins, cycles of pain, muscle guarding, fatigue, inactivity, loss of range of motion and reduced circulation can set in. These symptoms can be accompanied by emotional cycles of fear, anxiety, depression and avoidance. In time, people who experience chronic pain can end up believing that they will never get better. If they can break these cycles by eliminating or reducing the causes of the disorder and treating their symptoms and receiving the emotional support they need, they may well be able to move from a chronic state back to a self-limiting one.

It is still not clear why some conditions become chronic, while others do not. Conditions such as bulging discs in the spine that press on nerve roots, loss of joint cartilage that results in inflammation as part of degenerative joint disease, or overused tendons that remain irritated and painful, all have specific, physiological causes that can be identified and treated. However, a significant minority of MSDs have no identifiable cause: these conditions are often described as *non-specific, insidious or idiopathic*. It may be that many of these idiopathic conditions are the result of self-perpetuating pain signals due to chronic pain left untreated, or are due to subtle physiological changes that are difficult to detect, diagnose and treat. While a great deal of research is being conducted on the underlying causes of these non-specific conditions, it may take some time until effective treatments are developed. You can see why prevention and early treatment of symptoms is so critical.

That does not mean that nothing can be done about non-specific or chronic conditions. First of all, stay in touch with your PCP so they can continue to monitor your health and suggest possible treatments. Treatments can focus on reducing symptoms to a tolerable level, and

Common Symptoms of Depression

Just as with MSDs, it is important to treat depression early and appropriately so it doesn't worsen or become chronic. If you experience any of these symptoms for more than two weeks, consult your primary healthcare provider (PCP) or a mental health professional to be evaluated for depression.

- Feelings of hopelessness, worthlessness or guilt

- Lack of interest in your usual activities or pastimes

- Difficulty carrying out daily activities

- Loss of appetite

- Feelings of sadness or frequent spells of crying

- Thoughts of death or suicide

- Fatigue, lethargy or lack of energy

- Feeling down or empty

- Feeling agitated or restless

- Sleep disturbances

- Trouble concentrating

making changes at work and at home can help you avoid aggravating your symptoms. There is always hope that, given enough time and proper treatment, your symptoms will resolve to the point that they no longer prevent you from doing the things you want to do. In some cases, you may be plagued by symptoms for several years, and suddenly realize that the cycle of pain has simply stopped on its own and you feel much better. In the meantime, there are a number of practical steps you can take that can help you cope with your symptoms.

Coping With a Chronic Injury

An injury is considered chronic when symptoms continue beyond the normal duration of healing for a particular condition. Obviously an injury that continues that long is going to result in physical, emotional and financial concerns. MSDs can be particularly difficult to cope with emotionally, because there may be no outward signs of injury. Colleagues and family members may forget about the condition, or worse, begin to doubt the level of your symptoms. If your MSD prevents you from returning to work, you may feel alienated from your social network of colleagues and clients, and worried about your ability to make a living. If work caused the injury, you may be fearful and anxious about returning. All of these factors can reduce your motivation to take an active role in your recovery and rehabilitation.

A chronic injury can affect nearly every aspect of your life. You may be in pain some or all of the time, making you irritable, short-tempered or preoccupied. Your work may be interrupted, causing serious economic hardship and fear of losing career momentum or seniority. Your family may be less than completely supportive of your situation, which can leave you feeling abandoned. You may not be able to do your share of chores around the house, or become less involved in family activities, which can cause additional tension in your household. If your recovery is slow, you may lose hope at times.

As a result of these situations, you may experience a number of conflicting emotions—anger, sadness, frustration, despair—that can lead to anxiety and depression. Depression is, in fact, a very common side effect of injury. Symptoms of depression include feelings of hopelessness, lethargy, inability to carry out daily activities, frequent spells of crying, and loss of interest and enthusiasm for life. These symptoms should be carefully monitored. If they last more than two weeks, you should seek professional help. Left untreated, depression can worsen or become chronic; it can also interfere with your body's ability to heal, make you more attuned to pain, and hinder the treatment of your physical symptoms.

Staying proactive and seeking support for the emotional fallout of your condition can help you cope with the ups and downs of treating and living with a chronic injury. There are several steps you can take to keep your spirit in good shape as you move toward better health during treatment.

Keep a Symptoms Diary

People who have chronic conditions may begin to worry that they will never get better. One way to avoid this feeling is to keep a symptoms diary, in which you record your overall feelings and rate your symptoms on a numerical scale or another scale of your choice. Over time, you will notice that even though there are some days that are worse than others, on the whole you begin to have more good days than bad and your symptoms ratings show a trend toward improvement. Remember, some chronic conditions will resolve over time, but this can take months or even years. And as stated before, as time goes on you may start feeling better only to experience a setback, and then start feeling better again. During that time you will be better able to cope if you can keep a positive outlook. For those conditions that do not resolve, keeping a diary can help you keep track of activities that aggravate your symptoms, as well as activities and treatments that alleviate your symptoms.

Make a Plan for Dealing with Flare-Ups

One of the more frustrating aspects of recovering from an MSD can be the occasional flare-up of symptoms. Symptoms may recur for any number of reasons, including:

- You were beginning to feel better and overdid an activity
- A virus or other infection re-activated trigger points and caused muscle spasm
- Emotional distress caused an overall increase in muscle tension
- You had an accident, like a fall or playing a sport, involving the injured body part and aggravated your injury.

If you can identify the cause of the flare-up, you can try to avoid that exposure in the future. But often there are as many different factors that combine to cause a flare-up as there were in the original injury. In cases like these, the best you can do is to fall back on the coping methods that work best for you and remind yourself that symptom flare-ups are usually of short duration and will pass. Frequent or lengthy flare-ups indicate that further medical treatment is required. If you have gone back to work, you may need to take a break or cut back on your sessions until the flare-up subsides. Work with your PCP and your employer (if you have one) to develop a plan for dealing with flare-ups as they occur.

Treat Chronic Pain

Pain relief is important for your comfort level and recovery. If you have been in constant pain for a considerable amount of time, you may have nearly forgotten what it feels like to be pain free. Your muscles and nervous system may be in a continuous state of vigilance, waiting to defend you when the next wave of pain hits. Relieving pain, even if it is only for an hour or two, reminds your body what "normal" and "healthy" feel like. Once you remember that feeling, you can work more effectively toward health and normalcy.

Not enough is known at this time about the causes of chronic pain. There are often multiple risk factors involved in causing the disorders that result in chronic pain, and pain has numerous physical, psychological and emotional effects (see page 227). For these reasons, it does not make sense to approach the treatment of chronic pain by using just one modality; in fact, single modality treatments are often ineffective. It may be more effective to use a multidisciplinary team to deal with the causes and effects of chronic pain. This team often consists of a physician who is a pain specialist, a rehabilitation therapist, a psychologist, a vocational counselor, an anesthesiologist, and a massage practitioner, acupuncturist, or other complementary medicine practitioner.

Treatments may include medications to reduce the sensation of pain, injections to reduce inflammation or treat trigger points, rehabilitative exercises to maintain or improve conditioning and function, counseling to deal with the emotional and psychosocial aspects of pain, and massage to reduce stress and reduce muscle tension and address trigger points.

In cases where patients have become hypersensitive to pain signals, pain specialists can prescribe stronger medications, or use nerve blocks in cases of localized pain. Pain specialists are more likely to keep up on the latest research on pain, and may be able to provide newer and more effective treatments that other physicians may not be aware of.

Research into the physiological basis of chronic pain may yield new treatments that are more effective at addressing the specific causes of the pain, rather than just blocking all pain signals as many current pain medications do. For more information on pain treatment, see Chapter 15.

If you have good health insurance and access to a treatment center for chronic pain, you should take advantage of the services they offer. These centers specialize in complex cases, and often have multidisciplinary teams that can help you cope with the physical and emotional impacts of chronic pain. Treatments like these also exist for people who have limited resources: check with your municipality to see what's available. Even if you do not have access to this type of treatment facility, you should still plan on using multiple modalities as you arrange for healthcare and your own home care. Methods used to reduce inflammation, such as medication and ice therapy, are also very effective at relieving pain. Massage can relax stiff, tense, sore muscles and restore a feeling of well-being. Biofeedback, guided imagery, meditation and/or MBSR, breathwork and other relaxation techniques can help you deal with pain and stress. Many people swear by acupuncture for its pain-relief benefits. You can learn more about MBSR in Appendix C.

See a Counselor

It is impossible to properly treat your body without also addressing your emotions. Recent studies have proven that the body and mind cannot be separated: what happens to one affects the other. A counselor can help you bring these two pieces of the puzzle together. A well-trained counselor or psychotherapist can help you work out your feelings about your injury and how it is affecting your life. During a difficult or lengthy recovery period, it can be very reassuring to have someone in your life that is focused exclusively on your well-being and is always on your side. A good counselor can offer you encouragement, perspective, and compassion more consistently and objectively than even the best-meaning friend or family member. Chronic injury can be very upsetting. Having someone to rely on as you deal with it is invaluable. A sympathetic counselor can help you keep a positive attitude that can speed your healing process.

A counselor can also help you deal with your feelings about how and why you were injured. It is common for injury sufferers to feel that their injury happened because of some failing on their part. The information in this book should help you realize that injury is an occupational hazard of doing manual treatment work, and that a majority of manual therapists experience injury at some point in their careers. It is certainly not a sign of incompetence in your work and definitely not an indication that you are a bad person or that you did something "wrong." These attitudes can damage your self-esteem, or indicate that your self-esteem was not very strong to begin with. A skilled counselor can help you sort out these feelings, so you can regain a healthy self-image.

Your counselor can also help you identify deep-seated emotions that may have contributed to your injury, or may be keeping you from healing properly. Emotional issues like needing to prove your self-worth, difficulty setting boundaries with others, or expecting too much of yourself can all increase your risk of injury. A good psychotherapist, particularly one who has psychoanalytic training, can help you get at the root causes of these issues and overcome them. As a result, you will be better able to heal and avoid future situations that could cause re-injury.

If you are under a great deal of stress, your counselor may suggest some relaxation techniques such as meditation or guided imagery in addition to your sessions. Appendix C provides several techniques you can easily learn and then use to help reduce stress and regain a sense of well-being. The counselor may also recommend that you ask your doctor to prescribe a tranquilizer, anti-depressant or muscle relaxant to help you cope. Stress impedes healing, and should be reduced as much as possible while you are recuperating. If you have been feeling anxious and/or depressed consistently for more than two weeks, consider asking your doctor whether other medication or treatment approaches could be helpful. You are suffering enough just by being injured; don't hesitate to get the emotional help you need.

Your PCP may be able to refer you to a counselor in your area. Many pain centers and hospitals have mental health professionals on staff. Some communities have public health centers that offer psychological counseling at affordable prices; depending on your financial situation, there may be programs that will pay for part or all of this treatment. Licensure requirements vary for mental health professionals, but generally a Master of Social Work (MSW) trained in psychotherapy, a doctor of psychology (PhD) or a psychotherapist with recognized credentials and training are best suited to offer effective psychological services.

Join or Form a Support Group

Another way of coping emotionally is to join or form a support group. You may feel alone with your injury, and it is reassuring to know that there are many other therapists in your field who are going through the same experience. You may be able to find other injured therapists by putting a notice in your school's newsletter, website or on their bulletin board. Look in social media for groups you can join that may be helpful (note: *Save Your Hands!* will have a Facebook group shortly for this purpose). You can also contact the state or city chapter of your professional association and enlist their help in your search. Since injury is common among manual therapists, it should not be difficult to find others who will be willing to get together with you and share their experiences and feelings. Think about organizing a monthly in-person meeting, or an online meeting if that's more convenient.

Take Care of Yourself

While you are undergoing treatment for a chronic condition, do everything possible to take good care of yourself in general. It is common for people suffering from chronic injury to feel quite tired. Fatigue is a natural reaction to the ongoing pain and physical and emotional stress of chronic injury. Get plenty of sleep, eat well and exercise lightly to facilitate your healing. If you don't already have one, develop a good support network of family and friends, and let them know that you need their help to keep your morale up and cheer you on toward recovery. Give yourself a break, be good to yourself and let yourself heal.

Continuing to Work with a Chronic Injury

Chronic injuries are not necessarily debilitating. There were many practitioners in the survey of American massage therapists who reported ongoing symptoms that recurred frequently, but at a low level. These practitioners made changes to the way they practiced, including avoiding stressful techniques, reducing the number of treatments they gave in a week, and focusing more on their body mechanics and the ergonomics of their workspace. Physical therapists, physical therapist assistants and chiropractors all reported similar responses to their symptoms. The one thing they all had in common is that they were still involved enough in their respective professions to receive and respond to the surveys.

Working with a chronic condition is not out of the question, but may require considerable changes to the amount and intensity of work you do. You will also need to evaluate your condition periodically to make sure that your work does not aggravate your symptoms. If you start to feel better, after consultation with your PCP and your employer if you have one, you can try very slowly increasing your workload while remaining on the lookout for a recurrence of symptoms.

Making Long-Term Decisions About Your Career

At some point you may realize that you need to take a significant amount of time off from working as a manual therapist. Perhaps your symptoms are persistent enough to prevent you from keeping up with a regular schedule. Your flare-ups may be frequent or severe enough to make you worry about doing serious or permanent damage to your body if you continue to work. Perhaps the emotional strain of working coupled with the persistent threat of re-injury has taken its toll on you. Whatever the reason, you may be facing a long-term, and possibly permanent, change in the nature of your work.

Two issues may cause injured manual therapists to question whether they want to continue in their career. The first is that prior injury is a risk factor for future injury, and this is a very real concern. The second is the natural tendency to develop associations of fear and anxiety related to activities that cause pain. In some instances, work activities may truly be aggravating your symptoms, and avoiding them would help prevent re-injury. On the other hand, you may be needlessly avoiding work and other activities that would not be harmful to you and might actually be beneficial, due to anxiety about resuming them. If you believe that your work has caused your symptoms, then the idea of continuing to do the same type of work may be understandably unappealing. At the same time, the idea of embarking on a new career can be stressful in itself.

Remember, there are often a number of underlying risk factors that result in MSDs, and your work may be just one of those factors. If you can modify your risk factors at work and outside of work, you may be able to avoid re-injury and continue in your career. On the other hand, MSDs can become severe enough to result in permanent disability, and that risk needs to be balanced against the rewards that your work brings you. In the end, the decision about whether or not to continue in your profession is yours and yours alone.

You may not need to make an all-or-nothing choice at this point. You may decide to take a break for a while, or greatly scale back your workload to allow your body time to heal. You may decide to learn one or several modalities that would not aggravate your symptoms and recenter your career around those modalities. You may embark on another career, or go back to school with the idea that you can always return to hands-on treatment once your symptoms have resolved.

A minority of people, despite their best efforts, will end up becoming injured to the point that they can no longer perform the physically demanding tasks required of a manual therapist. As you read in the Introduction to this book, this happened to the author. At that point, it may help to remind yourself that you are more than your career. If it comes down to a choice between permanent pain and/or disability as a result of continuing in your current profession or changing careers, your long-term health is the obvious priority. It may also help to remember that people in many physically demanding careers find themselves in the same circumstances at some time in their lives. There are many allied professions in which you can use your training and experience in a different aspect of your field. Many PTs and OTs make a transition to working in an occupational health field, such as ergonomics. Many of them find that it is rewarding to help prevent injuries rather than treating them after the fact. Massage therapists can switch to lighter types of treatment, teach subjects not involving hands-on work, do research and write articles or books, or go into administration of a massage school, spa or clinic.

If you need to change careers, identify what drew you to your profession in the first place. Was it the satisfaction of helping your clients relieve their stress? If so, then a career in biofeedback, Reiki or breathwork may appeal to you. Was it the ability to make a difference in someone's overall health and well-being? Then perhaps working in nutrition or stress reduction might suit you. Was it the opportunity to work for yourself and the independence that gave you? There are many other careers that offer these advantages but do not rely as much or at all on doing physical work.

If hands-on treatment is what you really want to do, remember that there are many different modalities available to manual therapists, and a number of them are not physically demanding. The idea is to find the ones that allow you to continue using the knowledge, training and experience you have accumulated, but which do not continue to tax you physically or cause a recurrence of your symptoms. By staying close to the profession, you can use your abilities, stay current and continue to learn. You may also want to share your knowledge and experience by teaching it to others. Being injured enough to stop practicing in your original field does not take away your knowledge, your teaching or writing abilities, nor your authority in your field. Others in your profession should have the maturity to understand that.

Try not to think of your injury as the end of your career, but instead as an opportunity to make a transition to something new. You will always have the opportunity to return to hands-on treatment if your symptoms eventually resolve.

17

Conclusion: You Are Not Alone

njury prevention is a concern you share with all manual therapists. Get together with your colleagues and discuss ways you can support each other in your injury prevention efforts. The camaraderie will help you maintain perspective about this challenging subject. Your colleagues' encouragement will help you stay disciplined and consistent about staying in shape and taking care of yourself. Both students and professionals can benefit from group interaction about injury prevention and ergonomics.

Meet with each other regularly for discussion and hands-on practice sessions. Talk openly about your injury concerns, any symptoms you have developed, situations with clients that made you feel pressured or tense, or employers who are not adequately responsive to therapists' needs for better scheduling or improved workplace ergonomics. Support each other's attempts to advocate for yourselves and protect your musculoskeletal health at work. Encourage each other to not take life and work too seriously, and to make your own health and career longevity as important as your clients' or patients' health and comfort. In your hands-on practice sessions, watch each other work and point out potentially stressful or harmful habits. Offer constructive criticism about technique, and share new, less stressful techniques you pick up in your work or in continuing education courses. Use this book as a guide in your discussions, and refer to it as you evaluate each other's hands-on work.

Learn to Be Good to Yourself

The work of a manual therapist is challenging, demanding and rewarding. It is certainly possible to have a long, successful career as a manual therapist if you give your own physical and emotional needs the same care and consideration that you do your clients'. Allow yourself to be human, to have strengths and weaknesses, to make mistakes, and to learn and grow from those mistakes. When you develop compassion for yourself, your compassion for your clients or patients will deepen as well. The point where technique and compassion meet is where healing begins. Human beings have physical limits, and get injured if they push themselves too far past those limits for too long. Have enough respect for yourself to seek appropriate professional help when you are hurting, whether it is physically or emotionally. Listen to your body, and become aware of the messages it sends you from moment to moment. Become flexible in your thoughts and techniques, and you will be able to modify and adapt them quickly and easily in response to signals from your body and your client's body.

Redesigning your life and work to prevent injury is really about learning to be good to yourself. Taking responsibility for your own health and well-being is part of enhancing your self-respect and self-esteem. The best manual therapists are those who practice what they preach, who exude the kind of confidence and healthfulness that they are trying to instill in their clients. It is difficult to convince your clients or patients to make health and well-being a priority if it is not a priority for you. Adapting your work and personal life to allow room for health, relaxation and peace of mind are challenges that all human beings face as modern life becomes increasingly complex and demanding. If you allow the well-being that your healing profession promotes to permeate your own life, you have a bright future ahead of you.

Appendix A:
Risk Factor Worksheet

Use this worksheet to note and evaluate your exposures to risk factors in your work, home life and other activities, and find strategies to reduce those exposures. Review this worksheet every 6 months to 1 year, or anytime there's a change in your work situation to re-evaluate your risk.

I regularly perform **repetitive movements**:

	Doing what?	For how long?
In my practice		
At my other job		
At home, or during hobbies or sports		
I can reduce repetition by:		

I use a significant amount of **hand force** (gripping, pinching, pressing):

	Doing what?	For how long?
In my practice		
At my other job		
At home, or during hobbies or sports		
I can reduce hand force by:		

I repetitively move into or stay in **awkward postures**:

	Doing what?	For how long?
In my practice		
At my other job		
At home, or during hobbies or sports		
I can reduce awkward postures by:		

I hold positions that require **static loading**:

	Doing what?	For how long?
In my practice		
At my other job		
At home, or during hobbies or sports		
I can reduce static loading by:		

I place **contact stress** on my soft tissues:

	Doing what?	For how long?
In my practice		
At my other job		
At home, or during hobbies or sports		
I can reduce contact stress by:		

I regularly perform heavy, awkward or frequent **lifting**:

	Doing what?	How heavy?	In what posture?
In my practice			
At my other job			
At home, or during hobbies or sports			
I can reduce lifting by:			

I am frequently **carrying** objects:

	Doing what?	How heavy?	How far?
In my practice			
At my other job			
At home, or during hobbies or sports			
I can reduce carrying by:			

I am regularly **pushing** or **pulling**:

	Doing what?	For how long?
In my practice		
At my other job		
At home, or during hobbies or sports		
I can reduce pushing or pulling by:		

I exert myself to the point of **fatigue**:

	Doing what?	For how long?
In my practice		
At my other job		
At home, or during hobbies or sports		
I can reduce fatigue by:		

I am exposed to **vibration** (such as when operating power tools or vehicles):

	Doing what?	For how long?
In my practice		
At my other job		
At home, or during hobbies or sports		
I can reduce vibration exposure by:		

My **emotional state** recently is:

	How am I feeling?	How long have I felt this way?
In my practice		
At my other job		
At home, or during hobbies or sports		
How am I working on my emotional state?		

My physical condition recently is (include any symptoms or injuries):

	How am I feeling?	How long have I felt this way?
In my practice		
At my other job		
At home, or during hobbies or sports		
How am I working on my physical condition?		

Appendix B:
Ergonomics for Your Computer Workstation

Follow these guidelines for setting up your computer and using it in neutral posture at work and at home. Even in the best posture, you should not use the computer for more than an hour at a time without taking a break to stand up and walk around.

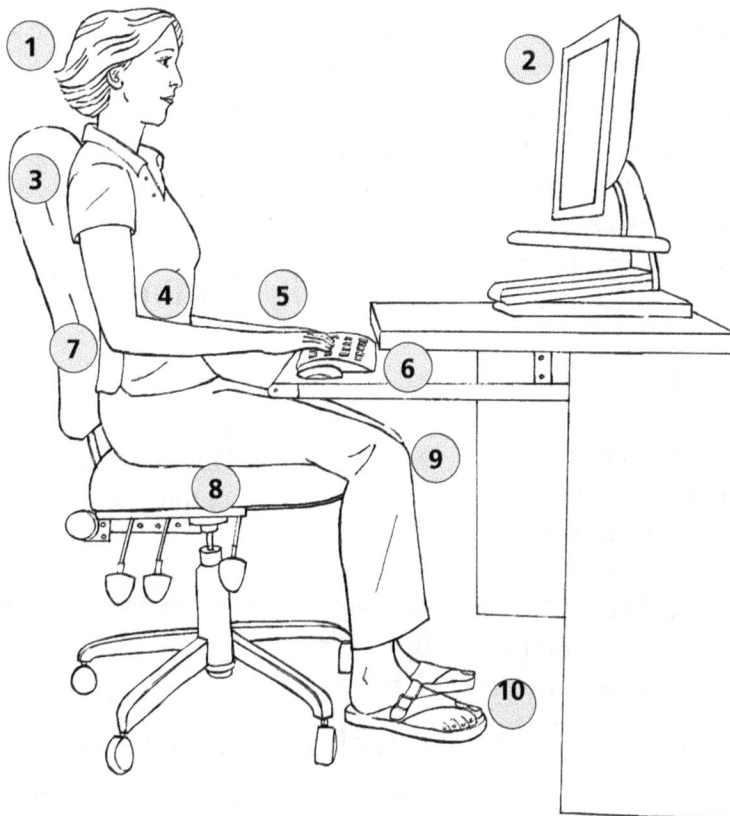

1	Head level, facing straight ahead, eyes gazing slightly downward.	**6**	Keyboard and mouse at your elbow level and close to each other.
2	Monitor centered in front of keyboard, top of screen at eye level.	**7**	Backrest slightly tilted back, and lumbar curve supported.
3	Shoulders relaxed, back and down.	**8**	Seat is level or tilted slightly forward, with thighs parallel to floor.
4	Elbows at your sides with forearms parallel to the floor.	**9**	Knees slightly lower than hips.
5	Wrists straight and not resting on any surface.	**10**	Feet flat on the floor or supported by a footrest.

Appendix C:
Daily Mindset and Self-Care Routine

You've read quite a bit about developing your self-awareness so far in this book. It is a challenge to maintain self-awareness, both emotional and physical, throughout your workday. Since physical and/or emotional tension is a risk factor for injury, it takes a certain mindset to make self-awareness a priority every day, so you can help prevent injury and support your general self-care.

In this Appendix, you'll find a routine to set in motion a healthy mindset, to reduce stress, increase well-being, and kickstart your daily self-awareness. The best time to do the following routine is first thing in the morning, before you have to deal with (and get distracted by) the activities of the day. Hopefully this routine will become a habit that you look forward to and which gives you more ease and well-being during your day and your work.

Goals

- Reduce stress and anxiety, physical and emotional tension, and enhance well-being and self-esteem
- Grounding/Centering—letting go of everything else that may be going on in your life so you can be totally present in the moment.
- Open and expand your mind to new ideas and possibilities

- Increase your ability to access your authentic self, without judgment
- Help you achieve self-awareness, self-acceptance and peaceful loving kindness toward yourself and others.

Your Daily Routine Includes:

1. Check-In and Assessment
2. A session of Mindfulness Based Stress Reduction
3. Gratefulness: Find three things for which you are grateful today and say them out loud

This routine should take 15–20 minutes to complete.

Check-In and Assessment

Take a few minutes to assess how you're feeling today. Note if there are any areas of your body that feel tight, achy, stiff, or where you have any discomfort or pain. Check in with yourself emotionally as well. Do you feel happy and peaceful, or anxious, or stressed-out? If you feel great, that's wonderful!

Otherwise, make a plan for how you're going to deal with these sensations during your workday. Perhaps between work sessions you can do some stretches of those tight areas. If you feel discomfort or pain, you can plan on trying to avoid using those parts of your body as you work, or at least not use them in every session. If there is pain, perhaps you need to plan on fewer sessions that day. Make a mental note to be extra-careful with your posture, breathing and body mechanics as you work today. If you feel upset in any way, call a friend and meet for lunch, or plan on taking a break to breathe with those feelings during your day.

Mindfulness Based Stress Reduction (MBSR)

MBSR is an evidence-based stress reduction practice based on Buddhist meditation. It was started by Jon Kabat-Zinn in 1979. It was then made into a formal program that has been taught for decades in hundreds of hospitals and clinics. Its goal is to help people reduce stress, anxiety, depression, chronic pain and much more. Many studies have been done by universities and researchers on MBSR, which have shown that it has a measurable effect on our brains, and helps us to relax and let go of stress.

The practice of MBSR, particularly on a regular basis, helps you ground and center yourself in the present moment where your awareness is the sharpest and the most natural. By concentrating on your breath, your thoughts are quieted and you make a deeper connection with who you are and what you feel. It effectively "calms down" your amygdala (the part of your brain that produces the "fight or flight" instinct that makes the adrenal glands pump out cortisol, one of the hormones that causes anxiety). MBSR has been shown to have long-term, positive effects on your mind and health even when you're not in a mindfulness session.

MBSR is also easy to learn, and will become easier and faster to do once you've practiced it a few times.

MBSR Instructions

- Go to a quiet, private place where you won't be interrupted.
- Set a timer. Start with 5 minutes per session and over a few weeks work up to at least 10 minutes. 20 minutes is ideal.
- Settle into a comfortable chair or sit on a yoga cushion, sitting tall in a dignified position with both feet on the ground.
- Become conscious of the weight of your back against the back of the chair, the weight of your body on the seat or cushion, and the feel of the ground under your feet.
- Gently close your eyes and keep them closed until the end of the session.
- Take a big breath in through your nose on a slow count of 5; hold your breath for 1 second at the top; then release it through your mouth on a count of 5. If you feel you'd like to, feel free to make a sound as you release the breath. Repeat two more times for a total of three "cleansing breaths."
- Continue to breathe normally and keep your attention on your breath as much as you can.
- Make no judgment of yourself. There is no "right" or "wrong" way to do this
- You will hear sounds, in your home, outside—notice them casually and let them fade. Return your attention to your breath.
- Thoughts will come into your mind. Let go of them. Don't judge them. Think of them

like leaves in a stream that slowly make their way downstream and out of your view until they are gone. Return your attention to the breath.

- If emotions come up, let yourself feel them fully. Don't push them down—let them be present. Then let go of them for this moment and return to concentrating on the breath.

- Feel again your back against the chair, the weight of your body against the seat of the chair or cushion, the feel of the ground beneath your feet.

- Open your eyes slowly. Take a moment to feel the difference in awareness and relaxation the session has brought you.

Gratitude

Expressing gratitude has been shown to lead to greater happiness. It improves your ability to deal with adversity, encourages positive feelings and improves your ability to enjoy life. It helps provide perspective: even when you feel dissatisfied or upset, there are still positive things in your life for which you can be grateful. Feeling bad and being grateful can exist at the same time—if that's the case for you, that's fine.

Instructions

- After your MBSR session, say out loud three things for which you feel grateful at that moment. If you prefer, you can write them in a Gratefulness Journal. But express them, either with your voice or by writing them down.

As you complete this morning routine, visualize a relaxed and confident you who is ready to face the day and all it will bring.

For more information on MBSR, here is a very interesting interview with Jon Kabat-Zinn: https://www.mindful.org/everyday-mindfulness-with-jon-kabat-zinn/

During the Day: Take Breathing, Stretching and/or MBSR Breaks

Find moments whenever possible to take mini-breaks. Even if you only have time to take three "Cleansing Breaths" (see above), you will let out some amount of stress (physical or emotional) or anxiety. If you do this several times a day, or you manage to do this during each work session, you will notice a cumulative effect over time. Get your client to breathe with you if you notice that they are breathing shallowly or holding their breath. Breathing fully is a habit that is beneficial to everyone—it may be a good way to begin and/or end a session, breathing together and creating that connection.

Ideally, take at least a ½ hour break from work every day. Go outside and breathe in the (hopefully) fresh air and see the light of day. Massage therapists and spa workers tend to work in rooms with low lighting, and light deprivation can exacerbate feelings of tension, anxiety and depression. Be sure to find a few times to see the daylight during your work day.

Stretch out your upper body and upper extremities as much as possible during your day. Between sessions is a great time to get some stretches into your day.

Maintaining Your Awareness During the Day

- If you find that your mind has wandered during a session and you feel less present or more tense, concentrating on your breath for even a few moments will bring you back to the present moment so you are there for yourself and for your client or patient.

- Ask yourself periodically throughout the day:
  - Do my arms or hands feel tight? If so, consciously relax them as you breathe deeply, and then find a different way of using them that feels better to you.
  - Do I feel any pain or discomfort? If so, check that you're in a healthy posture, try a different technique, watch your body mechanics, and make a mental note of it so you can address it fully later on.
  - Do I feel tired? Take three cleansing breaths, and choose some easier techniques for that particular session, so you don't tire yourself even more. You don't have to be "Super Therapist" in every session! See if you can find a time to close your eyes for 10 minutes during you workday as you breathe deeply. You can also splash some water on your face, or keep a spray bottle of water with sliced lemon in it to spray on your face and body to restore your energy.
  - Do I feel anxious or disturbed about something? Breathe through those feelings and try to let go of them, as they are likely causing some amount of physical tension in your body and you'll want to break that cycle. You may need a break to step outside, stretch, or visit the bathroom or break room so you can breathe deeply, gather yourself and try to alleviate that tension.

Appendix D:
Recommendations for Massage Schools

This is a challenging time for massage schools. The profession is growing rapidly, and there is increasing pressure upon schools to produce professional massage therapists who are skilled and ready to meet the demands of the workplace. It is no longer enough to teach Swedish relaxation massage, hygiene and professional ethics in school. To stay competitive, schools must now include curricula on everything from trigger point therapy and shiatsu, to deep tissue and sports massage, to hydrotherapy and spa treatments. They must also work many hours of anatomy, physiology, kinesiology and clinical treatment into the students' already hectic schedules.

School administrators and instructors may feel they have barely enough time to cover this information, let alone to get into the complex issue of injury prevention. When students complain of pain or discomfort, instructors can feel that there is not enough time to find out what is causing the problem. Without guidance from instructors, these symptoms can turn into injuries that can interfere with a student's training and possibly impact their budding career. Studies have shown that students are more likely to be injured than more experienced professionals. Without adequate information on injury prevention, all students remain at risk of injury, during their remaining time at school and later as professionals.

Schools and faculty want to provide the best training in the time available in the program. They also care about their students, and want to help them adjust physically and emotionally to the demands of doing massage. How can schools train good massage therapists who can compete in today's challenging massage market, and arm them with the knowledge to prevent injury at the same time?

The answer for schools and faculty is much like the answer for individual massage therapists: find a way to balance client care with self-care. In massage school, students learn to promote health, to encourage their clients to take time out for self-awareness, self-care and rest. Students need to learn to do the same for themselves, and the best place to start learning this important lesson is in massage school.

Administrators and educators can accomplish this goal by including the best possible information about injury prevention and ergonomics in their curricula. In a profession where the majority of practitioners experience symptoms of injury at some point in their careers, dealing with the possibility of injury during a professional training program is essential. According to the American Massage Therapy Association, the average massage therapist practices less than 8 years. With the number of risk factors involved in hands-on treatment, massage is a physically demanding profession that can take a physical and emotional toll on the practitioner. Surveys of massage therapists and other manual practitioners show that the first 5 years following graduation are the most critical ones, when inexperienced practitioners have more symptoms and injuries than their more experienced counterparts. Successful, actively practicing graduates provide one of the best forms of word-of-mouth marketing and referrals for massage schools. It is in the best interest of any school to graduate students who are equipped with the knowledge necessary to have successful careers and understand what they can do to prevent injury during their careers.

Students look to instructors for guidance about much more than just how to do massage techniques. They are too involved in their studies and not sufficiently aware of what awaits them in the professional arena to have any real perspective. They need their instructors to help them gain objectivity and a sense of proportion about their work. Just as instructors teach students to have respect for their clients' boundaries and safety, they must teach them to have respect for their own boundaries and safety. As instructors teach students to understand and treat injury in their clients, they must teach them to do the same for themselves. Taking care of oneself is a learned behavior that can be taught in massage school. Massage educators can be important mentors who help their students grow both professionally and personally in this manner.

Recommendations

There are a number of specific measures that school administrators and faculty can take to help their students prevent injury.

Speak Openly About Injury

Students need to hear directly from instructors that massage therapy is a physically demanding activity with risk factors for injury. At the same time, instructors can provide perspective by pointing out that many professions have inherent risks, and yet many people are able to enter those professions and have healthy, long-term careers. Instructors who are able to discuss this issue openly with students will reassure them and help them feel confident in their ability to prevent injury. Bringing this issue out into the daylight will also counteract the feelings of shame and inadequacy that often keep students from telling their instructors about symptoms, and keep them from seeking proper treatment for incipient injury.

Train Instructors about Injury Prevention

Make sure instructors are well-informed about massage-related injury, and that they receive the necessary training to be able to adequately teach students the most important aspects of of injury physiology, MSD prevention, ergonomics and body mechanics. Don't assume your instructors already know this information - it may not have been taught in their own training programs. By familiarizing themselves with the principles set forth in this book, instructors can provide students with the comprehensive, evidence-based information they need. Ideally, further training should be undertaken by instructors to enable them to reinforce and expand upon the principles and advice presented here.

Instructors should also watch for warning signs of injury in their students. Students tend not to speak up when they start experiencing symptoms, so instructors should look for subtle signs and unspoken signals of pain or discomfort. These can take the form of wincing or grimacing while doing a particular technique, constantly massaging their hands or forearms during class, seeing their hands shake or tremble while performing techniques or wearing splints or supports to school. Students who ask to be excused from doing massage exchanges should be asked if they are having pain or other symptoms that make these exchanges difficult for them.

Instructors are often unsure what and how much to say to students about injury. School administrators can help by giving instructors a protocol to use in these cases. It can be as simple as telling them to ask students periodically if they are experiencing symptoms, to take all complaints seriously, and to recommend that students who are having symptoms see an appropriate healthcare professional for evaluation. This protocol is succinct, but it can make the difference between a student remaining healthy or suffering a debilitating injury.

Most importantly, instructors can let their students know on the first day of school that they are available to help students find solutions if they begin to experience discomfort, tension or pain as they learn or perform techniques during their training. It is extremely important to avoid any stigma or embarrassment about admitting they are having any amount of difficulty.

Introduce Injury Prevention Information Early in the Program

New massage students generally do not have sufficient knowledge about injury or injury prevention to be able to adequately protect their musculoskeletal health while they are in school. They may not understand their own symptoms, know when and if they should see a healthcare provider, or understand the potential for chronic injury if they continue to stress their bodies. Students can become injured at the very beginning of their training, before they have acquired this knowledge. Equip students with the facts they need early in your program so they can start protecting themselves from injury from the beginning. It is far easier to prevent injury in the first place than to treat it once it occurs.

Training for students should include information on risk factors, the types of injuries that are common among practitioners, common symptoms, and the importance of dealing with symptoms immediately before they worsen. This knowledge can help students prevent a minor injury from becoming a major one. Many of the musculoskeletal disorders that students can encounter themselves are the same ones they will someday treat in their clients, so this information is entirely pertinent to their studies. Covering injury physiology and prevention early in the curriculum may help students be better prepared when clinical techniques are taught later on.

Integrate Injury Prevention into All Aspects of the Curriculum

Some massage schools create a separate course to present injury prevention and body mechanics information to their students. While dedicating a course to injury prevention is commendable, isolating the information in this way may send a message to students that these are special considerations that can be set aside when it is time to really focus on treatment work. The ideal choice would be to incorporate practical information on safe ways to do hands-on work right from the beginning, in all aspects of the students' school experience. Teach students the best way to lift and carry a massage table, how to set it up without getting into awkward postures, and how to find the proper table heights for various techniques. Give frequent, positive feedback on good body mechanics, and gently correct poor body mechanics before bad habits develop. Teach students a number of different ways of treating each part of the client's body, using different parts of the hand or arm, so they can choose the one they find most comfortable rather than being obligated to use ones that may cause pain or discomfort. Let shorter students know how to properly adjust their tables, and that they can ask a client to move closer to the edge of the table to avoid reaching out or bending forward too far.

By the time students graduate, they should think of working safely simply as the way massage is done, not as a separate piece of information that they have to try to remember along with everything else they have just learned.

Good Body Mechanics are Not Enough

Teaching students good body mechanics is not the same thing as teaching them injury prevention. As this book explains, body mechanics is an important component of injury prevention, but using good body mechanics does not prevent injury by itself. Injury prevention is a complex subject, and an effective injury prevention program must be multifaceted. Instructors and directors will find guidelines for a comprehensive approach to injury prevention in this book. For further information, or help in developing a comprehensive (and therefore effective) injury prevention program, please do not hesitate to contact Illuminate Press/Save Your Hands! (see contact information on the first and last pages of the book).

Don't Overload Students

Ideally, all students will enter school with the necessary level of physical conditioning to start doing hands-on massage work. Unfortunately, this is not always the case. Even for those who are already in good physical condition, it is important to slowly work up the endurance and specific muscle conditioning necessary to do intensive massage work. Hands-on work time, both in school and in extra-curricular massages, should be limited at first, and increase gradually over time. Be aware that with any increase in the amount of hands-on work that students are required to perform, there is the possibility that symptoms may arise. Check in with students to make sure they are comfortable with the new workload. This is particularly important in the first few weeks of teaching subjects that place new physical demands on students, such as when first teaching clinical or deep tissue massage. Checking in with students is also important if their workload increases when first working on the public in the student clinic, which can be an emotionally as well as physically stressful time.

For the same reason, exercise caution in suggesting volunteer opportunities, workshops and internships/externships. Before accepting students into an internship or externship program, find out if they have experienced any pain or discomfort while in school. Since students may be hesitant to admit problems, instructors may want to check with their other teachers and see if they have noticed any symptoms. Ideally, one instructor would be assigned to monitor each student's progress with weekly check-in meetings and watch out for any symptoms that may arise as they take on additional work while in school.

Review and Evaluate the Techniques Taught in Your Curriculum

Massage therapists who have a good level of awareness about injury prevention constantly evaluate and re-evaluate their techniques to make sure that they correspond with the principles of ergonomics and body mechanics they have been taught. It is useful for massage schools to review the techniques they teach in the same manner. Eliminate any technique that requires students to bend more than 20 degrees forward or deviate their wrists as they work; discourage lifting to as great a degree as possible; minimize the use of the thumbs as pressure tools. Using guidelines like these, and others presented in *Save Your Hands!*, can help instructors and school directors ensure that all techniques they teach are safe for students to perform.

Teach Technique in Context

In a well-meaning attempt to teach students as many techniques as possible, instructors can end up producing massage therapists who have a large repertoire of techniques and little judgment about how to use them properly and safely. These therapists may end up over-treating their clients and overusing their own bodies, increasing their risk of injury. In addition, there has been a recent emphasis on "treatment" massage that targets small areas of the client's body using hand force (which is hard on the therapist's hands and upper extremity), and a subtle move away from "relaxation" massage, which emphasizes lighter touch and larger muscle groups (easier on the therapist's body). Schools sometimes send a subtle message to students that treatment massage is better and relaxation massage is only for lazy or less well-trained therapists. From an injury prevention perspective this is not helpful, and we are not necessarily helping clients with this approach, either. Many clients don't like deep work, or want to have deep work on only one or two places on their bodies, or not at all. Emphasizing humanity, listening and artistry along with technique will help students become mature, well-rounded professionals, and help clients understand that there are many ways to benefit from massage, both with treatment massage and with relaxation massage (which is quite therapeutic in and of itself). In this way, their expectations of their therapist will become more realistic.

Schools and faculty can counteract a reliance on treatment technique in several ways. The first is by teaching technique in context from the very beginning of the training program. Many massage schools teach "routines," a series of specific techniques for each part of the body. Since these routines are not taught in the context of a particular client's complaints, students get the message that this is the only way to work on that part of the body. By the time the school curriculum starts asking students to match techniques to their client's real needs, the routines may already be ingrained. If students are limited to an hour session in a professional setting, they may spend so much time doing all their routines that they never get to the parts of the body that their clients came to them for. They may also end up exhausting themselves with each client. If a particular technique in the routine causes them symptoms, students may feel obligated to include the technique anyway. The clients end up dissatisfied, and the students end up overusing their bodies, which can set the stage for injuries to occur.

It may seem obvious to the seasoned professional that routines are meant to be suggestions, not set in stone. However, when students are tested on these routines and rewarded with a good grade if they do routines by rote, the routines are reinforced in the students' minds as simple, arbitrary solutions to every problem.

To give a more contextual view of technique, the instructor can mention a common client complaint and then show various techniques (not a routine) that can be used to address the complaint. Encourage students to be flexible and adaptive in their approach by asking them to name other techniques, including at least one not using their hands, that would work equally well for these complaints. Techniques that address the affected area in terms of the whole body can be taught alongside more area-specific techniques. Have students say out loud what complaint they are addressing with each technique. This method encourages critical thinking, and immediately connects techniques with helping the client, counteracting the tendency of students to perform the same techniques indiscriminately on every client.

Teach Relaxation Massage as Part of Treatment

Many students and professionals are confused about what constitutes a "relaxation" technique and what constitutes a "treatment" technique. This confusion often arises in school. Some school curricula teach "Swedish relaxation" techniques for a while before introducing their students to "clinical treatment." Treatment is often taught later in the program because the students learn about injury physiology only after they have learned more basic aspects of anatomy and physiology. The techniques used in the clinical curriculum may be new or different from those that students learned earlier in the program. These techniques also tend to be repetitive, specific and pressure-intensive, qualities that make them potentially risky for the students.

This method of teaching draws a distinction between techniques that are meant to relax the client and those that are meant to be therapeutic for the client. In students' minds, relaxation techniques are broader, lighter strokes that cover large areas and tie in the whole body; treatment techniques are small, hand-intensive, repetitive movements that are applied to smaller areas. Since treatment techniques are often taught as more advanced or professional ways of addressing client complaints, students receive the message that these techniques are more valuable. The fact that insurance reimburses "treatment" further encourages students to do mostly or exclusively treatment-related techniques in professional practice. Of course, many clients do schedule a massage to address a particular ache, pain or injury and want specific therapeutic treatment in small areas. The problem is that clients think these deep, specific treatments are the only or "best" way to treat their symptoms, and they undervalue the healing effects of lighter, broader types of massage. There are also clients who don't like very specific, deep techniques and find them too painful or just unpleasant.

To avoid this distinction between "relaxation" massage and "treatment" massage, design your curriculum to present relaxation as part of treatment. Impress upon students that inducing a state of relaxation is actually therapeutic, and an important part of encouraging healing. It helps soften muscles, reduce tension, warm up the tissues, and lessen muscle guarding. Going deeper afterward will be much more effective if it is needed and the client wants that type of treatment. Remind them that relaxation massage may be very helpful for clients that don't like or want deep or very specific work. If this concept can be clarified in the students' minds, it can help counteract the tendency of massage therapists to feel they must use techniques that are stressful to their own bodies to have a therapeutic effect on their clients.

Help Students Avoid Overusing Their Upper Extremity

Students often get into the habit of doing a particular technique with a particular part of their bodies. For example, if they were taught to use their thumbs to friction down the erector spinae group, they may always use their thumbs for this purpose on this part of the back. Varying the parts of their body they use in doing massage helps decrease the risk that any one part of the hand or arm will be overused and possibly lead to injury.

Try this exercise: have everyone start massaging as they usually do. When you say "change," everyone must do the technique they were just doing, but using a different part of their hand or arm to do it. For example, tell everyone they must now use their elbow to do the technique they were just doing. If students feel it is not appropriate to use the elbow in the particular area they were just massaging, ask them to explain why. Repeat this exercise a number of times during the session. It will help your students develop flexibility and avoid habitually overusing the same part of the arm or hand as they work.

Encourage Students to Think First, Then Massage

Help students understand that coming up with another technique to use is not the solution to every problem. Encourage your students to tell you "I don't know what to do next" while you are watching them practice, instead of rushing into another rote technique. Then you can discuss together the different options available to them. Reassure them that it is fine to do some broad effleurage strokes while they are thinking, strokes which are easy on their own body, feel good to the client, and aid in lymphatic drainage. Help them focus on their client's needs in moments of indecision more than on their own fear of seeming hesitant. Let them know that they don't always have to be "doing" something during a massage. They might need to simply rest for a moment and take a deep breath when they are feeling unsure how to proceed, particularly since muscular tension, a risk factor for injury, can set in during these moments of self-doubt. Finding opportunities for rest and recovery as they work is an important injury prevention concept for students to learn. It may also be a time to ask the client how they're feeling; for example, if the technique the therapist is doing is having the desired effect. Looking for options instead of seizing on technique introduces students to the subtleties of massage and encourages creativity, communication and flexibility, elements that will help them stay healthy and enhance their skill as professionals.

Teach Treatment Planning, Not Just Treatment

It is important to teach students how to create a treatment plan to counteract the tendency to do too much in one massage. Instructors should impress upon their students that they cannot, and should not, try to resolve every one of the client's complaints in one session. With the idea that complaints need to be addressed over a period of time, massage therapists have the freedom to pace themselves and space intensive treatments over a series of massages. This is also a moment to explain to the client that one massage cannot solve all their issues, and get them to commit to coming back another time or multiple times to get the resutls they want. This point should be made not only to maintain the student's health, but also to counteract the public's idea that massage can be a "quick fix." Massage

therapists can offer the public a tremendous service by helping them become more realistic about what it takes to stay healthy. If our clients understand that maintaining health takes self-awareness and effort on their parts, they will have more realistic demands of massage therapists, relieving some of the pressure that causes massage therapists to become injured.

Help Students Develop Healthy Attitudes about Massage

Massage therapists often have unrealistic expectations of themselves and their work. These attitudes are sometimes picked up in massage school. Just as medical schools are getting away from handing down the "all-knowing doctor" attitude from one generation of physicians to another, massage schools need to balance the "massage therapist as healer" message with some reality checking. Help your students understand that they are only human, that they cannot "cure" all of their clients' ills, and that clients must participate in their own healing. Most importantly, make sure they get a very strong message about setting limits and maintaining boundaries with clients. Too many massage therapists feel that hurting themselves is an unavoidable part of helping their clients. By counteracting this unhealthy idea from the very first days of massage training, schools can produce massage therapists who are capable of setting healthy boundaries and dealing with clients in a professional manner over a long career.

Continue to Stress a Whole-Body Approach to Massage

Educators and school administrators are in a good position to help shape the massage profession. There is concern in some circles that the growing emphasis on area-specific treatment instead of whole-body treatment in this profession may make massage indistinguishable from some kinds of physical therapy. The difference is that most physical therapists do not spend an hour doing manual treatment work during their sessions. The growing emphasis in massage on performing area-specific treatment, often with deep pressure and for an hour at a time, places greater demands on the therapist's body and increases the risk of injury.

It would be a shame to lose the integrity of massage as a separate, legitimate approach to health and wellbeing. Instead of giving in to societal pressure to pigeonhole massage and make it more easily quantifiable, massage therapists can educate the public that massage and bodywork in their many forms have much to offer, physically, emotionally and spiritually, in ways that are different than other modalities. Students need to learn the same thing, since they will be representing the massage profession to the public in the future.

Students can be trained to balance time spent on individual techniques with time spent incorporating those techniques into a full-body massage. In testing situations, students can be tested for the ability to incorporate techniques holistically, not just for the ability to demonstrate techniques in isolation. What has always made massage unique and popular is its ability to treat specific complaints and address the whole body at the same time. Eventually, the industry will need to find a happy balance between the specific and the holistic, since a career that concentrates on performing hour-long sessions of repetitive, intensive, specific treatment may well lead to injury for many therapists. We see evidence of a large number of massage therapists getting injured (see Chapter 1), and need to keep this fact in mind as we look at the massage industry.

Preparing Students for a Challenging Career

School administrators and instructors already do a great deal to help students get through school successfully. It makes sense to include injury awareness and prevention as part of these efforts. Students can either leave school ready to take on a challenging career, or develop symptoms that impede their success. Either will affect the school's reputation, and possibly its legal liability.

All the classes and training will be meaningless if symptoms or injury make it impossible for students to practice massage after they graduate or at some future time. There is, of course, a limit to how much students can be protected from injury; ultimately, it is their responsibility to look after their own health. By providing students with comprehensive information and conscientious guidance on ergonomics and injury prevention, you'll have the satisfaction of knowing that you have armed them with the knowledge to protect their health and the investment they have made in their training. In the long term, students will tell others about the school's caring approach to educating tomorrow's massage professionals, which can only reinforce the school's reputation and potentially attract more students.

Creating or Expanding Your School's Injury Prevention Program

We encourage school administrators and faculty to work together to incorporate comprehensive information on ergonomics, risk factor awareness and injury prevention strategies into their school's curriculum. *Save Your Hands!* is widely used as required or recommended reading at massage schools in the U.S., Canada, and a number of other countries. It has been designed to be used as the textbook for coursework on injury prevention and ergonomics for students, and as a guide for instructors to complete or expand their knowledge of MSD prevention for manual therapists as well as for clients.

Our associates are available to help schools create an injury prevention curriculum, to train an in-house instructor or administrator to teach injury prevention, to perform ergonomic evaluations of class and student clinic workspaces, and to train instructors and administrators to identify and help students manage symptoms and injury if they occur. It is a simple, cost-effective kindness to your students to institute a program to protect their musculoskeletal health during their training. For more information, please contact us at info@saveyourhands.com.

Appendix E:
Recommendations for Spas and Clinics

Spa and clinic management face the challenge of providing the best possible experience for their clients while also safeguarding the health of the massage therapists who work for them. Creating a space that is beautiful and relaxing while remaining functional and ergonomically sound for massage and esthetics professionals is not an easy task. The designer's selections for the decor or the wishes of management often dictate the choice and placement of equipment, and maintaining client comfort can seem to be in conflict with ensuring these workers' comfort and safety. Reconciling these often competing and conflicting priorities can seem complex and daunting.

When management joins forces with practitioners and ergonomics professionals to find solutions, these conflicts become much easier to overcome. Each spa or clinic has its own particular set of challenges, due to the physical setup of the treatment facilities and the types of services they offer. All spas and clinics have the same goals for their staff: to reduce turnover, to minimize workers' compensation claims, to improve productivity, and to enhance morale. All of these factors come together to make any spa or clinic more successful, and more attractive to potential hires.

Many spas and clinics provide ongoing training in different modalities, or in using good body mechanics. But massage therapists and estheticians can only use proper body mechanics if the treatment rooms or equipment are set up in a way that allows them to do so. Attention to scheduling and breaks is also extremely important, since overuse and fatigue can lead to injury. Massage work is particularly physically demanding on the practitioner's body, and symptoms and injury can occur even when therapists practice good prevention techniques. Spas and clinics need to have systems in place to deal with symptoms, injury and absences when they occur, and to facilitate a return to work for those therapists who need to take time off for recovery.

To adequately protect their massage therapists and estheticians, and thereby retain them, spas and clinics need to create a comprehensive program that encourages hands-on personnel, front desk/scheduling staff and management to work hand-in-hand on an ongoing basis to mitigate risk factors. The recommended components of such a program are:

- A commitment from management to make injury prevention a priority, understanding that developing an injury is common in this industry and that preventing injury will involve an investment of time and resources.
- Ongoing training for massage therapists and estheticians on body mechanics, ergonomics, awareness of risk factors,

knowledge of injury symptoms and injury prevention strategies. *Save Your Hands!* is an ideal reference text for these efforts. Treatment managers and supervisors can participate in our Certified Injury Prevention Instructor (CIPI) training and certification to ensure they are also aware of the issues involved in helping their staff in their efforts to prevent injury.

▪ Regular meetings with the staff to identify ergonomic issues and other concerns.

▪ A walk-through ergonomic evaluation of the facility by an ergonomist (which we can provide) to identify potential hazards related to equipment and treatment room layout.

▪ A process for finding and implementing solutions that involves the massage therapy and esthetician staff and includes follow-up to evaluate the effectiveness of the solutions.

▪ A medical management plan that encourages practitioners to report symptoms early, and establishes protocols to deal with symptoms, injury treatment, time off for recovery, and return to work.

All of the concepts in *Save Your Hands!* are applicable to workers who do any amount of manual treatment at spas or massage clinics, including massage therapists, estheticians, reflexologists, and practitioners of other modalities that involve risk factors for injury. Most of them are also applicable to other types of clinics, including physical therapy, chiropractic, and more, as well as day spas and hotel spas.

The following are some guidelines to help management mitigate injury risk factors for their hands-on personnel. The ones that are applicable only to spas have an asterisk (*) at the beginning.

▪ Train new employees on injury prevention as part of their new employee orientation. You can only protect your staff up to a point; they have equal responsibility to apply what they learn to protect themselves. Arm them with the information they need to do so, and reinforce the information periodically.

▪ When arranging work schedules, allow at least a 15-minute break between clients so practitioners can adequately recover from the physical exertion. Whenever possible, avoid scheduling deep tissue or other challenging treatments back-to-back for the same worker. Work with individual practitioners to develop schedules that allow them to earn the salary they need, while avoiding a workload that exceeds their capabilities and places them at risk for injury. Start new therapists with a lighter workload while they build endurance, and be prepared to move experienced practitioners to a lighter workload if they begin experiencing symptoms of injury, to give them an opportunity to heal.

▪ Evaluate treatment room dimensions and layout to ensure there is adequate space around the treatment table. Massage therapists will adopt much more dynamic working positions than estheticians or reflexologists, so they need at least three feet of open space around all sides of the table.

▪ When purchasing equipment, keep ergonomics principles in mind: the size, weight, dimensions and placement of equipment can either create a risk for injury, or help to reinforce good posture and body mechanics.

▪ Table width: There is a growing trend, particularly at spas, to purchase tables that are quite wide. Normal table width is 29 to 30 inches (74 to 76 cm); some spas buy tables as wide as 36 inches (91 cm). While it is true that clients can sometimes be quite large, wider tables result in more reaching with the arms and bending at the waist, particularly for shorter therapists. Instead, narrower tables are available with side extensions that can be added as needed.

- Hot towel cabinets, hydroculators, hot stone heaters, and similar pieces of equipment can be heavy and awkward to move. Place them in locations where they do not need to be lifted for cleaning or maintenance. For example, place stone heaters close to a sink where they can be drained with a short length of tubing. When equipment does need to be moved, use a rolling cart and two people to move it. When possible, equipment should be located between waist and shoulder level so that it can be accessed without bending or stooping.
- *Foot bath basins should be placed on casters if they are portable, since lifting a heavy, unstable bowl full of liquid from floor level could cause back injury. Emptying the basin into a floor drain allows it to be lifted without the weight of the water, or could even eliminate lifting altogether.
- *Floors in a wet spa environment tend to be tile or stone—surfaces that are durable, waterproof and aesthetically-pleasing, but also tiring to stand on for long durations. Anti-fatigue mats around the tables or other treatment areas help considerably, as can visco-elastic insoles for therapist's shoes. When planning a new facility, consider floor surfaces that have a cushioning layer

underneath them, but are still waterproof and easy to clean.

- *Carrying large bundles of linens and towels, particularly when they are wet, can be fatiguing and create a risk for upper extremity and back injury. Carts or wheeled hampers can make this task easier. You can also instruct staff to take smaller bundles at a time.
- Establish procedures for working with clients who have limited mobility and require assistance getting on and off treatment tables. Lifting these clients manually places both the client and the practitioner at risk for injury. Even if a therapist simply attempts to catch a client as they fall, there is a very real risk that both will go down. Local hospitals or nursing homes with rehabilitation departments, or a qualified ergonomist, should be able to help you identify the necessary equipment and training to safely move these clients. These procedures should be communicated to all staff, including those who work at the front desk and in scheduling, as they should notify the manager if a client needs to be moved from a wheelchair to the treatment table, for example, and make sure a second person is available to assist.
- Encourage open communication about symptoms and about making changes to improve working conditions. Make a suggestion box available, and check in with staff frequently, to see if they have any concerns or are experiencing any symptoms or discomfort. Have a protocol in place for practitioners who have symptoms or become injured, including ways to reduce

their workload, such as not scheduling them for deep tissue treatments. There should also be clear guidelines to determine at what point injured practitioners should take time off to recover, or work in a non-treatment capacity temporarily, perhaps assisting with supervisory duties. These modifications to work duties should also be considered when practitioners return to work following injury treatment so they can slowly and gradually increase the number of hands-on treatments they do.

Ergonomics Consultation During Spa or Clinic Design Process

Perhaps the most important recommendation is to take ergonomics into consideration in the design phase of creating a spa or clinic, before it is ever built. It is much cheaper and easier to build facilities and treatment rooms with ergonomics in mind than to have to change or retrofit equipment, rooms or flooring later. The relatively minimal cost of working with an ergonomist during the design process is trivial compared to the costs of making changes afterward. Solutions can be found that successfully reunite aesthetics for clients with staff safety and comfort and your design or build budget. Treatment staff can be more productive in a space that is designed for their comfort as well as the clients', and the savings on workers' compensation claims and missed days due to injury can be quite significant.

Of course, many spa or clinic directors, managers and staff find themselves working in existing facilities that may not be ergonomi-

cally ideal. When management joins forces with staff to find solutions, guided by the principles of ergonomics, these conflicts can be much easier to overcome. Spas and clinics have the same goals for their personnel: to make their facility a pleasant and comfortable place to work, to reduce turnover, to minimize workers' compensation claims, and to enhance morale. Happy therapists and estheticians provide the highest level of service to clients, so everyone wins!

Please contact us at info@saveyourhands. com for information about Save Your Hands! injury prevention training and ergonomics consulting services, which can provide assistance and guidance in your efforts to protect the health of your workers. We can provide professional consultants and ergonomists who can assist you during the design and construction phase of your facility, to create a safe work environment from the start. Be sure to also ask us about our Certified Injury Prevention Instructor certification, which enables spas and clinics to train a lead therapist or other staff member how to watch out for risk factors and teach and advise practitioners on staff about the many aspects of preventing injury. Of course, we also recommend that you provide each of your practitioners (and perhaps management as well) with a copy of this book, which offers the most complete, evidence-based information and recommendations available on injury prevention and ergonomics for spa and clinic staff.

Glossary

Body mechanics: The use of proper posture and body movements to minimize stress on muscles, joints and connective tissues.

Chronic pain: Pain that lasts beyond the normal duration of healing for a particular condition.

Contact stress: Pressure on soft tissues in the body from hard or sharp surfaces.

Ischemia: Lack of oxygen in tissues cause by a considerable reduction of blood flow to those tissues.

Ergonomics: The scientific study of the interaction between humans, the workplace, and the tools and equipment used at work. When applied in the workplace, the principles of ergonomics can help to reduce the risk of injury while improving performance.

Joint protection: Injury prevention techniques designed to help reduce aggravation of arthritis pain, which may also help to prevent osteoarthritis and other gradual-onset musculoskeletal disorders.

Manual therapist: A healthcare practitioner who uses hands-on techniques when treating the musculoskeletal system. Practitioners who do manual treatment work include massage therapists, physical therapists, physical therapist assistants, occupational therapists, hand therapists, osteopaths, chiropractors, nurses and athletic trainers.

Metabolic by-products: Side products of metabolism that collect in the muscles, including acidic substances, free radicals, depleted ATP and electrolytes.

Microtrauma: Microscopic tearing of the fibers of muscle or connective tissue, typically accompanied by inflammation and scarring. Scar tissue can accumulate to form adhesions. Repeated microtrauma to the same tissues can result in musculoskeletal disorders.

Musculoskeletal disorder (MSD): An injury of the soft tissues of the body, such as the muscles, tendons, ligaments, cartilage, intervertebral discs, blood vessels and nerves. While these injuries can occur suddenly, manual thera-pists commonly develop gradually-occurring MSDs, which are sometimes referred to by older terms like repetitive strain injuries (RSIs), cumulative trauma disorders (CTDs) or overuse injuries.

Neutral posture: The body position in which muscles can work the most efficiently, while joints, tendons, ligaments and nerves are under a minimum amount of stress or compression.

Non-specific pain: Pain that cannot be linked to any identifiable physiological cause. Also referred to as idiopathic or insidious pain.

Pain memory: A phenomenon in which the sensation of pain persists well after the initial trauma has healed, due to physiological changes in the nervous system.

Physical conditioning: A holistic approach to maintaining fitness levels, incorporating endurance, strength, flexibility, stability, balance, proprioception, circulation and lack of adhesions.

Primary Care Provider (PCP): The healthcare provider chosen by a patient to develop their treatment plan, provide ongoing evaluation, and coordinate care throughout a course of injury treatment.

Risk factor: Any aspect of one's work or home life, or inherent personal characteristics that increases the risk of injury. Includes both physical and emotional factors.

Scapular stabilization: A postural technique involving lifting the sternum while allowing the scapulae (shoulder blades) to drop down along the ribs, and maintaining this position while using the upper extremity. This technique allows manual therapists to more easily engage the larger muscles in the chest and back to help move their upper extremities.

Static loading: Maintaining a posture or effort that requires muscular contraction to the degree that circulation, flushing of metabolic by-products, and oxygenation of the tissues is impeded.

Bibliography

Books

Mary Beth Braun and Stephanie J. Simonson, *Introduction to Massage Therapy* (Philadelphia: Lippincott Williams & Wilkins, 2007).

Sharon J. Butler, *Conquering Carpal Tunnel Syndrome and Other Repetitive Strain Injuries: A Self Care Program* (Oakland, Calif.: New Harbinger Publications, 1996).

René Cailliet, *Soft Tissue Pain and Disability, 2nd Edition* (Philadelphia: F.A. Davis Company, 1991).

Don B. Chaffin, Gunnar B. J. Andersson and Bernard J. Martin, *Occupational Biomechanics, 3rd Edition* (New York: John Wiley and Sons, 1999).

Leon Chaitow, *Positional Release Techniques, 2nd Edition* (London, England: Churchill Livingstone, 2002).

Clair Davies, *The Trigger Point Therapy Workbook, 2nd Edition* (Oakland, Calif.: New Harbinger Publications, 2004).

Guy Fragala, *Ergonomics: How to Contain On-the-Job Injuries in Health Care* (Oakbrook Terrace, Ill.: Joint Commission on the Accreditation of Healthcare Organizations, 1996).

Tarek M. Khalil, Elsayed M. Abdel-Moty, Renee S. Rosomoff and Hubert L. Rosomoff, *Ergonomics in Back Pain: A Guide to Prevention and Rehabilitation* (New York: Van Nostrand Reinhold, 1993).

John D. Loeser, ed. and Steven H. Butler, C. Richard Chapman and Dennis C. Turk, assoc. ed., *Bonica's Management of Pain, 3rd Edition* (Philadelphia: Lippincott, Williams & Wilkins, 2001).

National Institute for Occupational Safety and Health (NIOSH); Department of Health and Human Services, *Musculoskeletal Disorders and Workplace Factors: A Critical Review of Epidemiologic Evidence for Work-Related Musculoskeletal Disorders of the Neck, Upper Extremity, and Low Back* (Washington, D.C.: 1997).

National Research Council and the Institute of Medicine, *Musculoskeletal Disorders and the Workplace: Low Back and the Upper Extremities* (Washington, D.C.: National Academies Press, 2001).

Emil Pascarelli, *Dr. Pascarelli's Complete Guide to Repetitive Strain Injury* (Hoboken, New Jersey: John Wiley & Sons, Inc., 2004).

Richard H. Rossiter and Sue Macdonald, *Overcoming Repetitive Motion Injuries the Rossiter Way* (Oakland, Calif.: New Harbinger Publications, 1999).

Mark S. Schwartz and Frank Andrasik, ed., *Biofeedback: A Practitioner's Guide, 3rd Edition* (New York: Guilford Press, 2003).

Devin J. Starlanyl and Mary Ellen Copeland, *Fibromyalgia and Chronic Myofascial Pain: A Survival Manual, 2nd Edition* (Oakland, Calif.: New Harbinger Publications, 2001).

Janet G. Travell and David G. Simons, *Myofascial Pain and Dysfunction: The Trigger Point Manual, Volumes 1 & 2, 2nd Edition* (Baltimore: Lippincott, Williams and Wilkins, 1992).

Journal Articles (Other than Already Footnoted Articles)

Wayne J. Albert, et al., "Biomechanical Assessment of Massage Therapists," *Occupational Ergonomics*, 2006; 6(1), 1–11.

Jeremy D.P. Bland, "Treatment of Carpal Tunnel Syndrome," *Muscle & Nerve*, 2007; 36(2), 167–171.

Fearon A. Buck, et al., "Muscular and Postural Demands of Using a Massage Chair and Massage Table," *Journal of Manipulative and Physiological Therapeutics*, 2007; 30(5): 357–364.

Daniel C. Cherkin, et al., "A Review of the Evidence for the Effectiveness, Safety, and Cost of Acupuncture, Massage Therapy, and Spinal Manipulation for Back Pain," *Annals of Internal Medicine*, 2003; 138(11), 898–906.

Irene L. D. Houtman, et al., "Psychosocial Stressors at Work and Musculoskeletal Problems," *Scandinavian Journal of Work, Environment & Health*, 1994; 20(2): 139–145.

Christopher A. Moyer, James Rounds and James W. Hannum, "A Meta-Analysis of Massage Therapy Research," *Psychological Bulletin*, 2004; 130(1): 3–18.

Berit Schiottz-Christensen, et al., "The Role of Active Release Manual Therapy for Upper Extremity Overuse Syndromes—A Preliminary Report," *Journal of Occupational Rehabilitation*, 1999; 9(3): 201-211.

Anne Wajon and Louise Ada, "Prevalence of Thumb Pain in Physical Therapists Practicing Spinal Manipulative Therapy," *Journal of Hand Therapy*, 2003 Jul–Sep; 16(3): 237–44.

Anne Wajon, Louise Ada and Kathryn Refshauge, "Work-Related Thumb Pain in Physiotherapists is Associated with Thumb Alignment During Performance of PA Pressures," *Manual Therapy*, 2006; 12(1): 12–16.

Online Articles (Other than Already Footnoted Articles)

Mayo Clinic Staff, Water: How Much Should You Drink Every Day? MayoClinic.com, *www.mayoclinic.com/health/water/NU00283*, 2006.

National Institute of Mental Health, Depression, NIMH Web site, *www.nimh.nih.gov/health/publications/depression/complete-publication.shtml*, 2008.

Open eOrthopod, Various Patient Guides (Medical Multimedia Group, LLC, 2007), *www.eorthopod.com/public/*

Thomas Trumble and Carol Recor, University of Washington Orthopaedic Grand Rounds: Hand and Wrist Arthritis, University of Washington Medical Center, Seattle, Wash., July 22, 2003, University of Washington Television Web site, *www.uwtv.org/programs/*

Cleveland Clinic Staff, Muscle Relaxers, https://my.clevelandclinic.org/health/treatments/24686-muscle-relaxers

Electronic Presentations

Elizabeth Vukovic Gartlan, Repetitive Strain Injuries: Nutrition in Treatment & Prevention (presented at New York University, New York, NY, 2007).

George Piligian, Nutrition and Musculoskeletal Disorders (presented at Mount Sinai School of Medicine, New York, NY, 2007).

Other Publications

Dennis M. J. Homack, "Occupational Injuries to Chiropractors in New York State," (Masters' Thesis, Graduate School of Cornell University, 2004).

Handouts on Health: Back Pain (National Institute of Arthritis and Musculoskeletal and Skin Diseases, National Institutes of Health, U.S. Department of Health and Human Services, Bethesda, MD, September 2005).

Washington State Department of Labor and Industries, Lessons for Lifting and Moving Materials (Olympia, Wash., 1996).

Index

Tables are indicated by "t"; figures are indicated by "f"

About the Authors

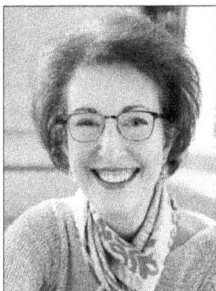

Lauriann Greene, has been a leading writer, speaker and researcher on injury prevention and ergonomics for manual therapists since 1995. She studied at Brown and Harvard Universities and attended the Mannes College of Music before graduating in 1993 with honors from Seattle Massage School. As a former professional orchestral conductor and pianist, Lauriann was interested in working with other musicians to reduce playing-related upper extremity injury. This interest led her to write an article on musculoskeletal disorders among musicians that appeared in *Massage Therapy Journal* in 1994.

Lauriann used this research, as well as her own experience with an MSD while at massage school to develop the Save Your Hands! Workshops for massage therapists. After passing her state boards in 1993, she taught these in-person workshops to hundreds of students and professionals across the U.S. and Canada. Based on the anecdotal evidence she obtained from workshop participants and existing research on musculoskeletal disorders, the first edition of *Save Your Hands!* was published by Infinity Press in 1995. It was the first comprehensive book on injury prevention for massage therapists ever published.

Since that time, Lauriann has written numerous articles for publications including *Massage Therapy Journal, Massage Magazine, ISPA Pulse Magazine, Massage & Bodywork* and *Positive Health Magazine*. She also wrote a regular column in *Massage Magazine* called "Helping the Healers" for two years. In 2005, Lauriann joined forces with ergonomist and massage therapist Rick Goggins and the ABMP on a a survey that produced the first reliable statistics on the prevalence of injury among massage therapists and bodyworkers. The results were published in 2006 in *Massage & Bodywork*. Lauriann also completed training to become a Certified Ergonomics Assessment Specialist (CEAS) at that time. Lauriann now offers a range of injury prevention and ergonomics consulting and educational services to therapists, schools, clinics and spas.

Richard W. Goggins, MS, CPE, LMP, is Board Certified as a Professional Ergonomist, and is a Licensed Massage Practitioner in Washington State. He has a bachelor's degree in biology from Columbia University, and a master's degree in Human Factors/Ergonomics from the University of Southern California (USC). During and following his time at USC, Rick worked for Hughes Space and Communications in El Segundo, Calif., helping them to establish their ergonomics program. From there, he moved north to work for the Washington State Department of Labor and Industries, where he is now Senior Ergonomist with their Division of Occupational Safety and Health.

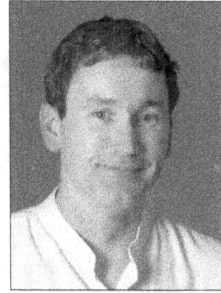

Through his work at Labor and Industries, Rick has helped employers in a variety of industries prevent injuries among their employees. He is frequently asked to present talks and workshops on ergonomics at conferences around the country, and has written several articles on the subject for publications including *Professional Safety, Journal of Safety Research* and *Massage & Bodywork*. He is a past president of the Puget Sound Human Factors and Ergonomics Society, and worked with that group on a project to educate schoolchildren on computer ergonomics.

Rick first became interested in massage after receiving excellent treatment from several different massage therapists. He did his massage training at Alexandar's School of Natural Therapeutics in Tacoma, Wash., an experience that he still counts as one of his favorites. He is a professional member of the American Massage Therapy Association. Rick combined his in-depth knowledge of injury prevention and manual treatment work in his collaboration with Lauriann Greene on the first-ever injury survey among massage therapists, and on the 2008 second edition of *Save Your Hands!*

Contributor

Janet M. Peterson, PT, DPT, has been performing injury prevention services for for over twenty-five years; she has had her own practice in ergonomics consulting since 1998 in Seattle, Wash. Janet earned her master's degree in physical therapy from Stanford University and her doctorate in physical therapy through Temple University. She was on the Board of Directors for the American Physical Therapy Association and is a past president of the Physical Therapy Association of Washington, receiving the 2003 "Physical Therapist of the Year" award. She is a member of the Puget Sound Human Factors and Ergonomics Society and the Pacific Northwest Ergonomic Roundtable.

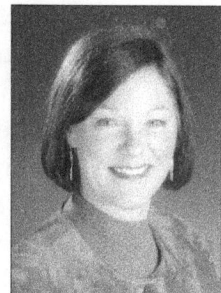

Save Your Hands! Training and Consulting Services

Save Your Hands! offers a full range of injury prevention and ergonomics services in the U.S., Canada and worldwide, to practitioners, businesses that hire manual therapists, and schools that train them. Our team of experienced ergonomics and injury prevention specialists provides workshops, seminars, instructor training, ergonomics consulting and turn-key injury prevention solutions using the proven methods and techniques described in this book.

Workshops

Save Your Hands! Workshops provide practical information and useful techniques to help manual healthcare students and professionals prevent musculoskeletal injury, reduce fatigue and discomfort, and extend their careers. Attendees learn to reduce the physical demands of their work on their own bodies while still providing a thorough hands-on treatment to their clients. Each attendee receives a copy of *Save Your Hands! Revised and Updated Second Edition*.

Combining lecture and discussion with plenty of hands-on practice, the workshops are taught in an informal style that encourages active participation. Attendees come away from the workshop with an excellent overview of ergonomics and injury prevention principles, and a self-care action plan including recommended changes to their practice based on what they have learned.

Save Your Hands! Workshops are currently available for massage therapists and bodyworkers. A continuing education course for 10 contact hours will be available soon. Workshops for other manual healthcare professionals are in development.

Certified Instructor Training

Qualified massage therapists can attend special, four-part training to become Certified Injury Prevention Instructors and teach Save Your Hands! Workshops to massage therapy and other manual therapy professionals and students. With the best-known name in injury prevention for manual therapists behind you, you will be able to help others in the manual therapy professions protect themselves from injury while obtaining a valuable credential and post-nominal (CIPI) and creating a new source of income for yourself. Continuing education credits will be available for this in-depth training. The CIPI training is ideal for lead therapists working in a spa or clinic, so they can help their practioners learn how to prevent work-related MSDs. We encourage spas and clinics to designate a lead therapist to take this training to lead the injury prevention effort for their facility.

Seminars, Lectures and Roundtables

Lauriann Greene, author of *Save Your Hands!* is available to speak at meetings and conferences of professional associations, as well as schools and businesses about all aspects of injury prevention and ergonomics for manual therapists. Seminars, lectures, media appearances including podcasts and informal talks or roundtable discussions can be customized as needed. Topics include injury prevention and ergonomics for the individual practitioner, best practices for schools, clinics and spas, and creation of standards for the profession as a whole.

Ergonomics Consulting

Manual therapists can only work optimally in an environment that is designed for their comfort and safety, and with a comprehensive program in place to help them prevent injury. Save Your Hands! Ergonomics Consulting specializes in optimizing the work environment for manual therapists and implementing effective programs and protocols to protect hands-on practitioners from work-related injury.

Our trained ergonomics specialists understand the issues and challenges present in settings where manual therapists work and train, and can help businesses create a workplace that provides comfort and safety for practitioners while providing the best possible client experience. We work closely with clinics, group practices, spas, clinics and other facilities to find cost-effective solutions to help decrease workers' compensation claims, minimize missed days of work due to injury, enhance morale, and reduce staff turnover. All of our consulting services are customized to meet the specific needs of your organization.

Turn-Key Injury Prevention Solutions for Schools

A successful, career-long approach to injury prevention begins in school, where students acquire good work habits, healthy attitudes, and a thorough understanding of injury risk factors, ergonomics concepts and injury prevention strategies. Save Your Hands! offers schools a multifaceted turn-key solution to help them minimize risk exposure for students and prepare them for the demanding profession that awaits them. We work closely with each school to develop an effective, self-sustaining, comprehensive injury prevention program. Using a train-the-trainer approach, we provide school staff with the necessary tools to integrate this program into their own, with follow-up and support. Schools that use *Save Your Hands!* as a recommended or required textbook and/or train an instructor to teach the principles and suggestions in the book have access to an Instructors' Guide and Curriculum Guides, as well as custom-designed curricula if desired. Ergonomic evaluation of class and clinic workspaces is also highly recommended to optimize workspaces for student safety and comfort as they learn.

Benefits for schools include lowering the incidence of symptoms among students (who have been shown to be quite prone to injury), increasing students' satisfaction with the program, and enhancing the image of the school for potential students.

For more information on all
Save Your Hands! services,
please see our website at
www.SaveYourHands.com, or
contact us at *info@saveyourhands.com*
or *hello@illuminatepress.com*.

For More Information

E-mail: hello@illuminatepress.com
Website: www.saveyourhands.com, www.illuminatepress.com

For practitioners interested in our Continuing Education open-book, 100+ question quiz, please scan this QR code to access it:

Interested in ordering multiple books for your school, spa, clinic or library? Please scan the following QR code for more information:

Interested in hiring Lauriann and her team for consulting, during design/build or for an existing facility? Please scan the following QR code for more information:

www.ingramcontent.com/pod-product-compliance
Lightning Source LLC
Chambersburg PA
CBHW080244030426
42334CB00023BA/2689